Student Handbook and Solutions Manual

Harry Nickla

Creighton University

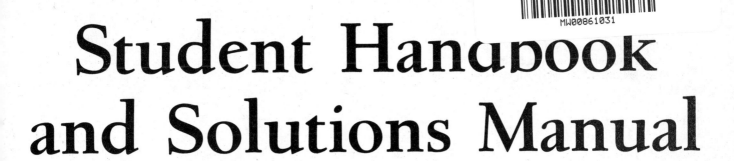

ESSENTIALS OF
Genetics

SIXTH EDITION

William S. Klug • Michael R. Cummings • Charlotte A. Spencer

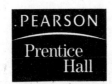

PEARSON

Prentice
Hall

Upper Saddle River, NJ 07458

Editor-in-Chief: Dan Kaveney
Executive Editor: Gary Carlson
Project Manager: Crissy Dudonis
Executive Managing Editor: Kathleen Schiaparelli
Assistant Managing Editor: Karen Bosch Petrov
Production Editor: Traci Douglas
Supplement Cover Manager: Paul Gourhan
Supplement Cover Designer: Victoria Colotta
Manufacturing Buyer: Ilene Kahn
Manufacturing Manager: Alexis Heydt-Long

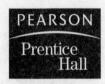

Printed in the United States of America

10 9 8 7 6 5 4 3 2 1

ISBN 0-13-224140-4

Pearson Education Ltd., *London*
Pearson Education Australia Pty. Ltd., *Sydney*
Pearson Education Singapore, Pte. Ltd.
Pearson Education North Asia Ltd., *Hong Kong*
Pearson Education Canada, Inc., *Toronto*
Pearson Educación de Mexico, S.A. de C.V.
Pearson Education—Japan, *Tokyo*
Pearson Education Malaysia, Pte. Ltd.

Contents

Introduction: Students, Read this Section First   Page   1

Solutions to Text Problems

Essentials of Genetics (6th edition)

Chapter 1: Introduction to Genetics   7
Chapter 2: Mitosis and Meiosis   12
Chapter 3: Mendelian Genetics   27
Chapter 4: Modification of Mendelian Ratios   43
Chapter 5: Sex Determination and Sex Chromosomes   64
Chapter 6: Chromosome Mutations: Variation in Number and Arrangement   72
Chapter 7: Linkage and Chromosome Mapping in Eukaryotes   84
Chapter 8: Genetic Analysis and Mapping in Bacteria and Bacteriophages   97
Chapter 9: DNA Structure and Analysis   105
Chapter 10: DNA Replication and Synthesis   117
Chapter 11: Chromosome Structure and DNA Sequence Organization   127
Chapter 12: The Genetic Code and Transcription   134
Chapter 13: Translation and Proteins   147
Chapter 14: Gene Mutation, DNA Repair, and Transposition   157
Chapter 15: Regulation of Gene Expression   170
Chapter 16: Cell-Cycle Regulation and Cancer   184
Chapter 17: Recombinant DNA Technology   191
Chapter 18: Genomics and Proteomics   199
Chapter 19: Applications and Ethics of Genetic Engineering   206
Chapter 20: Developmental Genetics   212
Chapter 21: Quantitative Genetics   219
Chapter 22: Population Genetics   228
Chapter 23: Evolutionary Genetics   238
Chapter 24: Conservation Genetics   246

Sample Test Questions   253

Sample Test Answers   276

How to Increase Your Chances of Success in Genetics:

1. Attend Class
2. Read the Book
3. Do the Assigned Problems
4. Don't Cram
5. Study When There Are No Tests
6. Develop Confidence from Effort
7. Set Disciplined Study Goals
8. Learn Concepts
9. Be Careful with Old Exams
10. Don't "Second Guess" the Teacher

A first course in genetics can be a humbling experience for many students. The intent of this book is to help you understand introductory genetics as presented in the text **Essentials of Genetics** (6th edition). It is possible that the lowest grades received in one's major, or even in one's undergraduate career, may be in genetics. It is not unusual for some students to become frustrated with their own inability to succeed in genetics. This frustration is felt by teachers as they field the following types of student comments.

"I studied all the material but failed your test."

"I must have a mental block to it. I just don't get it. I just don't understand what you are asking."

"Where did you get that question? I didn't see anything like that in the book or in my notes."

"This is the first test I have **ever** failed."

"I helped three of my friends last night and I got the lowest grade."

"I am getting a 'D' in your course and I have never received less than a 'B' in my whole life."

"I stayed up all night studying for your exam and I still failed."

Similar to Algebra

Think back to the first time you encountered "word problems" in your first algebra class. How many times did you ask yourself, your parents, or to your teacher the following classic question?

> "I hate word problems, I just can't understand them, and why do I need to learn this anyway, I'll never use it?"

At that time you had two choices, drop out and be afraid of problem solving for the rest of your life (which unfortunately happens too often) or regroup, seek help, strip away distractions, and focus in on learning something new and powerful. Because you are taking genetics, you probably succeeded in algebra, perhaps with difficulty at first, and you will probably succeed in genetics.

In algebra you were forced to convert something real and dynamic (two trains leaving at different times from different stations at different speeds, when do they meet?) to a somewhat abstract formula which can be applied to an infinite number of similar problems. In genetics you will again learn something new. It will involve the conversion of something real and dynamic (genes, chromosomes, hereditary elements, gamete formation, gene splicing, and evolution) to an array of general concepts (similar to mathematical formulas) which will allow you to predict the outcome of an infinite number of presently known and yet to be discovered phenomena relating to the origin and maintenance of life.

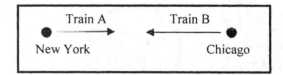

1

Mental Pictures and Symbols

When working almost any "word" problem it is often helpful to make a simple drawing, which relates, in space, the primary participants. From that drawing one can often predict or estimate a likely outcome. A mathematical formula and its solution provide the precise outcome. To understand genetics it is often helpful to make drawings of the participants whether they be crosses (Aa X Aa), gametes (A or a), or the interactions of molecules (anticodon with codon).

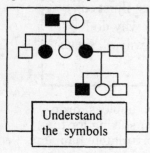

Understand the symbols

As with algebra, symbols used to represent a multitude of structures, movements, and interactions, are abstract, informative, and fundamental to understanding the discipline. It is the set of symbols and their interrelationships that comprise the concepts that make up the framework of genetics. Test questions and problems exemplify the concepts and may be completely unfamiliar to the student, nevertheless they refer directly to the basic concepts of genetics.

Attendance and Attention Are Mandatory

Many professors do not take attendance in lectures; therefore, it is likely that some students will opt to take a day off now and then. Unless those students are excellent readers and excellent students in general, continual absences will usually result in failure.

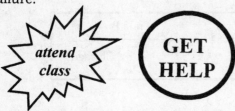

attend class · GET HELP

Remember how difficult it was to set up and understand the first algebra word problem on your own. It is likely that your ultimate source of understanding came from the course instructor. While using the text is important in your understanding of genetics, the teacher can walk you through the concepts and strategies much more efficiently than a text because a text is organized in a sequential manner. A good teacher can "cut and paste" an idea from here and there as needed.

To benefit from the wisdom of the instructor, the student must concentrate during the lecture session rather than sit, passively taking notes, assuming that the ideas can be figured out at a later date. Too often the student will not be able to relate to notes passively taken weeks before. In addition, the instructor will not be able to cover all the material in the text. Parts will be emphasized while other areas may be omitted entirely.

There is no magic formula for understanding genetics or any other discipline of significance. Learning anything, especially at the college level, requires time, patience, and confidence. First, a student must be willing to focus on the subject matter for an hour or so each day over the entire semester (quarter, trimester, *etc.*). Study time must be free of distractions and pressured by realistic goals.

The student must be patient and disciplined. It will be necessary to study when there are no assignments due and no tests looming.

Since it is the instructor who writes and grades the tests, who is in a better position to prepare the students for those tests?

The majority of successful students are willing to read the text ahead of the lecture material, spend time thinking about the concepts and examples, and work as many sample problems as possible. They study for a period of time, stop, then return to review the most difficult areas. They do not try to cram information into marathon study sessions a few nights before the examinations. While they may get away with that practice on occasion, more often than not, understanding the concepts in genetics requires more mature study habits and preparation.

Perhaps a Different Way of Thinking

Because the acquisition of problem-solving ability requires that students rely on new and important ways of seeing things rather than memorizing the book and notes, some students find the transition more difficult than others.

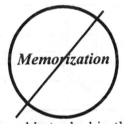
Memorization

Some students are more able to deal in the abstract, concept-oriented framework than others. Students who have typically relied on "pure memory" for their success, will find a need to focus on concepts and problem-solving. They may struggle at first just as they may have struggled with the first word problem in algebra. But the reward for such struggle is intellectual growth. That's what college is supposed to stimulate. With such growth will come an increased ability to solve a variety of problems beyond genetics. Problem-solving is a process, a style, which can be applied to many disciplines. Few people are actually born with the touch of synthetic brilliance. Success comes from probing deeply into a few areas to see how problems are approached in a given discipline. Then, because problems are usually approached in a fairly consistent manner, a given problem-solving approach can often be applied to a variety of activities.

Read ahead. You have been told that it is important to read the assigned material before attending lectures. This allows you to make full use of the information provided in the lecture and to concentrate on those areas that are unclear in the readings. An opportunity is often provided for asking questions. Your questions will be received much more favorably if you can say that after reading the book and listening to the lecture a particular point is still unclear. It is very likely that your question will be quickly dealt with to your benefit and the benefit of others in the class.

Ask Questions and Don't Tune Out!

How to Study

Genetics is a science that involves symbols (A, b, p), structures (chromosomes, ribosomes, plasmids), and processes (meiosis, replication, translation) that interact in a variety of ways. Models describe the manner in which hereditary units are made, how they function, and how they are transmitted from parent to offspring. Because many parts of the models interact both in time and space, genetics can not be viewed as a discipline filled with facts that should be memorized. Rather, one must be, or become, comfortable with seeking to understand not only the components of the models but also how the models work.

One can memorize the names and shapes of all the parts of an automobile engine, but without studying the interrelationships among the parts in time and space, one will have little understanding of the real nature of the engine.

Time, Work, Patience

It takes time, work, and patience to see how an engine works and it will take time, work, and patience to understand genetics.

Don't cram. A successful tennis player doesn't learn to play tennis overnight; therefore, you can't expect to learn genetics under the pressure of night-long cramming. It will be necessary for you to develop and follow a realistic study schedule for genetics as well as the other courses you are taking. It is important that you focus your study periods into intensive, but short sessions each day throughout the entire semester (quarter, trimester). Because genetics tests often require you to think "on the spot" it is very important that you get a good night's sleep before each test. Avoid caffeine in the evening before the test because a clear, rested, well-prepared mind will be required.

Study when there are no tests

Study goals. The instruction of genetics is often divided into large conceptual units. A test usually follows each unit. It will be necessary for you to study genetics on a routine basis long before each test. To do so, set specific study goals. Adhere to these goals and don't let examinations in one course interfere with the study goals of another course. Notice that each course being taken is handled in the same way - study ahead of time and don't cram.

Study each subject at least every other day --- especially when there are no tests!

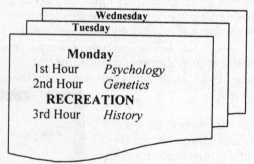

Wednesday		
Tuesday		
Monday		
1st Hour	*Psychology*
2nd Hour	*Genetics*
RECREATION		
3rd Hour	*History*

Develop a Realistic Monthly Schedule

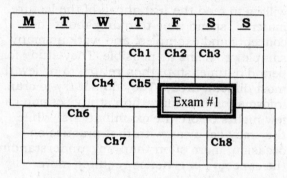

M	T	W	T	F	S	S
				Ch1	Ch2	Ch3
		Ch4	Ch5			
				Exam #1		
	Ch6					
		Ch7				Ch8

Develop a Plan for the Semester

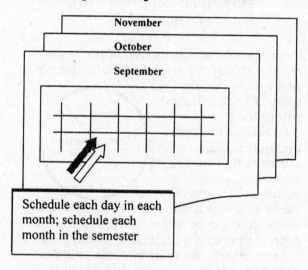

November

October

September

Schedule each day in each month; schedule each month in the semester

Work the assigned problems. The basic concepts of genetics are really quite straightforward but there are many examples that apply to these concepts. To help students adjust to the variety of examples and approaches to concepts, instructors often assign practice problems from the back of each chapter. If your instructor has assigned certain problems, finish working them *at least* one week before each examination. Before starting a set of problems, read the chapter carefully and consider the information presented in class.

4

Suggestions for working problems:

(1) Work the problem without looking at the answer. Commit each answer to paper!

(2) Check your answer in this book.

(3) If incorrect, work the problem again.

(4) If still incorrect, you don't understand the concept.

(5) Re-read your lecture notes and the text.

(6) Work the problem again.

(7) If you still don't understand the solution, mark it, and go to the next problem.

In your next study session, return to those problems that you have marked. Expect to make mistakes and learn from those mistakes. Sometimes what is difficult to see one day may be obvious the next. If you are still having problems with a concept, schedule a meeting with your instructor. Usually the problem can be cleared up in a few minutes.

You will notice that in this book, I have presented the solution to each problem. I provide different ways of looking at some of the problems. Instructors often take a problem directly from those at the end of the chapters or they will modify an existing problem. Reversing the "direction" of a question is a common approach. Instead of giving characteristics of the parents and asking for characteristics of the offspring, the question may provide characteristics of the offspring and ask for particulars on the parents. Think as you work the problems.

Separate examples from concepts. As mentioned earlier, genetics boils down to a few (perhaps 15 to 20) basic concepts. However, there are many examples that apply to those concepts. Too often students have trouble separating examples from the concepts. Notice that in the "Sample Test" section in this book, I have made such separations clear. Examples allow you to picture, in concrete terms, various phenomena but they don't exemplify each phenomenon or concept in its entirety.

Be careful when using old examinations. Often it is customary for students to request or otherwise obtain old examinations from previous students. Such a practice is loaded with pitfalls. First, students often, albeit unconsciously, find themselves "second guessing" about questions on an upcoming examination. They forget that an examination usually only

> *Old examinations may help, but............*

tests over a subset of the available information in a section. Therefore entire "conceptual areas" may be available that have not appeared on recent exams.

Often the reproductions of old examinations are of poor quality (having been copied and passed around repeatedly) and it is difficult to determine whether the answer provided is correct. In addition, if a question has the same general structure as one on a previous examination, but is modified, students often provide an answer for the "old" question rather than the one being asked. Granted, it is of value to see the format of each question and the general emphasis of previous examinations, but remember that each examination is potentially a new production capable of covering areas that have not been tested before. This is especially likely in a course such as genetics where the material changes very rapidly.

Students: Read All Of This Section First!!!

Structure of this book

The intent of this book is to help you understand the concepts of genetics as given in the text and most likely in the lectures, then to apply these concepts to the solution of all problems and questions at the ends of each chapter. Rather than merely provide you with the solutions to the problems, I have tried to walk you through each component of each question so that you can see where information is obtained and how it can be applied in the solution. At the beginning of each chapter is a section that relates general concept areas to particular problems. This should help you practice certain conceptual areas as needed.

Vocabulary: Organization and listing of terms and concepts. Understanding the vocabulary of a discipline is essential to understanding the discipline. Throughout the text by Klug et al. you will find terms in bold print. Such terms generally refer to structures or substances, processes/methods, and concepts. I have separated these terms and *other important terms* into these categories.

> *Structures and Substances*
>
> *Processes/Methods*
>
> *Concepts*

Those terms or concepts which require special explanation or are more complex or intimately related to other terms are denoted with a code (**F2.1**, **F23.2**, *etc.*) which refers you to the figures immediately following each **Concepts** section of this book.

Use the listings as checklists to make certain that you understand the meaning of each term in each chapter. Also, by a given term's category, you can begin to understand whether it refers to a structure or substance, a process or method, or a more general concept. Notice that the various terms are not redefined. It is important that you use the text for the original definitions.

> ***Understand the words and phrases of the discipline***

Concepts. In the section *Vocabulary: Organization and Listing of Terms and Concepts* you will find a section called *Concepts* after which there may be a simple sketch or two to help you focus on a particular concept. Such sketches are oversimplifications and you should fill in the details by examining the textbook and the lecture notes.

Solved problems. Each of the problems at the end of each chapter is solved from a beginner's point of view. There are other features of this section. Many of the answers to the questions and problems will refer you to the text. Be certain that you fully understand the solution to each of the questions suggested or assigned by your instructor.

Supplemental questions. A series of solved sample test questions supplement the questions provided in the text and help you determine your level of preparation. These sample test questions are located at the end of this book. Concepts relating to each question as well as common errors are presented in boxes before and after each answer.

> *Supplemental Questions*
> *Concepts*
> *Comprehensive Solution*
> *Common Errors*

Chapter 1: Introduction to Genetics

Concept Areas	Corresponding Problems
Mendelism	1, 3, 4
Homologous Chromosomes	6
Chromosome Theory of Inheritance	1, 2, 6
Central Dogma of Genetics	5, 7, 8, 9
Model Organisms and Methods	10, 14
Genetics and Social Issues	11, 12, 13, 15

Vocabulary: Organization and Listing of Terms and Concepts

Historical

Genetics

   Mendel (1866)

   Rediscovery (1900)

      Correns

   Avery, MacLeod, McCarty (1944)

   Watson and Crick (1953)

Structures and Substances

Model Organisms

   Escherichia coli

   Saccharomyces cerevisiae

   Neurospora crassa

   Caenorhabditis elegans

   Arabidopsis thaliana

   Danio rerio

Gene

   allele

   phenotype

genotype

protein

Bacteriophage (phage)

Genetic material

   DNA (deoxyribonucleic acid)

   RNA (ribonucleic acid)

   nucleotide

      A, T, G, C

   amino acids (20)

   messenger RNA

   ribosome

   transfer RNA

   enzymes

      restriction enzymes

   energy of activation

Sickle cell anemia

   α, β

Dolly

Chapter 1   Introduction to Genetics

Transgenic organism

DNA (chip) microarray

Processes/Methods

deCode

Mitosis, Meiosis

Transcription

Translation

    ribosome, tRNA

Coding

    complementarity, hydrogen bonds

Transmission genetics

Molecular genetic analysis

  sequencing

  genomics

  recombinant DNA technology

  gene therapy

Genetics and Society

  Human Genome Project

  human genetic engineering

  cloning

Concepts

Genealogy in Iceland

Genetics

  variation, alleles

  genotype, phenotype

Chromosome

  diploid number (2n)

  haploid number

  homologous chromosomes

Chromosome theory of inheritance

Genetic variation

  gene mutations

Genetic information

  genetic code

  protein synthesis

Central dogma of genetics

Human Genome Project

Model organisms

Genetics and social issues

F1.1 Simple diagram of the relationships among major components of the *Trinity of Molecular Genetics*

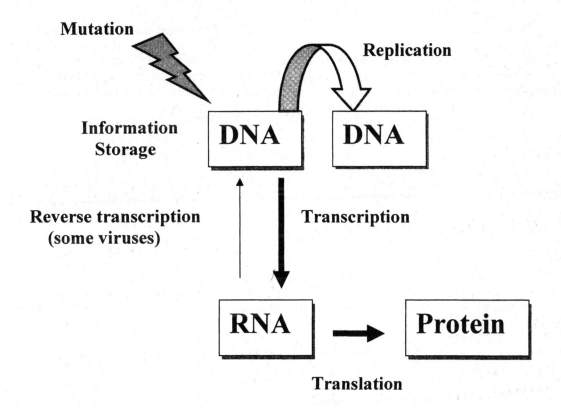

Solutions to Problems and Discussion Questions

1. Mendel proposed that traits are passed from one generation to the next by following certain predictable patterns. He hypothesized that traits in peas are controlled by discrete units, which are now called genes. He also suggested that factors occur in pairs and that members of each gene pair separate from each other during gamete formation.

2. Based on the parallels between Mendel's model of heredity and the behavior of chromosomes, the chromosome theory of inheritance emerged. It states that inherited traits are controlled by genes residing on chromosomes that are transmitted by gametes.

3. The genotype of an organism is defined as the specific allelic or genetic constitution of an organism, often, the allelic composition of one or a limited number of genes under investigation. The observable feature of those genes is called the phenotype.

4. A gene variant is called an allele. There can be many such variants in a population, but for a diploid organism, only two such alleles can exist in any given individual.

5. Genes possess a variety of functions. Since proteins can contain up to twenty different amino acids, each being structurally unique, a vast amount of functional variation is possible. In addition, proteins can engage in a variety of enzymatic activities. DNA is made up of only six different components (sugar, phosphate, and four bases) arranged in a rather monotonous, linear fashion. It seemed likely that proteins, given their cellular abundance and versatility, should be the genetic material.

6. *Genes*, linear sequence of nucleotides, usually exert their influence by producing polypeptides through the process of transcription and translation. Genes are the functional units of heredity. They associate, sometimes with proteins, to form *chromosomes*. During the cell cycle, chromosomes and therefore genes, are duplicated by a variety of enzymes so that daughter cells inherit copies of the parental hereditary information. Genes of eukaryotes and prokaryotes are composed of DNA.

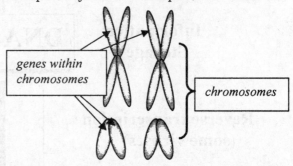

7. Genetic information is encoded in DNA by the sequence of bases. This sequence is transcribed into RNA products, most of which are then translated into polypeptides.

8. The central dogma of molecular genetics refers to the relationships among DNA, RNA, and proteins. The processes of *transcription* and *translation* are integral to understanding these relationships. See F1.1 above in this book. Because DNA and RNA are discrete chemical entities, they can be isolated, studied, and manipulated in a variety of experiments that define modern genetics.

9. If a protein chain is 5 amino acids long, at each position, there can be 20 amino acids; therefore, there would be

$$20^5$$

different possible combinations.

10. Restriction enzymes (endonucleases) cut double-stranded DNA at particular base sequences. Often, short single-stranded overhangs are generated so that ends from one fragment can anneal with ends from another (assuming the same enzyme is used). When a vector is cleaved with the same enzyme, complementary ends are created such that ends, regardless of their origin, can be combined and ligated to form intact double-stranded structures. Such recombinant forms are often useful for industrial, research, and/or pharmaceutical efforts.

11. In the last forty years, human traditional transmission, cytological, and molecular genetics have provided an understanding of many aspects of both plant and animal biology including development of pest resistant crops and identification of hazardous organisms in our food (*E. coli,* for example). Recently, biotechnology has allowed genes to be moved in a variety of ways to generate transgenic plants. Such plants can be engineered to increase their ecological breadth, disease resistance, and/or nutrient value. Wheat, rice, corn, beans, and cassava are being modified to enhance nutritional value by increasing vitamin and mineral content.

12. Unique transgenic plants and animals can be patented as ruled by the United States Supreme Court in 1980. Supporters of organismic patenting argue that it is needed to encourage innovation and allow the costs of discovery to be recovered. Capital investors assume that there is a likely chance that their investments will yield positive returns. Others argue that natural substances should not be privately owned and that once owned by a small number of companies, free enterprise will be stifled. Individuals and companies needing vital, but patented products, may have limited access. Such concentration of products may reduce genetic variation as farmers are forced to grow a limited suite of crops.

13. Some mechanism should be in place to protect the investments of individuals and institutions that develop needed and useful products. However, safeguards, both ethical and economic, need to be developed to ensure that relatively free and fair access exists when vital issues are in question. Any mechanism needs to protect investors as well as consumers.

14. Model organisms are not only useful, but necessary for understanding genes that influence human diseases. Given that many genetic/molecular systems are highly conserved across broad phylogenetic lines, what is learned in one organism is usually applied to all organisms. In addition, most model organisms have peculiarities, such as ease of growth, genetic understanding, or abundant offspring, that make them straightforward and especially informative in genetic studies.

15. This question is open to many "answers" depending on the individual. Although it may be difficult to put yourself in this position, consider not only what your decision would be, but also why you would make such a decision. Often, as a person ages, their perspective changes; for instance, how would the possibility of children under your care influence your decision?

Chapter 2: Mitosis and Meiosis

<u>Concept Areas</u>	<u>Corresponding Problems</u>
Cell Structure	1
Homology of Chromosomes	2, 3
Cell Division	8
Mitosis	4, 5, 6, 7
Meiosis	9, 10, 11, 12, 13, 14, 15, 16, 17, 18, 19, 20, 21, 22, 27, 28, 29, 30, 31
Chromosome Structure	6, 23, 24, 25, 26

Vocabulary: Organization and Listing of Terms and Concepts

Structures and Substances

Cells

  plasma membrane

  cell wall

    cellulose, peptidoglycan

  capsule

Diplococcus pneumoniae

    cell coat

    AB, MN antigens

  histocompatibility antigens

  receptor molecules

Nucleus, nucleoid

  genetic material (DNA)

  genes

  chromatin

  histones

  chromosomes

nucleolus

nucleolar organizer (NOR)

Cytoplasm

  organelles

  cytosol

  endoplasmic reticulum (ER)

  ribosomes

  cytoskeleton

  mitochondria

  chloroplasts

  centrosome

  basal body

  centrioles, spindle fibers

  microtubules, microfilaments

  tubulin

  kinetochore

Chapter 2 Mitosis and Meiosis

Chromosomes

    chromatin

    chromomere

    centromere

    metacentric

    submetacentric

    acrocentric

    telocentric

        p arm, *q* arm

        karyotype

        locus (loci)

        allele

        sex-determining chromosomes

          X, Y

    genome

Mitosis

    zygotes

        centrosome

        spindle fibers

        chromatid

          sister chromatid

          metaphase plate

            daughter chromosome

          molecular motors

      cell plate

   middle lamella

cell furrow

Meiosis

    synapsis

    chromomere

    bivalent

    tetrad

    dyad

    monad

        sister chromatids

        nonsister chromatids

        chiasma (chiasmata)

    spermatogonium

    primary spermatocyte

    secondary spermatocyte

    spermatid

    spermatozoa (sperm)

    oogonium

    primary oocyte

    secondary oocyte

    first polar body

    ootid

    second polar body

    ova (ovum)

Processes/Methods

Oxidative phases of cell respiration

Photosynthesis

Karyokinesis

Cytokinesis

Mitosis

    prophase

    prometaphase

    metaphase

    anaphase

    telophase

  Cell cycle

    cytokinesis

    interphase

    S phase (replication)

    G1, G2, G0

Meiosis

    reductional

    equational

    prophase I

      leptonema

        homology search

      zygonema

      pachynema

        synapsis

diplonema

diakinesis (terminalization)

  metaphase I

  anaphase I

    disjunction, nondisjunction

  telophase I

    random segregation

    independent assortment

Meiosis II

  prophase II

  metaphase II

  anaphase II

  telophase II

Spermatogenesis

Spermiogenesis

Oogenesis

First meiotic division

Second meiotic division

Nondisjunction

Sexual reproduction

  reshuffle chromosomes

  provides for crossing over and variation

Sporophyte

Gametophyte

Folded-fiber model

Concepts

Prokaryotic

Eukaryotic

Endosymbiont hypothesis

Homologous chromosomes (F2.2)

    diploid number (2n) (F2.1)

    loci, locus (F2.2)

    haploid genome (haploid number, *n*)

        biparental inheritance

        alleles (F2.2)

Crossing over

Mitosis (F2.3)

    identical daughters

    equivalent genetic information

Meiosis (F2.4)

    produces haploid gametes or spores

    reshuffles genetic combinations

    genetic recombination

    constant amount of genetic material

    production of variation

Nondisjunction

Fertilization

    reconstitution of genetic material

Segregation

Independent assortment

Primary nondisjunction (meiosis I)

Secondary nondisjunction (meiosis II)

Gametophyte stage

Sporophyte stage

Sexual reproduction

F2.1 Diagram illustrating relationships among stages of interphase. Also illustrated are chromosomes, chromosome number and structure in an organism with a diploid chromosome number of 4 (2*n* = 4). Individual chromosomes cannot be seen at interphase, therefore the chromosomes pictured here are hypothetical. In mitosis there is no change in chromosome number even though the DNA content doubles during the S phase. The chromosomes become doubled structures as a result of S phase.

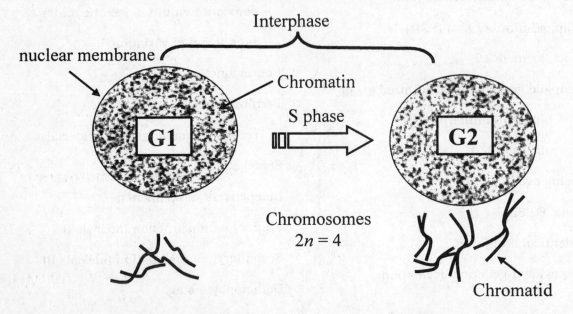

F2.2 Important nomenclature referring to chromosomes and genes in an organism where the diploid chromosome number is 4 (2*n* = 4). There are two pairs of chromosomes, one large metacentric, one small telocentric. Sister chromatids are identical to each other while homologous chromosomes are similar to each other in terms of overall size, centromere location, function, and other factors described in the text.

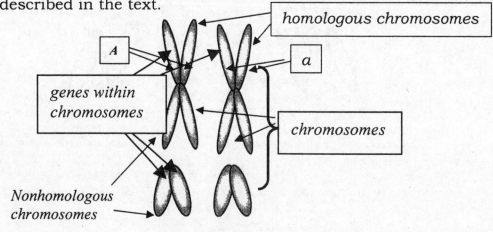

F2.3 Illustration of chromosomes of mitotic cells in an organism with a chromosome number of 4 ($2n = 4$).

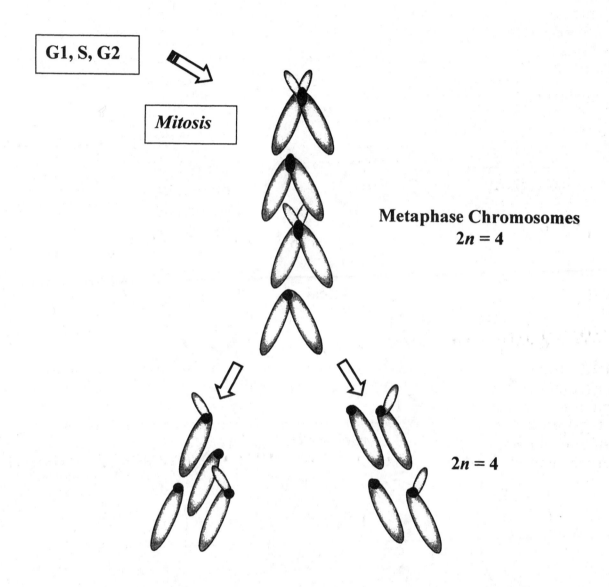

G1, S, G2

Mitosis

Metaphase Chromosomes
$2n = 4$

$2n = 4$

F2.4 Illustration of chromosomes of meiotic cells in an organism with a chromosome number of 4 (2*n* = 4).

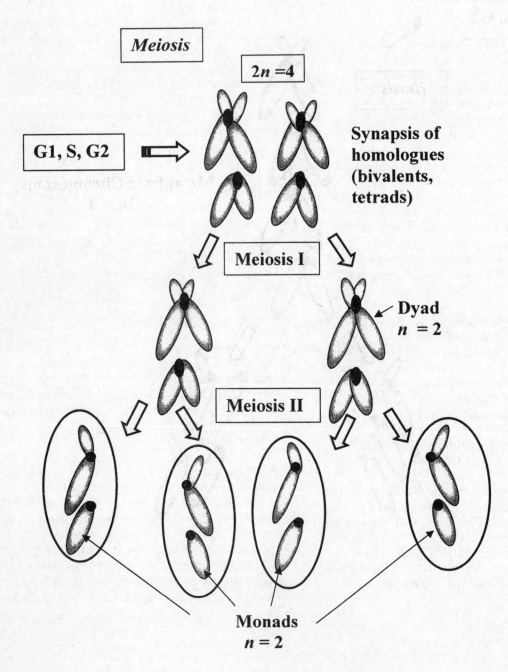

Solutions to Problems and Discussion Questions

1. (a) During interphase of the cell cycle (mitotic and meiotic), chromosomes are not condensed and are in a genetically active, spread out, form. In this condition, chromosomes are not visible as individual structures under the microscope (light or electron). See F2.1 for a sketch of what *chromatin* might look like. Chromatin contains the genetic material which is responsible for maintaining hereditary information (from one cell to daughter cells and from one generation to the next) and production of the phenotype.

(b) The *nucleolus (pl. nucleoli)* is a structure which is produced by activity of the nucleolar organizer region in eukaryotes. Composed of ribosomal RNA and protein, it is the structure for the production of ribosomes. Some nuclei have more than one *nucleolus*. Nucleoli are not present during mitosis or meiosis because in the condensed state of chromosomes, there is little or no RNA synthesis.

(c) The *ribosome* is the structure where various RNAs, enzymes, and other molecular species assemble the primary sequence of a protein. That is, amino acids are placed in order as specified by messenger RNA. Ribosomes are relatively non-specific in that virtually any ribosome can be used in the translation of any mRNA. The structure and function of the ribosome will be described in greater detail in later chapters of the text.

(d) The *mitochondrion (pl. mitochondria)* is a membrane-bound structure located in the cytoplasm of eukaryotic cells. It is the site of oxidative phosphorylation and production of relatively large amounts of ATP. It is the trapping of energy in ATP which drives many important metabolic processes in living systems.

(e) The *centriole* is a cytoplasmic structure involved (through the formation of spindle fibers) in the migration of chromosomes during mitosis and meiosis of animal cells.

(f) The *centromere* serves as an attachment point for sister chromatids (see F2.3, 2.4) and a region where spindle fibers attach to chromosomes (kinetochore). The centromere divides during mitosis and meiosis II, thus aiding in the partitioning of chromosomal material to daughter cells. Failure of centromeres or spindle fibers to function properly may result in nondisjunction.

2. One of the most important concepts to be gained from this chapter is the relationship which exists among chromosomes in a single cell. Chromosomes which are homologous normally share many properties including:

Overall length: look carefully at the figures above to see that each cell, prior to anaphase I, contains two chromosomes in which a homolog is of approximately the same overall length.

Position of the centromere (metacentric, submetacentric, acrocentric, telocentric): again, look carefully at F2.2 and F2.3. Notice that in each if there is one metacentric chromosome, there will be another metacentric chromosome.

Banding patterns: Using various cytological techniques, bands can be induced in chromosomes. Homologous chromosomes of pair #1 for example will have the same banding pattern. While the overall length of chromosome pairs #16 and #17 appear to be the same, the banding patterns of these non-homologous chromosomes will be different.

Sister chromatids have identical banding patterns, as would be expected since sister chromatids are, with the exception of mutation, identical copies of each other. We would expect that homologous chromosomes would have banding patterns which are very similar (but not identical) because homologous chromosomes are genetically similar but not genetically identical.

Type and location of genes: notice in F2.2 that a locus signifies the location of a gene along a chromosome. What that really means is that for each characteristic specified by a gene, like blood type, eye color, skin pigmentation, there are genes located along chromosomes. The *order* of such loci is identical in homologous chromosomes, but the genes themselves, while being in the same order, may not be identical. Look carefully at the inset (box) in the upper portion of F2.2 and see that there are alternative forms of genes, *A* and *a*, at the same location along the chromosome. *A* and *a* are located at the same place and specify the same *characteristic* (eye color, for example) but there are slightly different manifestations of eye color (*brown* vs. *blue* for example). Just as an individual may inherit gene *A* from the father and gene *a* from the mother, each zygote inherits one homologue of each pair from the father and one homologue of each pair from the mother.

Autoradiographic pattern: homologous chromosomes tend to replicate during the same time of S phase.

Diploidy is a term often used in conjunction with the symbol $2n$. It means that both members of a homologous pair of chromosomes are present. Refer to F2.1 in this book. Notice that during mitosis, the normal chromosome complement is $2n$ or diploid. In humans, the diploid chromosome number is 46 while in *Drosophila melanogaster* it is 8. The text lists the *haploid* chromosome number for a variety of species.

Notice that in man and flies, the haploid chromosome number is one-half the diploid number. This applies to other organisms as well. However, it is very important to realize that *haploidy* specifically refers to the fact that each haploid cell contains *one chromosome of each homologous pair of chromosomes.*

Compare the nuclear contents of a spermatid and a cell at zygonema in the text. Note that each spermatid contains one member of each of the original chromosome pairs (seen at zygonema). Haploidy is usually symbolized as *n*.

The change from a diploid ($2n$) to haploid (n) occurs during *reduction division* when tetrads become dyads during meiosis I. Referring to the number of human chromosomes, the primary spermatocyte ($2n = 46$) becomes two secondary spermatocytes each with $n = 23$.

3. As you examine the criteria for *homology* in question #2 above, you can see that overall length and centromere position are but two factors required for homology. Most importantly, genetic content in non-homologous chromosomes is expected to be quite different. Other factors including banding pattern and time of replication during S phase would also be expected to vary among non-homologous chromosomes.

4. Because a major section of Chapter #2 deals with mitosis, it would be best to deal with this question by reading the appropriate section in the text and examining corresponding figures. Understanding mitosis and all the related terms is essential for an understanding of genetics. There are several sample test questions at the end of this book which will help you determine your understanding of mitosis.

5. The first sentence tells you that $2n = 16$ and it is a question about mitosis. Since each chromosome in prophase is doubled (having gone through an S phase) and is visible at the end of prophase, there should be 32 chromatids. Because the centromeres divide and what were previously sister chromatids migrate to opposite poles during anaphase, there should be 16 chromosomes moving to each pole. If you refer to F2.2 you will see an example with $2n = 4$ and that there are four doubled chromosomes in prophase. Notice that there are eight chromatids visible at late prophase.

6. Refer to the text figures for an explanation. Notice the different anaphase shapes of chromosomes as they move to the poles: metacentric (a), submetacentric (b), acrocentric (c), telocentric (d). Your understanding of these structures will be determined by several of the sample test questions at the end of this book.

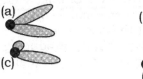 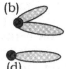

7. Because of a cell wall around the plasma membrane in plants, a cell plate, which was laid down during anaphase, becomes the middle lamella where primary and secondary layers of the cell wall are deposited.

8. Carefully read the section on mitosis and cell division in the text. Major divisions of the cell cycle include Interphase and Mitosis. Interphase is composed of three phases: G1, S, and G2. (Some cells have a temporary or permanent G0 phase between G1 and S.) During the S phase, chromosomal DNA doubles. Karyokinesis involves nuclear division while cytokinesis involves division of the cytoplasm. Refer to F2.1 for information pertaining to the interphase. Refer to the text figures for a diagram of mitosis. Notice that, in contrast to meiosis, there is no pairing of homologous chromosomes in mitosis and the chromosome number does not change.

9. Not necessarily. If crossing over occurred in meiosis I, then the chromatids in the secondary oocyte are not identical. Once they separate during meiosis II, dissimilar chromatids reside in the ootid and the second polar body.

10. Compared with mitosis which maintains a chromosomal constancy, meiosis provides for a reduction in chromosome number, and an opportunity for exchange of genetic material between homologous chromosomes. In mitosis there is no change in chromosome number or kind in the two daughter cells whereas in meiosis numerous potentially different haploid (n) cells are produced. During oogenesis, only one of the four meiotic products is functional; however, four of the four meiotic products of spermatogenesis are potentially functional.

11. (a) *Synapsis* is the point-by-point pairing of homologous chromosomes during prophase of meiosis I.

(b) *Bivalents* are those structures formed by the synapsis of homologous chromosomes. In other words, there are two chromosomes (and four chromatids) which make up a bivalent. If an organism has a diploid chromosome number of 46, then there will be 23 bivalents in meiosis I.

(c) *Chiasmata* is the plural form of chiasma and refers to the structure, when viewed microscopically, of crossed chromatids. Notice figures in the text, the exchange of chromatid pieces in diplonema and diakinesis.

(d) *Crossing over* is the exchange of genetic material between chromatids. If there are allelic differences between the two homologs, crossing over results in genetic recombination. It is a method of providing genetic variation through the breaking and rejoining of chromatids.

(e) *Chromomeres* are bands of chromatin which look different from neighboring patches along the length of a chromosome.

(f) Examine F2.1 in this book. Notice that *sister chromatids* are "post-S phase" structures of replicated chromosomes. Sister chromatids are genetically identical (except where mutations have occurred) and are originally attached to the same centromere. Identify sister chromatids in the figures in the text. Note that sister chromatids separate from each other during anaphase of mitosis and anaphase II of meiosis.

(g) *Tetrads* are synapsed homologous chromosomes thereby composed of four chromatids. There are as many tetrads as the haploid chromosome number.

(h) Actually, each tetrad is made of two dyads which separate from each other during anaphase I of meiosis. Note that *dyads* are composed of two chromatids joined by a centromere.

(i) At anaphase II of meiosis, the centromeres divide and sister chromatids (*monads*) go to opposite poles.

12. Sister chromatids are genetically identical, except where mutations may have occurred during DNA replication. Nonsister chromatids are genetically similar if on homologous chromosomes or genetically dissimilar if on nonhomologous chromosomes. If crossing over occurs, then chromatids attached to the same centromere may no longer be identical.

13. During meiosis I chromosome number is reduced to haploid complements. This is achieved by synapsis of homologous chromosomes and their subsequent separation. It would seem to be more mechanically difficult for genetically identical daughters to form from mitosis if homologous chromosomes paired. By having chromosomes unpaired at metaphase of mitosis, only centromere division is required for daughter cells to eventually receive identical chromosomal complements.

14. Look carefully at F2.4 in this book and notice that for a cell with 4 chromosomes, there are two tetrads each comprised of a homologous pair of chromosomes.

(a) If there are 16 chromosomes there should be 8 tetrads.

(b) Also note that, after meiosis I and in the second meiotic prophase, there are as many dyads as there are pairs of chromosomes. There will be 8 dyads.

(c) Because the monads migrate to opposite poles during meiosis II (from the separation of dyads) there should be 8 monads migrating to *each* pole.

15. Examine appropriate figures in the text. Notice that major differences include the sex in which each occurs, and that the distribution of cytoplasm is unequal in oogenesis but considered to be equal in the products of spermatogenesis. Chromosomal behavior is the same in spermatogenesis and oogenesis except that the nuclear activity in oogenesis is "off-center" thereby producing first and second polar bodies by unequal cytoplasmic division.

In humans, each spermatogonium and primary spermatocyte produces four spermatids whereas each oogonium and primary oocyte produces one ootid. Because early development occurs in the absence of outside nutrients, it is likely that the unequal distribution of cytoplasm in oogenesis evolved to provide sufficient information and nutrients to support development until the transcriptional activities of the zygotic nucleus begin to provide products.

Polar bodies probably represent nonfunctional by-products of such evolution.

secondary spermatocytes and secondary oocytes) are genetically unique.

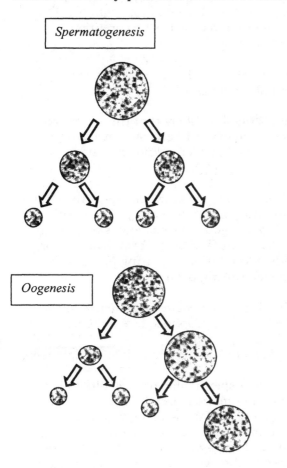

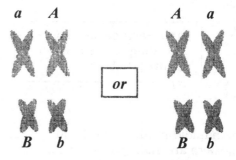

Notice that there are two different orientations of tetrads in meiosis. Independent assortment of nonhomologous chromosomes adds to genetic variability. Daughter cells resulting from the process of mitosis are usually genetically identical.

17. This question specifically tests your understanding of meiosis and the behavior of chromosomes during anaphase. In this question you must first visualize the alignment of the three homologous chromosome pairs C1/C2, M1/M2, and S1/S2 in mitosis where there is no synapsis of homologous chromosomes.

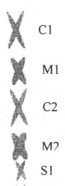

(a) After mitosis, when sister chromatids have migrated to opposite poles, each daughter cell will be genetically identical and have the same chromosomal content as the parent cell: C1/C2, M1/M2, and S1/S2

16. This answer contains several parts. First, through independent assortment of chromosomes at anaphase I of meiosis, daughter cells (secondary spermatocytes and secondary oocytes) may contain different sets of maternally- and paternally-derived chromosomes. Examine the diagram below. Notice that there are several ways in which the maternally- and paternally-derived chromosomes may align. Can you calculate the probability of all the maternally-derived chromosomes going to the "right-hand" pole? Second, crossing over, which happens at a much higher frequency in meiotic cells as compared to mitotic cells, allows maternally- and paternally-derived chromosomes to exchange segments thereby increasing the likelihood that daughter cells (that is,

(b) The first meiotic metaphase will have the following configuration:

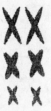

| Label each chromosome according to the symbols in part **(a)** above |

(c) For the haploid products of the above cell in part (b), there are eight possibilities, depending on the alignment of the homologous chromosomes:

 C1 **or** C2

 M1 **or** M2

 S1 **or** S2

18. If there are eight combinations possible for part (c) in the previous problem, there would be 16 combinations with the addition of another chromosome pair.

19. As you first read this question, think about an animal with $n = 6$, therefore there will be 6 tetrads. The question concerns one of these tetrads as it passes normally through meiosis I, but one dyad undergoes secondary nondisjunction. Secondary nondisjunction occurs during the second meiotic division.

(a) The mature ovum should contain $n+1$ chromosomes: the five chromosomes from normal disjunction and two (from one dyad) from the nondisjunctional chromosome.

(b) The second polar body did not receive one of the six monads it would normally receive, so it should have five monads (which are chromosomes).

(c) When the normal sperm with its n chromosome number combines with an $n+1$ ovum, it will produce a zygote with $2n+1$, or thirteen chromosomes. This condition is termed *trisomy*.

20. One half of each tetrad will have a maternal homolog: $(1/2)^{10}$.

21. (a) While it is likely that the molecular processes involved in crossing over occur earlier, crossing over is known to have occurred by pachynema.

(b) *Synapsis* begins at zygonema with continuation of the homology search and when homologous chromosomes align in a point-by-point fashion to form bivalents or tetrads. More intimate pairing (synapsis) is completed during pachynema.

(c) Chromosomes begin to condense at the earliest stage of prophase I, leptonema.

(d) *Chiasmata* are clearly visible at diplonema.

22. In angiosperms, meiosis results in the formation of microspores (male) and megaspores (female) which give rise to the haploid male and female gametophyte stage. Micro- and megagametophytes produce the pollen and the ovules respectively. Following fertilization, the sporophyte is formed.

23. The transition from chromatin to individual chromosomes occurs at the beginning of mitosis (or meiosis). During this time, chromatin fibers fold up and condense into the typical mitotic chromosome. The *folded-fiber model* depicts this transition.

24. The folded-fiber model is based on each chromatid consisting of a single fiber wound like a skein of yarn. Each fiber consists of DNA and protein. A coiling process occurs during the transition of interphase chromatin to more condensed chromosomes during prophase of mitosis or meiosis. Such condensation leads to a 5000-fold contraction in the length of the DNA within each chromatid. The transition is at the end of interphase and the beginning of prophase when the chromosomes are in the condensation process. This eventually leads to the typically shortened and "fattened" metaphase chromosome.

25. They would probably be homologous chromosomes and contain similar (but not identical) genetic information. Their centromeres would most likely be in the same position relative to chromosome arm lengths and any physical characteristics such as secondary constrictions or bands would be similar. They would have a similar sequence of nitrogenous bases. They would most likely replicate synchronously during the S phase of the cell cycle.

26. Duplicated chromosomes A^m, A^p, B^m, B^p, C^m, and C^p will align at metaphase, with the centromeres dividing and sister chromatids going to opposite poles at anaphase.

27. Side-by-side alignment of A^m, A^p, B^m B^p, C^m, C^p will occur in various arrangements at metaphase I. Eight possible combinations of products will occur at the completion of anaphase: A^m, B^p, C^m, for example (each with sister chromatids). In other words, after meiosis I, the two product cells would be as follows: A^m or A^p, B^m or B^p, C^m or C^p.

28. As long as you have accounted for eight possible combination in the previous problem, there would be no new ones added in this problem.

29. Eight (2 X 2 X 2) combinations are possible.

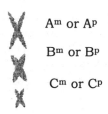

A^m or A^p

B^m or B^p

C^m or C^p

30. See the products of nondisjunction of chromosome C at the end of meiosis I as follows.

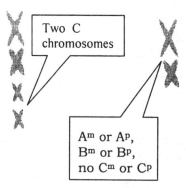

Two C chromosomes

A^m or A^p, B^m or B^p, no C^m or C^p

At the end of meiosis II, assuming that, as the problem states, the C chromosomes separate as dyads instead of monads during meiosis II, you would have monads for the A and B chromosomes, and dyads (from the cell on the left) for both C chromosomes as one possibility.

However, another possibility exists as shown below for the products of meiosis II:

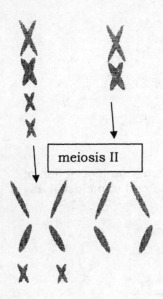

31. Taking this question exactly as it is described --- nondisjunction of the *C* chromosome at meiosis I and again, nondisjunction of the same chromosome at meiosis II, you will end up, after fertilization, with the following combinations under the first condition in problem 30.

zygote 1:   two copies of chromosome *A*
                two copies of chromosome *B*
                five copies of chromosome *C*

zygote 2-4:   two copies of chromosome *A*
                two copies of chromosome *B*
                one copy of chromosome *C*

Under the second possibility described in problem 30, one would expect the following zygotes after fertilization:

zygotes 1-2:   two copies of chromosome *A*
                two copies of chromosome *B*
                three copies of chromosome *C*

zygotes 3-4:   two copies of chromosome *A*
                two copies of chromosome *B*
                one copy of chromosome *C*

Chapter 3: Mendelian Genetics

Concept Areas	Corresponding Problems
Mendel's Model	3, 4, 9, 10, 12
Monohybrid Crosses	1, 2, 5, 17, 19
Homology	11
Dihybrid Crosses	6, 7, 8, 13, 30
Trihybrid Crosses	15, 21, 22, 23
Independent Assortment	14, 15, 16, 28
Chi-Square Analysis	17, 18, 19, 20, 31
Pedigree Analysis	24, 25, 26, 27, 29

Vocabulary: Organization and Listing of Terms and Concepts

Historical

Mendelian Genetics (Gregor Mendel)

Transmission genetics

Pisum sativum (1866)

units of heredity (particulate)

Punnett squares

Structures and Substances

Unit factors, genes

Alleles

Starch-branching enzyme (SBEI)

transposable element

Processes/Methods

Transmission genetics

true-breeding, "breed true"

monohybrid cross

selfing, self-fertilizing

reciprocal cross

testcross

parental generation (P_1)

first filial generation (F_1)

second filial generation (F_2)

ratios

3:1, 1:1

1:2:1

9:3:3:1, 1:1:1:1

27:9:9:9:3:3:3:1

product law

2^n (n = haploid chromosome number)

sum law

dihybrid cross (two-factor cross)

trihybrid cross (three-factor cross)

forked-line (branch diagram) method

Chapter 3 Mendelian Genetics

Statistical testing (analysis)

    predicted occurrences

    proportions

    sample size

    chance deviation

    random fluctuations

    null hypothesis

    measured (observed) values

    predicted values

    goodness of fit

    chi-square analysis (χ^2)

    degrees of freedom (*df*)

    probability value (*p*)

        reject the null hypothesis

        fail to reject the null hypothesis

        0.05 probability value

Pedigree

    sibs, sibship line

        monozygotic (identical) twins

        dizygotic (fraternal) twins

           proband

Concepts

Unit factors in pairs (F3.1)

Dominance/recessiveness (F3.1)

Symbolism (F3.2, F3.3)

Segregation

Chromosome theory of inheritance

Phenotype, genotype

Homozygous (homozygote)

Heterozygous (heterozygote)

Independent assortment

Product law, sum law

Genotypic ratio

Continuous variation

Discontinuous variation

Diploid number

Statistical testing

F3.1 Illustration of the union of maternal and paternal genes (*A* and *a*) to give two genes in the zygote. Mendelian "unit factors" occur in pairs in diploid organisms. Dominant genes are often given the upper case letter as the symbol while the lower case letter is often used to symbolize the recessive gene.

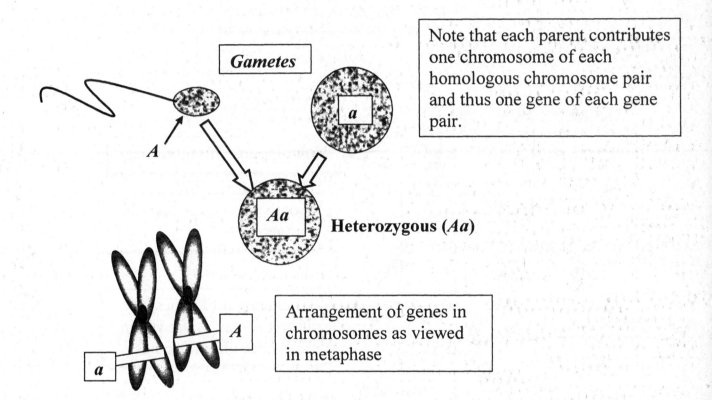

Gametes

a

Note that each parent contributes one chromosome of each homologous chromosome pair and thus one gene of each gene pair.

Aa   Heterozygous (*Aa*)

Arrangement of genes in chromosomes as viewed in metaphase

A

a

A

F3.2 Critical symbolism associated with genes and chromosomes. Below are positioned two different gene pairs (*Aa* and *Bb*) on non-homologous chromosomes. Note, with two different gene pairs two different characteristics may be involved such as seed shape (*A* and *a*) and seed color (*B* and *b*).

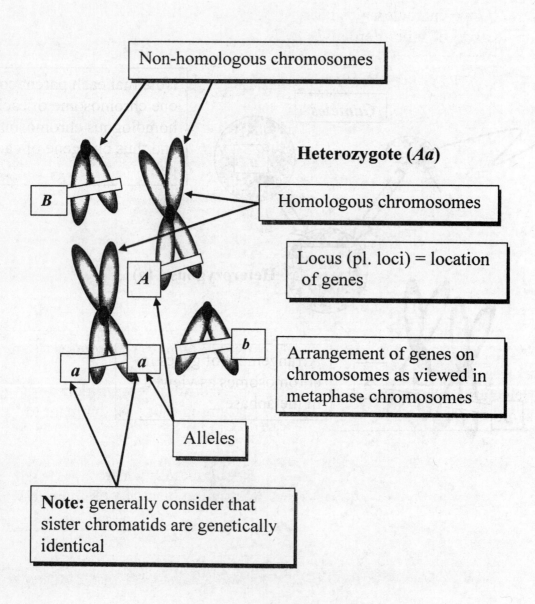

Non-homologous chromosomes

Heterozygote (*Aa*)

Homologous chromosomes

Locus (pl. loci) = location of genes

Arrangement of genes on chromosomes as viewed in metaphase chromosomes

B

A

b

a   *a*

Alleles

Note: generally consider that sister chromatids are genetically identical

F3.3 One of the most important concepts for this section is illustrated in the figure below. Two gene pairs (*W* and *B*) are presented, each representing a different characteristic, seed shape (*W* or *w*) and seed color (*B* or *b*). Different gene pairs may influence completely different characteristics (as indicated here) or the same characteristic (described in Chapter 4).

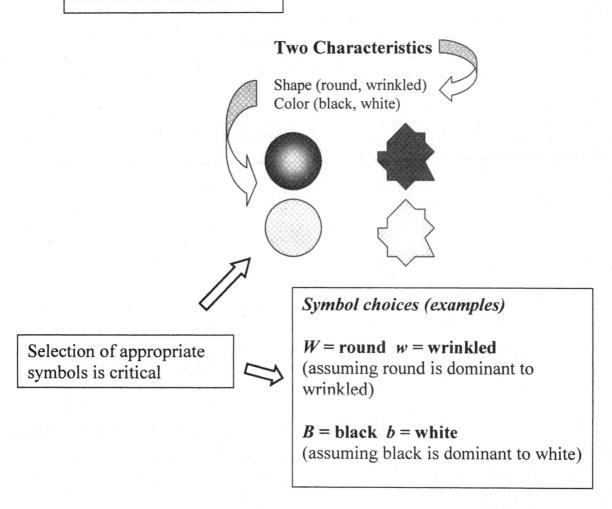

Two characteristics but a total of four alternatives

Two Characteristics

Shape (round, wrinkled)
Color (black, white)

Selection of appropriate symbols is critical

Symbol choices (examples)

W = **round** *w* = **wrinkled**
(assuming round is dominant to wrinkled)

B = **black** *b* = **white**
(assuming black is dominant to white)

Solutions to Problems and Discussion Questions

1. Several points surface in the first sentence of this question. First, two alternatives (black and white) of one characteristic (coat color) are being described, therefore a monohybrid condition exists.

Second, are the guinea pigs in the parental generation (P_1) homozygous or heterozygous? Notice in the introductory sentence, just after PROBLEMS AND DISCUSSION QUESTIONS, there is the statement "members of the P_1 generation are homozygous. . ."

Third, which is dominant, *black* or *white*? Note that all the offspring are black, therefore black can be considered dominant. The second sentence of the problem verifies that a monohybrid cross is involved because of the 3/4 black and 1/4 white distribution in the offspring. Referring to appropriate text figures and knowing that genes occur in pairs in diploid organisms, one can write the genotypes and the phenotypes requested in part (a) as follows:

(a)

P_1:			
Phenotypes:	Black	X	White
Genotypes:	*WW*		*ww*
Gametes:	(W)		(w)
F_1:		*Ww* (Black)	

Ww X *Ww*

¼ = *WW* black
½ = *Ww* black
¼ = *ww* white

2. Start out with the following gene symbols:

A = normal (not albino),
a = albino.

Since albinism is inherited as a recessive trait, genotypes *AA* and *Aa* should produce the normal phenotype, while *aa* will give albinism. **(a)** The parents are both normal, therefore they could be either *AA* or *Aa*. The fact that they produce an albino child requires that each parent provides an *a* allele to the albino child; thus the parents must both be heterozygous (*Aa*). **(b)** To start out, the normal male could have either the *AA* or *Aa* genotype. The female must be *aa*. Since all the children are normal, one would consider the male to be *AA* instead of *Aa*. However, the male could be *Aa*. Under that circumstance, the likelihood of having six children, all normal, is 1/64.

3. Three of Mendel's postulates are illustrated in a problem such as this one. Unit factors occur in pairs (postulate 1) and demonstrate dominance/recessive relationships (postulate 2). The fact that these unit factors separate from each other during gamete formation illustrates postulate 3.

4. *Pisum sativum* is easy to cultivate and it is naturally self-fertilizing, but it can be crossbred. It has numerous visible features (e.g. tall or short, red flowers or white flowers) which are consistent under a variety of environmental conditions yet contrast due to genetic circumstances. Seeds could be obtained from local merchants. Three excellent books give insight into Mendel's life and the context of his discoveries: Carlson, E. A. 1966. *The Gene: A Critical History*. Philadelphia: W. B. Saunders.; Sturtevant, A. H. 1965. *A History of Genetics*. New York: Harper and Row.; Voeller, B. R. 1968. *The Chromosome Theory of Inheritance*. New York: Appleton-Century-Crofts.

5. First, read the entire question and see that you are to determine the pattern of inheritance for "checkered and plain." Notice that there is reference to one characteristic, *pattern*, with two alternatives, checkered vs. plain. We should consider this to be a monohybrid condition unless complications arise.   Assignment of symbols:

P = checkered; p = plain.

Checkered is tentatively assigned the dominant function because in a casual examination of the data, especially cross (b), we see that checkered types are more likely to be produced than plain types.

Cross (a):
PP X *PP*   or   *PP* X *Pp*

Cross (b):
PP X *pp*

This assignment seems reasonable because among 38 offspring, no plain types are produced.

Cross (c):

Because all the offspring from this cross are plain, there is no doubt that the genotype of both parents is *pp*.

Genotypes of all individuals:

	F₁ Progeny	
P₁ Cross	Checkered	Plain
(a) *PP* X *PP*	*PP*	
PP X *Pp*	*PP, Pp*	
(b) *PP* X *pp*	*Pp*	
(c) *pp* X *pp*		*pp*

If you crossed the F₁ generation from cross (b), you would form ¾ checkered and ¼ plain.

6. In the first sentence you are told that there are two *characteristics* which are being studied: seed shape and cotyledon color. Expect, therefore, this to be a dihybrid situation with *two gene pairs* involved. One also sees the possible alternatives of these two characteristics: *seed shape*; wrinkled vs. round; *cotyledon color*; green vs. yellow. After reading the second sentence you can predict that the allele for round seeds is dominant to that for wrinkled seeds and the allele for yellow cotyledons is dominant to the allele for green cotyledons.

Symbolism:	
w = wrinkled seeds	g = green cotyledons
W = round seeds	G = yellow cotyledons

P₁:

WWGG   X   *wwgg*

Parents are considered to be homozygous for two reasons. First, in the introductory sentence, just after PROBLEMS AND DISCUSSION QUESTIONS, there is the statement "members of the P₁ generation are homozygous. . ." Second, notice that the only offspring are those with round seeds and yellow cotyledons.

Gametes produced: One member of each gene pair is "segregated" to each gamete.

WWGG   *wwgg*

(WG)   (wg)

F₁: *WwGg*

F_1 X F_1:

> *WwGg* X *WwGg*

Gametes produced: Under conditions of independent assortment, there will be four (2^n, where n = number of heterozygous gene pairs) different types of gametes produced by each parent.

Punnett Square:

	WG	Wg	wG	wg
WG	WWGG	WWGg	WwGG	WwGg
Wg	WWGg	WWgg	WwGg	Wwgg
wG	WwGG	WwGg	wwGG	wwGg
wg	WwGg	Wwgg	wwGg	wwgg

Collecting the phenotypes according the dominance scheme presented above, gives the following:

9/16 *W_G_* round seeds, yellow cotyledons
3/16 *W_gg* round seeds, green cotyledons
3/16 *wwG_* wrinkled seeds, yellow cotyledons
1/16 *wwgg* wrinkled seeds, green cotyledons

Notice that a dash (_) is used where, because of dominance, it makes no difference as to the dominant/recessive status of the allele.

Forked, or branch diagram:

Seed shape	Cotyledon color	Phenotypes

```
              3/4 yellow ⇨ 9/16 round,yellow
            /
3/4 round
            \
              1/4 green   ⇨ 3/16 round, green

              3/4 yellow ⇨ 3/16 wrinkled, yellow
            /
1/4 wrinkled
            \
              1/4 green   ⇨ 1/16 wrinkled, green
```

7. Symbolism as before:

w = wrinkled seeds	*g* = green cotyledons
W = round seeds	*G* = yellow cotyledons

Examine each characteristic (seed shape vs. cotyledon color) separately.

(a) Notice a 3:1 ratio for seed shape, therefore *Ww* X *Ww*; and no green cotyledons, therefore *GG* X *GG* or *GG* X *Gg*. Putting the two characteristics together gives

> *WwGG*   X   *WwGG*
>
> or
>
> *WwGG*   X   *WwGg*.

(b) Notice a 1:1 ratio for seed shape (8/16 wrinkled and 8/16 round) and a 3:1 ratio for cotyledon color (12/16 yellow and 4/16 green). Therefore the answer is

> *wwGg*   X   *WwGg*.

(c) This is a typical 1:1:1:1 test cross (or backcross) ratio and will signify that one parent is doubly heterozygous while the other is fully homozygous recessive. The answer is

> *WwGg*   X   *wwgg*.

8. A test cross involves a cross of an organism with an unknown genotype to a fully homozygous recessive organism. In Problem 7, (c) fits this description.

9. Because independent assortment may be defined as one gene pair segregating independently of another gene pair, one would need at least two gene pairs in order to demonstrate independent assortment. The problem satisfies criteria for Mendel's postulate of independent assortment.

10. Mendel's four postulates are related to the diagram below.

1. Factors occur in pairs. Notice *A* and *a*.
2. Some genes have dominant and recessive alleles. Notice *A* and *a*.
3. Alleles segregate from each other during gamete formation. When homologous chromosomes separate from each other at anaphase I, alleles will go to opposite poles of the meiotic apparatus.
4. One gene pair separates independently from other gene pairs. Different gene pairs on the same homologous pair of chromosomes (if far apart) or on nonhomologous chromosomes will separate independently from each other during meiosis.

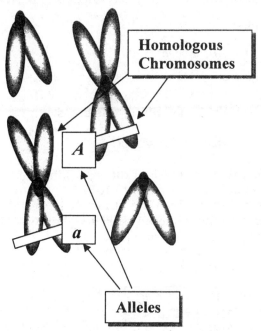

Homologous Chromosomes

A

a

Alleles

11. Carefully re-read the answer to Question #2 in Chapter #2. Briefly, the factors which specify chromosomal homology are the following:

overall length,
position of the centromere,
banding patterns,
type and location of genes,
autoradiographic pattern
function

12. Homozygosity refers to a condition where both alleles of a gene pair are the same (i.e., *AA* or *GG* or *hh*) whereas heterozygosity refers to the condition where members of a gene pair are different (i.e., *Aa* or *Gg or Bb*). Homozygotes produce only one type of gamete whereas heterozygotes will produce 2^n types of gametes where n = number of heterozygous gene pairs (assuming independent assortment).

13. There are two characteristics presented here, body color and wing length. First, assign meaningful gene symbols.

Body color	*Wing length*
E = gray body color	*V* = long wings
e = ebony body color	*v* = vestigial wings

(a)

P_1:

EEVV X *eevv*

F_1: *EeVv* (gray, long)

F_2: This will be the result of a Punnett square with 16 boxes as in the text.

Phenotypes	*Ratio*	*Genotypes*	*Ratio*
gray, long	9/16	*EEVV*	1/16
		EEVv	2/16
		EeVV	2/16
		EeVv	4/16
gray, vestigial	3/16	*EEvv*	1/16
		Eevv	2/16
ebony, long	3/16	*eeVV*	1/16
		eeVv	2/16
ebony, vestigial	1/16	*eevv*	1/16

(b)

> P₁:
>
>   *EEvv* X *eeVV*
>
> F₁: It is important to see that the results from this cross will be exactly the same as those in part (a) above. The only difference is that the recessive alleles are coming from both parents, rather than from one parent only as in (a). The F₂ ratio will be the same as (a) also. When you have genes on the autosomes (not X-linked), independent assortment, complete dominance, and no gene interaction (see later) in a cross involving double heterozygotes, the offspring ratio will be 9:3:3:1.

(c)

> P₁:
>
>   *EEVV* X *EEvv*
>
> F₁: *EEVv* (gray, long)
>
> F₂: Notice that all the offspring will have gray bodies and you will get a 3:1 ratio of long to vestigial wings. You should see this before you even begin working through the problem. Even though this cross involves two gene pairs, it will give a "monohybrid" type of ratio because one of the gene pairs is homozygous (body color) and *one* gene pair is heterozygous (wing length).
>
> | Phenotypes | Ratio | Genotypes | Ratio |
> |---|---|---|---|
> | gray, long | 3/4 | *EEVV* | 1/4 |
> | | | *EEVv* | 2/4 |
> | gray, vestigial | 1/4 | *EEvv* | 1/4 |

NOTE: After working through this problem, it is important that you try to work similar problems without constructing the time-consuming Punnett squares especially if each problem asks for phenotypic rather than genotypic ratios.

14. The general formula for determining the number of kinds of gametes produced by an organism is 2^n where n = number of *heterozygous* gene pairs.

   (a) 4: *AB, Ab, aB, ab*

   (b) 2: *AB, aB*

   (c) 8: *ABC, ABc, AbC, Abc, aBC, aBc, abC, abc*

   (d) 2: *ABc, aBc*

   (e) 4: *ABc, Abc, aBc, abc*

   (f) $2^5 = 32$

15. **(a)** When examining this cross

   AaBbCc X *AaBBCC*

expect there to be eight different kinds of gametes from one parent (*AaBbCc*), and two different kinds from the other (*AaBBCC*). Therefore there should be sixteen kinds (genotypes) of offpsring (8 X 2).

   Gametes: Gametes:

ABC
ABc
AbC
Abc
aBC
aBc
abC
abc

ABC
aBC

Offspring:

Genotypes	Ratio	Phenotypes
AABBCC	(1/16)	
AABBCc	(1/16)	
AABbCC	(1/16)	
AABbCc	(1/16)	
AaBBCC	(2/16)	A_B_C_ = 12/16
AaBBCc	(2/16)	
AaBbCC	(2/16)	
AaBbCc	(2/16)	
aaBBCC	(1/16)	
aaBBCc	(1/16)	aaB_C_ = 4/16
aaBbCC	(1/16)	
aaBbCc	(1/16)	

(b) There will be four kinds of gametes for the first parent (*AaBBCc*) and two kinds of gametes for the second parent.

Gametes: Gametes:

ABC	aBC
ABc	aBc
aBC	
aBc	

Offspring:

Genotypes	Ratio	Phenotypes	
AaBBCC	1/8	A_BBC_	= 3/8
AaBBCc	2/8		
AaBBcc	1/8	A_BBcc	= 1/8
aaBBCC	1/8	aaBBC_	= 3/8
aaBBCc	2/8		
aaBBcc	1/8	aaBBcc	= 1/8

(c) There will be eight (2^n) different kinds of gametes from each of the parents, therefore a 64-box Punnett square. Doing this problem by the forked-line method helps considerably.

1/4 AA —
- 1/4 BB —
  - 1/4 CC = 1/64 AABBCC
  - 2/4 Cc = 2/64 AABBCc
  - 1/4 cc
- 2/4 Bb —
  - 1/4 CC
  - 2/4 Cc
  - 1/4 cc
- 1/4 bb —
  - 1/4 CC
  - 2/4 Cc
  - 1/4 cc

etc.

2/4 Aa
- 1/4 BB
  - 1/4 CC
  - 2/4 Cc
  - 1/4 cc
- 2/4 Bb
  - 1/4 CC
  - 2/4 Cc
  - 1/4 cc
- 1/4 bb
  - 1/4 CC
  - 2/4 Cc
  - 1/4 cc

1/4 aa
- 1/4 BB
  - 1/4 CC
  - 2/4 Cc
  - 1/4 cc
- 2/4 Bb
  - 1/4 CC
  - 2/4 Cc
  - 1/4 cc
- 1/4 bb
  - 1/4 CC
  - 2/4 Cc
  - 1/4 cc

Simply multiply through each component to arrive at the final genotypic frequencies.

For the phenotypic frequencies, set up the problem in the following manner

3/4 A_ —
- 3/4 B_ —
  - 3/4 C_ = 27/64 A_B_C_
  - 1/4 cc = 9/64 A_B_cc
- 1/4 bb —
  - 3/4 C_
  - 1/4 cc

etc.

1/4 aa —
- 3/4 B_ —
  - 3/4 C_
  - 1/4 cc
- 1/4 bb —
  - 3/4 C_
  - 1/4 cc

16. In reading this question, notice that there are two characteristics being considered; seed color (yellow, green) and seed shape (round, wrinkled). At this point you should be able to do this problem without writing down each of the steps. The F_1 can be considered to be a double heterozygote (with round and yellow being dominant). See the cross this way:

Symbols:

Seed shape	Seed color
W = round	*G* = yellow
w = wrinkled	*g* = green

P_1:   *WWgg*   X   *wwGG*

F_1:   *WwGg* cross to *wwgg*

         (which is a typical testcross)

The offspring will occur in a typical 1:1:1:1 as

         1/4 *WwGg* (round, yellow)

         1/4 *Wwgg* (round, green)

         1/4 *wwGg* (wrinkled, yellow)

         1/4 *wwgg* (wrinkled, green)

Again, at this point it would be very helpful if you could do such simple problems by inspection.

17. Since these are F_2 results from monohybrid crosses a 3:1 ratio is expected for each. Referring to the text one can set up the analysis easily.

(a)

Expected ratio	Observed (o)	Expected (e)
3/4	882	885.75
1/4	299	295.25

Expected values are derived by multiplying the expected ratio by the total number of organisms.

$$\chi^2 = \sum (o - e)^2/e = .064$$

In looking in the χ^2 table with 1 degree of freedom (because there were two classes, therefore n-1 or 1 degree of freedom), we find a probability (p) value between 0.9 and 0.5.

We would therefore say that there is a "good fit" between the observed and expected values. Notice that as the deviations between the observed and expected values increase the value of χ^2 increases. So the higher the χ^2 value the more likely the null hypothesis will be rejected.

(b)

Expected ratio	Observed (o)	Expected (e)
3/4	705	696.75
1/4	224	232.25

$$\chi^2 = 0.39$$

The p value in the table for 1 degree of freedom is still between 0.9 and 0.5, however, because the χ^2 value is larger in (b) we should say that the deviations from expectation are greater. The deviation in each case can be attributed to chance.

18. (a) One must think of this problem as a dihybrid F_2 situation with the following expectations:

Expected ratio	Observed (o)	Expected (e)
9/16	315	312.75
3/16	108	104.25
3/16	101	104.25
1/16	32	34.75

$$\chi^2 = 0.47$$

Looking at the table in the text one can see that this χ^2 value is associated with a probability greater than 0.90 for 3 degrees of freedom (because there are now four classes in the χ^2 test). The observed and expected values do not deviate significantly.

To deal with parts **(b)** and **(c)** it is easier to see the observed values for the monohybrid ratios if the phenotypes are listed:

smooth, yellow	315
smooth, green	108
wrinkled, yellow	101
wrinkled, green	32

For the smooth: wrinkled *monohybrid component*, the smooth types total 423 (315 + 108), while the wrinkled types total 133 (101 + 32).

Expected ratio	Observed (o)	Expected (e)
3/4	423	417
1/4	133	139

The χ^2 value is 0.35 and in examining the text for 1 degree of freedom, the p value is greater than 0.50 and less than 0.90. We fail to reject the null hypothesis and are confident that the observed values do not differ significantly from the expected values.

(c) For the yellow:green portion of the problem, see that there are 416 yellow plants (315 + 101) and 140 (108 + 32) green plants.

Expected ratio	Observed (o)	Expected (e)
3/4	416	417
1/4	140	139

The χ^2 value is 0.01 and in examining the text for 1 degree of freedom, the p value is greater than 0.90. We fail to reject the null hypothesis and are confident that the observed values do not differ significantly from the expected values.

19. It would be best to set up two tables based on the two hypotheses:

(a)

Expected ratio	Observed (o)	Expected (e)
3/4	250	300
1/4	150	100

(b)

Expected ratio	Observed (o)	Expected (e)
1/2	250	200
1/2	150	200

For the test of a 3:1 ratio, the χ^2 value is 33.3 with an associated p value of less than 0.01 for 1 degree of freedom. For the test of a 1:1 ratio, the χ^2 value is 25.0 again with an associated p value of less than 0.01 for 1 degree of freedom. Based on these probability values, both null hypotheses should be rejected.

20. Use of the $p = 0.10$ as the "critical" value for rejecting or failing to reject the null hypothesis instead of $p = 0.05$ would allow more null hypotheses to be rejected. Notice in the text that as the χ^2 values increase, there is a higher likelihood that the null hypothesis will be rejected because the higher values are more likely to be associated with a p value which is less than 0.05.

As the critical *p* value is increased, it takes a smaller χ^2 value to cause rejection of the null hypothesis. It would take less difference between the expected and observed values to reject the null hypothesis, therefore the stringency of failing to reject the null hypothesis is increased.

21. Given the cross *AaBbCC* X *AABbCc* we can apply the product rule which states that when two or more events occur independently but simultaneously, their combined probability is equal to the product of their individual probabilities.

The probability of getting *AA* from

   Aa   X   *AA*   is 1/2

The probability of getting *Bb* from

   Bb   X   *Bb*   is 1/2

The probability of getting *Cc* from

   CC   X   *Cc*   is 1/2

The *overall* probability then is

$$1/2 \quad X \quad 1/2 \quad X \quad 1/2 = 1/8$$

22. The probability of getting *aabbcc* from the *AaBbCC* X *AABbCc* mating is zero because of homozygosity for *AA* and *CC*.

23. Because all the offspring will show the dominant A and C phenotypes and 3/4 will show the B phenotype, the probability of an offspring showing all three dominant traits would be 1 X 3/4 X 1 = 3/4.

24. While there are many different inheritance patterns which will be described later in the text (codominance, incomplete dominance, sex-linked inheritance, etc.) the range of solutions to this question is limited to the concepts developed in the first three chapters, namely dominance or recessiveness.

If an allele is dominant, it will not skip generations nor will it be passed to offspring unless at least one of the parents has the allele. On the other hand, alleles that are recessive can skip generations and exist in a carrier state in parents. For example, notice that II-4 and II-5 produce a female child (III-4) with the affected phenotype. On these criteria alone, the allele must be viewed as being recessive. Note: if an allele is recessive and X-linked (to be discussed later) the pattern will often be from affected male to carrier female to affected male.

To provide genotypes for each individual, consider that if the box or circle is shaded, the *aa* genotype is to be assigned. If offspring are affected (shaded), a recessive allele must have come from both parents.

I-1 (*Aa*), I-2 (*aa*), I-3 (*Aa*), I-4(*Aa*)

II-1 (*aa*), II-2 (*Aa*), II-3 (*aa*), II-4 (*Aa*), II-5 (*Aa*), II-6 (*aa*), II-7 (*AA* or *Aa*), II-8 (*AA* or *Aa*)

III-1 (*AA* or *Aa*), III-2 (*AA* or *Aa*), III-3 (*AA* or *Aa*), III-4 (*aa*), III-5 (probably *AA*), III-6 (*aa*)

IV-1 through IV-7 all *Aa*.

25. *Unit Factors in Pairs*: It is important to see that each time a phenotype (normal or abnormal) is being stated, genotypes are symbolized as pairs of genes; *AA*, *Aa* or *aa*. Review F3.2 to understand the need to assign appropriate symbols to genes.

Dominance and Recessiveness: Because the gene for normal pigmentation is completely dominant over the gene for albinism (*a* is fully recessive), it was necessary to consider, at first, whether normally pigmented individuals in the problem were homozygous normal (*AA*) or heterozygous (*Aa*). By looking at the frequency of expression of the recessive gene in the offspring (in *aa* individuals) one can often determine an *Aa* type from an *AA* type.

Segregation: During gamete formation when homologous chromosomes move to opposite poles, paired elements (genes) separate from each other.

26. The allele is inherited as an autosomal recessive. Notice that two normal individuals II-3 and II-4 have produced a daughter (III-2) with myopia.

I-1 (*aa*), I-2 (*Aa* or *AA*), I-3 (*Aa*), I-4 (*Aa*)
II-1 (*Aa*), II-2 (*Aa*), II-3 (*Aa*), II-4 (*Aa*), II-5 (*aa*),
II-6 (*AA* or *Aa*), II-7 (*AA* or *Aa*)
III-1 (*AA* or *Aa*), III-2 (*aa*), III-3 (*AA* or *Aa*)

27. (a) There are two possibilities. Either the trait is dominant, in which case I-1 is heterozygous as are II-2 and II-3, or the trait is recessive and I-1 is homozygous and I-2 is heterozygous. Under the condition of recessiveness, both II-1 and II-4 would be heterozygous, II-2 and II-3 homozygous.

    (b) Recessive: Parents *Aa, Aa*

    (c) Recessive: Parents *Aa, Aa*

    (d) Recessive or dominant: if recessive, parents *AA* (probably), *aa*. Second pedigree: recessive or dominant, not sex-linked, if recessive, parents *Aa, aa*

28. (a) First consider that each parent is homozygous (true-breeding in the question) and since in the F$_1$ only round, axial, violet, and full phenotypes were expressed, they must each be dominant. Because all genes are on nonhomologous chromosomes, independent assortment will occur.

(b) Round, axial, violet and full would be the most frequent phenotypes:

    3/4 X 3/4 X 3/4 X 3/4

(c) Wrinkled, terminal, white, and constricted would be the least frequent phenotypes:

    1/4 X 1/4 X 1/4 X 1/4

(d)

3/4 X 3/4 X 3/4 X 3/4 +
1/4 X 1/4 X 1/4 X 1/4 = 82/256

(e) There would be 16 different phenotypes in the test cross offspring just as there are 16 different phenotypes in the F$_2$ generation.

29. (a) The first task is to draw out an accurate pedigree (one of several possibilities):

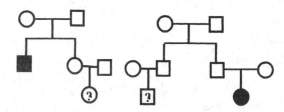

(b) The probability that the female (whose maternal uncle had TSD) is heterozygous is 1/3 because she is not TSD and her mother had a 2/3 chance of being heterozygous and she has a 1/2 chance of passing the TSD gene to her daughter (2/3 X 1/2 = 1/3). The male (whose paternal first cousin had TSD) has a 1/4 chance of being heterozygous, assuming that either (but not both, because the gene is said to be rare) his grandmother or grandfather was heterozygous. Therefore the probability that both the male and female are heterozygous is:

    1/3   X   1/4 = 1/12

(c) The probability that neither is heterozygous is:

    2/3   X   3/4 = 6/12

(d) The probability that one is heterozygous is:

    (1/3 X 3/4)   +   (2/3 X 1/4)   = 5/12

30. (a) Notice in cross #1 that the ratio of straight wings to curled wings is 3:1 and the ratio of short bristles to long bristles is also 3:1. This would indicate that straight is dominant to curled and short is dominant to long.

Possible symbols would be (using standard *Drosophila* symbolism):

straight wings = w^+ curled wings = w

short bristles = b^+ long bristles = b

(b)

Cross #1: w^+/w ; b^+/b X w^+/w ; b^+/b
Cross #2: w^+/w ; b/b X w^+/w ; b/b
Cross #3: w/w ; b/b X w^+/w ; b^+/b
Cross #4: w^+/w^+ ; b^+/b X w^+/w^+ ; b^+/b (one parent could be w^+/w)
Cross #5: w/w ; b^+/b X w^+/w ; b^+/b

31. (a) First, consider that the data represent a 3:1 ratio based on the information given in the problem: *Ss* X *Ss*. Compute the expected quantities for each class by multiplying the totals by 3/4 and 1/4.

Set I Expected Numbers:

    Tall = 26.25
    Short = 8.75

Set II Expected Numbers:

    Tall = 262.5
    Short = 87.5

For Set I the χ^2 value would be:

$(30-26.25)^2/26.25$ + $(5-8.75)^2/8.75$

= 2.15 with p being between 0.2 and 0.05

so one would accept the null hypothesis of no significant difference between the expected and observed values.

For Set II, the χ^2 value would be:

21.43 and $p<0.001$ and one would reject the null hypothesis and assume a significant difference between the observed and expected values.

(b) Clearly, with an increase in sample size a different conclusion is reached. In fact, most statisticians recommend that the expected values in each class should not be less than 10. In most cases, more confidence is gained as the sample size increases, however, depending on the organism or experiment, there are practical limits on sample size.

Chapter 4: Modification of Mendelian Ratios

<u>**Concept Areas**</u>	<u>**Corresponding Problems**</u>
Incomplete Dominance, Codominance	1, 2, 5, 6, 12, 13, 28, 28, 30
Multiple Alleles	3, 11, 21, 27, 30
Lethal Alleles	4, 31
Gene Interaction	8, 9, 14, 16, 18, 19, 20, 22, 26
Epistasis	7, 8, 9, 16, 17, 20, 25, 29
Complementation	25
X-Linkage	10, 11, 13, 14, 15, 16, 23, 24
Extranuclear Inheritance	32, 33, 34, 35, 36, 37

Vocabulary: Organization and Listing of Terms and Concepts

Structures and Substances

Wild-type, mutations

   null allele

Antigens

Antibodies

   isoagglutinogen

   H substance

White locus

Lethal allele

Ommatidia

   drosopterin

   xanthommatin

Hexosaminidase

Hypoxanthine-guanine
phosphoribosyl transferase (HGPRT)

Processes/Methods

Incomplete (partial) dominance

   pink flowers, 1:2:1

Codominance

   MN blood groups

Multiple allelism

   ABO blood types

   Bombay phenotype

   white eye in *Drosophila*

Lethal alleles

   recessive, dominant

     yellow coat color in mice

     Huntington's disease

Gene interaction: discontinuous variation

    epistasis (T4.1)

    epistatic

    homozygous recessive, 9:3:4

        coat color in mice

        Bombay phenotype

    dominant

        fruit color in squash, 12:3:1

    other

        white flowers in peas, 9:7

    novel phenotypes

    fruit shape in *Cucurbita*

    complementation

X-linkage, Chromosome Theory

    hemizygous

    crisscross pattern

Sex-limited inheritance

    feathering in chickens

Sex-influenced inheritance

    pattern baldness

Penetrance, Expressivity

Position effect

    heterochromatin

Conditional mutation

    temperature

Tay-Sachs, Lesch-Nyhan

Duchene muscular dystrophy (DMD)

Huntington Disease

Genetic anticipation

    myotonic dystrophy

Genomic (parental) imprinting

    Prader-Willi syndrome, Angelman syndrome

Extranuclear inheritance

    organelle heredity

        chloroplasts, mitochondria

        heteroplasmy

        Four O'clocks, *poky, petites*

        MERRF, LHON

    maternal effect

        Limnaea coiling

        bicoid (*bic*)

Concepts

Symbolism (F4.2)

Gene interaction (F4.1)

Allele (F4.2), wild type, mutation

    loss of function

    gain of function

Symbolism (F4.2)

    recessive trait (*e, e* ⁺)

    dominant trait *(Wr, Wr* ⁺*)*

    no dominance *(R1, R2) (L^{M}, L^{N})*

    leu-, leu+, dnaA, BRCA1

Modified ratios (T4.1), lethality

    3:1, 1:2:1, 9:3:3:1

    3:6:3:1:2:1, 9:3:4, 12:3:1, 9:7

Complementation

X-linked inheritance

Sex-limited inheritance

Sex-influenced inheritance

Phenotypic expression

    penetrance, expressivity

    genetic background

    environmental effects

Extranuclear inheritance (F4.3)

    organelle, maternal effect

T4.1 Examples of typical monohybrid and dihybrid ratios with several modifications.

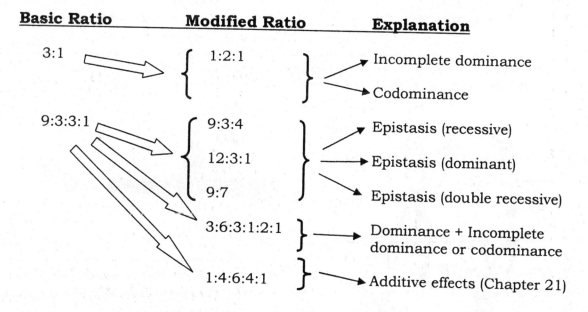

Basic Ratio	Modified Ratio	Explanation
3:1	1:2:1	Incomplete dominance
		Codominance
9:3:3:1	9:3:4	Epistasis (recessive)
	12:3:1	Epistasis (dominant)
	9:7	Epistasis (double recessive)
	3:6:3:1:2:1	Dominance + Incomplete dominance or codominance
	1:4:6:4:1	Additive effects (Chapter 21)

F4.1 Illustration of gene interaction where products from more than one gene pair influence one characteristic or phenotypic trait.

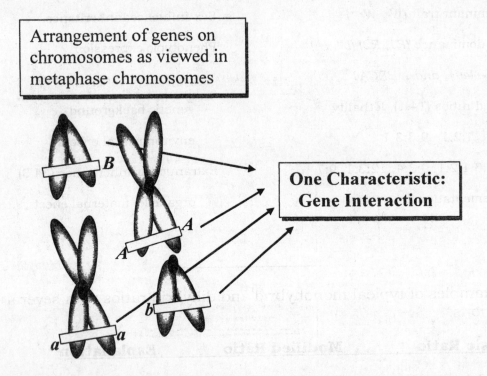

Arrangement of genes on chromosomes as viewed in metaphase chromosomes

B

A

A

b

a

a

One Characteristic: Gene Interaction

Example: Two gene pairs influencing the pigmentation pattern on the shark. Various gene products contribute in a variety of ways to generate a particular pigment pattern.

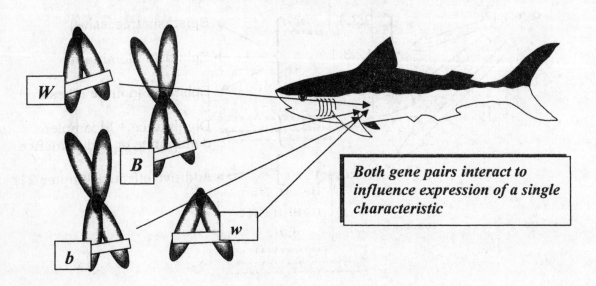

W

B

b

w

Both gene pairs interact to influence expression of a single characteristic

F4.2 Symbolism associated with the wild type activity of a gene and several possible outcomes of the mutant state: **A.** wild type; **B.** too much product; **C.** too little product; **D.** no product; **E.** both products expressed; **F.** reduced product.

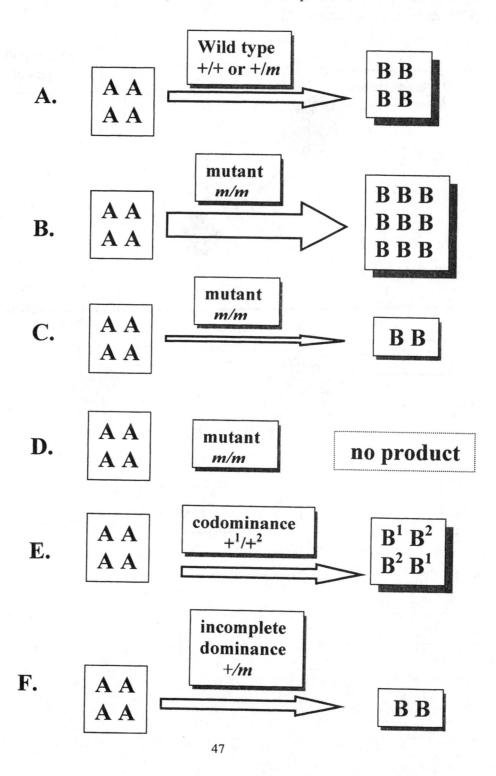

F4.3 Illustration of the common pattern seen in many cases of extranuclear inheritance. The condition of the female (egg) parent has a stronger influence on the phenotype of the offspring than the male (sperm/pollen) parent. Reciprocal crosses give different results in offspring.

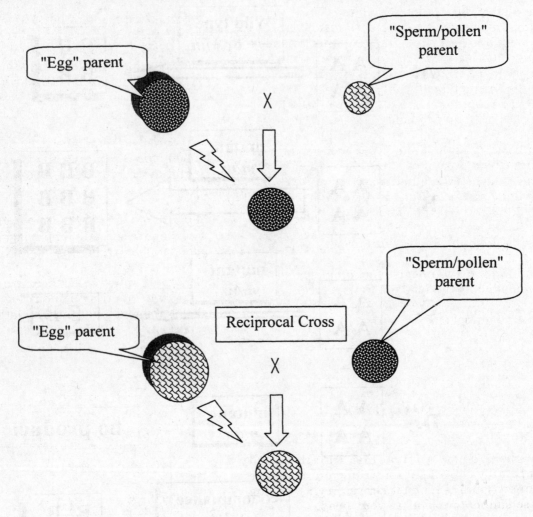

Solutions to Problems and Discussion Questions

1. In the first sentence of this problem, notice that there is one characteristic (coat color) and three phenotypes mentioned; red, white, or roan. The fact that roan is intermediate between red and white suggests that this may be a case of incomplete dominance, with roan being the intermediate and therefore the heterozygous type. If that is the case, then we should suspect a 1:2:1 phenotypic ratio in crosses of "roan to roan."

Looking at the data given, notice that a cross of the "extremes" (red X white) gives roan, suggesting its heterozygous nature and the homozygous nature of the parents. Seeing the 1:2:1 ratio in the offspring of

roan   X   roan

confirms the hypothesis of incomplete dominance as the mode of inheritance.

> Symbolism:
>
> AA = red,
>
> aa = white,
>
> Aa = roan

Crosses: It is important at this point that you not be fully dependent on writing out complete Punnett squares for each cross. Begin working these simple problems in your head.

> AA X AA ⟹ AA
>
> aa X aa ⟹ aa
>
> AA X aa ⟹ Aa
>
> Aa X Aa ⟹
>
> 1/4 AA; 2/4 Aa; 1/4 aa

2. *Incomplete dominance* can be viewed more as a quantitative phenomenon where the heterozygote is intermediate (approximately) between the limits set by the homozygotes. Pink is intermediate between red and white.

Codominance can be viewed in a more qualitative manner where both of the alleles in the heterozygote are expressed. For example, in the AB blood group, both the I^A and I^B genes are expressed. There is no intermediate class which is part I^A and I^B.

3. In this problem remember that individuals with blood type B can have the genotype $I^B I^B$ or $I^B I^o$ and those with blood type A, genotypes $I^A I^A$ or $I^A I^o$.

Male Parent: must be $I^B I^o$ because the mother is $I^o I^o$ and one inherits one homolog (therefore one allele) from each parent.

Female Parent: must be $I^A I^o$ because the father is $I^B I^o$ and one inherits one homolog (therefore one allele) from each parent. The father can not be $I^B I^B$ and have a daughter of blood type A.

Offspring:

$I^A I^o$ X $I^B I^o$

	I^B	I^o
I^A	$I^A I^B$ (AB)	$I^A I^o$ (A)
I^o	$I^B I^o$ (B)	$I^o I^o$ (O)

The ratio would be

1(A):1(B):1(AB):1(O).

4. Notice that there is one typical (coat color) and one atypical (lethality) characteristic mentioned. Often under this condition of two characteristics, we must decide if the problem involves one or more than one gene pair. Because the genotypes are given here, it is obvious that lethality is associated with expression of the coat color alleles and therefore one gene pair is involved. This is a monohybrid condition.

Pp X Pp ⇨

> 1/4 PP (**lethal**)
>
> 2/4 Pp (platinum)
>
> 1/4 pp (silver)

Therefore the ratio of surviving foxes is 2/3 platinum, 1/3 silver. The P allele behaves as a recessive in terms of lethality (seen only in the homozygote) but as a dominant in terms of coat color (seen in the homozygote).

5. Three independently assorting characteristics are being dealt with: flower color (incomplete dominance), flower shape (dominant/recessive), and plant height (dominant/recessive). Establish appropriate gene symbols:

> Flower color:
>
> RR = red ; Rr = pink; rr = white
>
> Flower shape:
>
> P = personate; p = peloric
>
> Plant height:
>
> D = tall; d = dwarf

(a)

> $RRPPDD$ X $rrppdd$ ⇨
>
> $RrPpDd$ (pink, personate, tall)

(b) Use *components* of the forked line method as follows:

> 2/4 pink X 3/4 personate X 3/4 tall
>
> = 18/64

6. There are two characteristics, flower color and flower shape. Because pink results from a cross of red and white, one would conclude that flower color is "monohybrid" with incomplete dominance.

In addition, because personate is seen in the F_1 when personate and peloric are crossed, personate must be dominant to peloric. Results from crosses (c) and (d) verify these conclusions. The appropriate symbols would be as follows

> Flower color:
>
> RR = red; Rr = pink; rr = white
>
> Flower shape:
>
> P = personate; p = peloric

(a)

> $RRpp$ X $rrPP$ ⟹ $RrPp$

(b)

> $RRPP$ X $rrpp$ ⟹ $RrPp$

(c)

> $RrPp$ X $RRpp$ ⟹ { $RRPp$
> $RRpp$
> $RrPp$
> $Rrpp$

(d)

> $RrPp$ X $rrpp$ ⟹ { $rrPp$
> $rrpp$
> $RrPp$
> $Rrpp$

In the cross of the F₁ of (a) to the F₁ of (b), both of which are double heterozygotes, one would expect the following:

$$RrPp \quad X \quad RrPp$$

1/4 red
⟋ 3/4 personate ---> 3/16 red, personate
⟍ 1/4 peloric ---> 1/16 red, peloric

2/4 pink
⟋ 3/4 personate ---> 6/16 pink, personate
⟍ 1/4 peloric ---> 2/16 pink, peloric

1/4 white
⟋ 3/4 personate ---> 3/16 white, personate
⟍ 1/4 peloric ---> 1/16 white, peloric

7. Notice that the distribution of observed offspring fits a 9:3:4 ratio quite well. This suggests that two independently assorting gene pairs with epistasis are involved. Assign gene symbols in the usual manner:

A = pigment; a = pigmentless (colorless)

B = purple; b = red

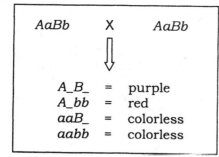

One may see this occurring in the following manner:

precursor ---↑-> cyanidin ---↑-> purple pigment

(colorless) *aa*   (red) *bb*

8. This is a case of gene interaction (novel phenotypes) where the yellow and black types (double mutants) interact to give the cream phenotype and epistasis where the *cc* genotype produces albino.

(a)

$$AaBbCc \implies \text{gray } (C \text{ allows pigment})$$

(b)

$$A\_B\_Cc \implies \text{gray } (C \text{ allows pigment})$$

(c) Use the forked line method for this portion

3/4 A_
  ⟋ 3/4 B_
    ⟋ 1/2 Cc ⟹ 9/32 gray
    ⟍ 1/2 cc ⟹ 9/32 albino
  ⟍ 1/4 bb
    ⟋ 1/2 Cc ⟹ 3/32 yellow
    ⟍ 1/2 cc ⟹ 3/32 albino

1/4 aa
  ⟋ 3/4 B_
    ⟋ 1/2 Cc ⟹ 3/32 black
    ⟍ 1/2 cc ⟹ 3/32 albino
  ⟍ 1/4 bb
    ⟋ 1/2 Cc ⟹ 1/32 cream
    ⟍ 1/2 cc ⟹ 1/32 albino

Combining the phenotypes gives (always count the proportions to see that they add up to 1.0):

16/32 albino;

9/32   gray;

3/32   yellow;

3/32   black;

1/32   cream

9. Treat each of the crosses as a series of monohybrid crosses, remembering that albino is epistatic to color and black and yellow interact to give cream.

(a) Since this is a 9:3:3:1 ratio with no albino phenotypes, the parents must each have been double heterozygotes and incapable of producing the *cc* genotype.

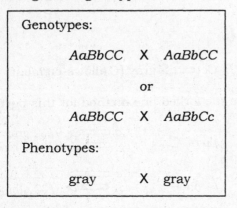

Genotypes:

    AaBbCC   X   *AaBbCC*

             or

    AaBbCC   X   *AaBbCc*

Phenotypes:

      gray   X   gray

(b) Since there are no black offspring, there are no combinations in the parents which can produce *aa*. The 4/16 proportion indicates that the *C* locus is heterozygous in both parents.

If the parents are

  AABbCc   X   *AaBbCc*

           or

  AABbCc   X   *AABbCc*

then the results would follow the pattern given. Phenotypes: gray   X   gray.

(c) Notice that 16/64 or 1/4 of the offspring are albino, therefore the parents are both heterozygous at the *C* locus. Second, notice that without considering the *C* locus, there is a 27:9:9:3 ratio which reduces to a 9:3:3:1 ratio. Given this information, the genotypes must be

  AaBbCc   X   *AaBbCc*.

Phenotypes: gray   X   gray

10. In order to solve this problem one must first see the possible genotypes of the parents and the grandfathers. Since the gene is X-linked, the cross will be symbolized with the X chromosomes.

RG = normal vision; *rg* = color-blind

     Mother's father: X^{rg}/Y

     Father's father: X^{rg}/Y

     Mother: $X^{RG}X^{rg}$

     Father: X^{RG}/Y

Notice that the mother must be heterozygous for the *rg* allele (being normal-visioned and having inherited an X^{rg} from her father) and the father, because he has normal vision, must be X^{RG}. The fact that the father's father is color-blind does not mean that the father will be color-blind. On the contrary, the father will inherit his X chromosome from his mother.

$$X^{RG} X^{rg} \quad X \quad X^{RG}/Y$$

$X^{RG}X^{RG}$	= 1/4 daughter normal
$X^{RG}X^{rg}$	= 1/4 daughter normal
X^{RG}/Y	= 1/4 son normal
X^{rg}/Y	= 1/4 son color-blind

Looking at the distribution of offspring:

(a) 1/4

(b) 1/2

(c) 1/4

(d) zero

11. The mating is $X^{RG}X^{rg}; I^AI^O$ X $X^{RG}Y; I^AI^O$

Based on the son who is color-blind and blood type O, the mother must have been heterozygous for the *RG* locus and both parents must have had one copy of the I^O gene. The probability of having a female child is 1/2, that she has normal vision is 1 (because the father's X is normal) and 1/4 type O blood. The final product of the independent probabilities is

$$1/2 \quad X \quad 1 \quad X \quad 1/4 \quad = \quad 1/8$$

12. In seeing that the distribution of phenotypes in the F1 is different when comparing males and females, it would be tempting to suggest that the gene is X-linked. However, given that the reciprocal cross gives identical results suggests that the gene is autosomal. Seeing the different distribution between males and females one might consider sex-influenced inheritance as a model and have males more likely to express mahogany and females more likely to express red. This situation is similar to pattern baldness in humans. Consider two alleles which are autosomal and let

> *RR* = red, *Rr* = red in females
>
> *Rr* = mahogany in males
>
> *rr* = mahogany
>
> P₁:
>
> female: *RR* (red) X male: *rr* (mahogany)
>
> F₁:
>
> *Rr* = females red; males mahogany
>
> 1/2 females (red)
>
> 1/2 males (mahogany)

F₂:

$$1/4 \; RR; \; 2/4 \; Rr, \; 1/4 \; rr$$

Because half of the offspring are males and half are females, one could, for clarity, rewrite the F₂ as:

	1/2 *females*	1/2 *males*
1/4 *RR*	1/8 red	1/8 red
2/4 *Rr*	2/8 red	2/8 mahogany
1/4 *rr*	1/8 mahogany	1/8 mahogany

13. The tortoise shell condition is caused by the phenomenon of dosage compensation where one of the two X chromosomes is randomly inactivated in mammalian females. Once inactivated, all cells descending from a given cell will have the same X chromosome inactive. A tortoise shell female is *Bb* and when crossed with a *BY* male produces the following offspring:

$$Bb \quad X \quad BY$$
$$\downarrow$$

females:　*BB* (black)
　　　　　Bb (tortoise shell)

males:　　*BY* (black)
　　　　　bY (yellow)

From the above information, it would seem impossible to get a tortoise-shell male, however, rare nondisjunction in the female can produce a tortoise-shell male with the a *BbY* genotype.

14. Symbolism: Normal wing margins = sd^+; scalloped = sd

(a)

P₁: $X^{sd}X^{sd}$ ✗ X^+/Y ⟱

F₁: 1/2 X^+X^{sd} (female, normal)

1/2 X^{sd}/Y (male, scalloped)

F₂: 1/4 X^+X^{sd} (female, normal)

1/4 $X^{sd}X^{sd}$ (female, scalloped)

1/4 X^+/Y (male, normal)

1/4 X^{sd}/Y (male, scalloped)

(b)

P₁: X^+/X^+ ✗ X^{sd}/Y ⟱

F₁: 1/2 X^+X^{sd} (female, normal)

1/2 X^+/Y (male, normal)

F₂: 1/4 X^+X^+ (female, normal)

1/4 X^+X^{sd} (female, normal)

1/4 X^+/Y (male, normal)

1/4 X^{sd}/Y (male, scalloped)

If the *scalloped* gene were not X-linked, then all of the F₁ offspring would be wild (phenotypically) and a 3:1 ratio of normal to scalloped would occur in the F₂.

15. Assuming that the parents are homozygous, the crosses would be as follows. Notice that the X symbol may remain to remind us that the *sd* gene is on the X chromosome. It is extremely important that one account for both the mutant genes and each of their wild type alleles.

P₁: $X^{sd}X^{sd}; e^+/e^+$ ✗ $X^+/Y; e/e$

F₁:

1/2 $X^+X^{sd}; e^+/e$ (female, normal)

1/2 $X^{sd}/Y; e^+/e$ (male, scalloped)

F₂:

	X^+e^+	X^+e	$X^{sd}e^+$	$X^{sd}e$
$X^{sd}e^+$				
$X^{sd}e$	Fill in box on your own.			
Ye^+				
Ye				

Phenotypes:

3/16 normal females

3/16 normal males

1/16 ebony females

1/16 ebony males

3/16 scalloped females

3/16 scalloped males

1/16 scalloped, ebony females

1/16 scalloped, ebony males

Forked-line method:

P₁: $X^{sd}X^{sd}; e^+/e^+$ ✗ $X^+/Y; e/e$

F₁: 1/2 $X^+X^{sd}; e^+/e$ (female, normal)
1/2 $X^{sd}/Y; e^+/e$ (male, scalloped)

F₂:

	Wings	Color	
1/4	females, normal	⟨ 3/4 normal	3/16
		1/4 ebony	1/16
1/4	females, scalloped	⟨ 3/4 normal	3/16
		1/4 ebony	1/16
1/4	males, normal	⟨ 3/4 normal	3/16
		1/4 ebony	1/16
1/4	males, scalloped	⟨ 3/4 normal	3/16
		1/4 ebony	1/16

16. It is extremely important that one account for both the mutant genes and each of their wild type alleles.

(a) P₁: $X^v X^v$; $+/+$ X X^+/Y; b^r/b^r ⟱

F₁:

1/2 $X^+ X^v$; $+/b^r$ (female, normal)
1/2 X^v/Y; $+/b^r$ (male, vermilion)

F₂:

Eye color (X)	Eye color (autosomal)	
1/4 females, normal	3/4 normal	3/16
	1/4 brown	1/16
1/4 females, vermilion	3/4 normal	3/16
	1/4 brown	1/16
1/4 males, normal	3/4 normal	3/16
	1/4 brown	1/16
1/4 males, vermilion	3/4 normal	3/16
	1/4 brown	1/16

3/16 = females, normal
1/16 = females, brown eyes
3/16 = females, vermilion eyes
1/16 = females, white eyes
3/16 = males, normal
1/16 = males, brown eyes
3/16 = males, vermilion eyes
1/16 = males, white eyes

(b)

P₁: $X^+ X^+$; b^r/b^r X X^v/Y; $+/+$ ⟱

F₁:

1/2 $X^+ X^v$; $+/b^r$ (female, normal)

1/2 X^+/Y; $+/b^r$ (male, normal)

F₂:

Eye color (X)	Eye color(autosomal)	
2/4	females, normal	3/4 normal
		1/4 brown
1/4	males, normal	3/4 normal
		1/4 brown
1/4	males, vermilion	3/4 normal
		1/4 brown

6/16 = females, normal
2/16 = females, brown eyes
3/16 = males, normal
1/16 = males, brown eyes
3/16 = males, vermilion eyes
1/16 = males, white eyes

(c)

P₁: $X^v X^v$; b^r/b^r X X^+/Y; $+/+$ ⟱

F₁: 1/2 $X^+ X^v$; $+/b^r$ (female, normal)
     1/2 X^v/Y; $+/b^r$ (male, vermilion)

F₂:

Eye color (X)	Eye color (autosomal)	
1/4	females, normal	3/4 normal
		1/4 brown
1/4	females, vermilion	3/4 normal
		1/4 brown
1/4	males, normal	3/4 normal
		1/4 brown
1/4	males, vermilion	3/4 normal
		1/4 brown

3/16 = females, normal
1/16 = females, brown eyes
3/16 = females, vermilion eyes
1/16 = females, white eyes
3/16 = males, normal
1/16 = males, brown eyes
3/16 = males, vermilion eyes
1/16 = males, white eyes

17. The key to dealing with this problem rests in seeing that there are two ways in which the sandy phenotype can be obtained. Notice that in cross 1, crossing sandy with sandy gives an F_1 with the all red phenotype. Since the problem states that all the strains are true-breeding, there is likely some sort of complementation between the two sandy strains to give the "all red" F_1 in cross 1. If you start out with that premise and assign the following genotypic possibilities, all the data fall into place.

> $A\_B\_$ = red
> A_bb or $aaB\_$ = sandy
> $aabb$ = white

For the lost data in crosses 1 and 4, use the following:

Cross 1: $aaBB$ X $AAbb$

F_1: $AaBb$

F_2:

> 9/16 = $A\_B\_$ (red)
> 6/16 $\begin{cases} 3/16 = A\_bb \text{ (sandy)} \\ 3/16 = aaB\_ \text{ (sandy)} \end{cases}$
> 1/16 = (white)

Cross 4: $aabb$ X $AABB$

F_1: $AaBb$

F_2:

> 9/16 = $A\_B\_$ (red)
> 6/16 $\begin{cases} 3/16 = A\_bb \text{ (sandy)} \\ 3/16 = aaB\_ \text{ (sandy)} \end{cases}$
> 1/16 = (white)

18. (a) Because the denominator in the ratios is 64 one would begin to consider that there are three independently assorting gene pairs operating in this problem. Because there are only two characteristics (eye color and croaking) however, one might hypothesize that two gene pairs are involved in the inheritance of one trait while one gene pair is involved in the other.

(b) Notice that there is a 48:16 (or 3:1) ratio of rib-it to knee-deep and a 36:16:12 (or 9:4:3) ratio of blue to green to purple eye color. Because of these relationships one would conclude that croaking is due to one (dominant/recessive) gene pair while eye color is due to two gene pairs. Because there is a (9:4:3) ratio regarding eye color, some gene interaction (epistasis) is indicated.

(c) Symbolism:

> Croaking: $R\_$ = utterer; rr = mutterer

> Eye color:

Since the most frequent phenotype is blue eye, let $A\_B\_$ represent the genotypes. For the purple class, "a 3/16 group" use the A_bb genotypes. The "4/16" class (green) would be the $aaB\_$ and the $aabb$ groups.

(d) The cross involving a blue-eyed, mutterer frog and a purple-eyed, utterer frog would have the genotypes:

> $AABBrr$ X $AAbbRR$

which would produce an F_1 of $AABbRr$ which would be blue-eyed and utterer. The F2 will follow a pattern of a 9:3:3:1 ratio because of homozygosity for the A locus and heterozygosity for both the B and R loci.

> 9/16 $AAB\_R\_$ = blue-eyed, utterer

> 3/16 AAB_rr = blue-eyed, mutterer

> 3/16 $AAbbR\_$ = purple-eyed, utterer

> 1/16 $AAbbrr$ = purple-eyed, mutterer

19. In doing these types of problems, take each characteristic individually, then build the complete genotypes. Notice that the ratio of purple-eyed to green-eyed frogs is 3:1, therefore expect the parents to be heterozygous for the A locus. Because the ratio of utterer to mutterer is also 3:1, expect both parents to be heterozygous at the R locus.

The *B* locus would have the *bb* genotype because both parents are purple-eyed as given in the problem. Both parents would therefore be *AabbRr*.

20. Notice that in a cross between the F₁'s in this problem that a 12:3:1 ratio is obtained which is a clear sign that epistasis has modified a typical 9:3:3:1 ratio. In this case cattle in one of the "3/16" classes has the same phenotype as cattle in the "9/16" class. Since the "9/16" class typically takes the genotype of *A_B_* it seems reasonable to think of the following genotypic classifications:

*A_B_* = solid white (9/16)
*aaB_* = solid white (3/16)
A_bb = black and white spotted (3/16)
aabb = solid black (1/16)

The selection of "*bb*" as giving the spotted phenotype is arbitrary. One could obtain *AAbb* true-breeding black and white-spotted cattle.

21. It is important to see that this problem involves multiple alleles, meaning that monohybrid type ratios are expected, and that there is an order of dominance which will allow certain alleles to be "hidden" in various heterozygotes. As with most genetics problems, one must look at the phenotypes of the offspring to assess the genotypes of the parents.

(a)

> Parents: sepia   X   cream

Because both guinea pigs had albino parents, both are heterozygous for the c^a allele.

> Cross:
>
> $c^k c^a$ X $c^d c^a$
>
> 2/4 sepia; 1/4 cream; 1/4 albino

(b)

> Parents: sepia   X   cream

Because the sepia parent had an albino parent it must be $c^k c^a$. Because the cream guinea pig had two sepia parents

$$(c^k c^d \ X \ c^k c^d \ or \ c^k c^d \ X \ c^k c^a),$$

the cream parent could be $c^d c^d$ or $c^d c^a$.

> Crosses: $c^k c^a$ X $c^d c^d$
>
> 1/2 sepia; 1/2 cream
> (if parents are assumed to be homozygous)
>
> or $c^k c^a$ X $c^d c^a$
>
> 1/2 sepia; 1/4 cream; 1/4 albino

(c)

> Parents: sepia X cream

Because the sepia guinea pig had two full color parents which could be

$$Cc^k, \quad Cc^d, \quad or \quad Cc^a$$

(not *CC* because sepia could not be produced), its genotype could be

$$c^k c^k, \quad c^k c^d, \quad or \quad c^k c^a.$$

Because the cream guinea pig had two sepia parents

$$(c^k c^d \ X \ c^k c^d \quad or \quad c^k c^d \ X \ c^k c^a),$$

the cream parent could be $c^d c^d$ or $c^d c^a$.

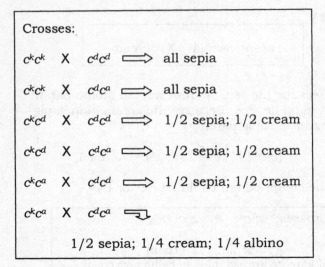

Crosses:

$c^k c^k$ X $c^d c^d$ ⟹ all sepia

$c^k c^k$ X $c^d c^a$ ⟹ all sepia

$c^k c^d$ X $c^d c^d$ ⟹ 1/2 sepia; 1/2 cream

$c^k c^d$ X $c^d c^a$ ⟹ 1/2 sepia; 1/2 cream

$c^k c^a$ X $c^d c^d$ ⟹ 1/2 sepia; 1/2 cream

$c^k c^a$ X $c^d c^a$ ⟹

1/2 sepia; 1/4 cream; 1/4 albino

(d)

Parents: sepia   X   cream

Because the sepia parent had a full color parent and an albino parent (Cc^k X $c^a c^a$), it must be $c^k c^a$. The cream parent had two full color parents which could be Cc^d or Cc^a; therefore it could be $c^d c^d$ or $c^d c^a$.

Crosses:

$c^k c^a$ X $c^d c^d$ ⟹ 1/2 sepia; 1/2 cream

$c^k c^a$ X $c^d c^a$ ⟹

1/2 sepia; 1/4 cream; 1/4 albino

22. One can envision two pathways leading to the production of green pigment:

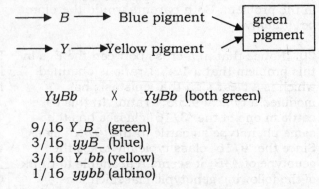

$YyBb$ X $YyBb$ (both green)

9/16 $Y\_B\_$ (green)
3/16 $yyB\_$ (blue)
3/16 Y_bb (yellow)
1/16 $yybb$ (albino)

Given that both parents are true-breeding and the sort of gene interaction described is occurring, one can come up with the following symbols:

P₁: $YYBB$ X $yybb$
     (green)   (albino)
                or

          $YYbb$ X $yyBB$
                      ↓
                   $YyBb$
                   (green)

Crossing these F₁'s gives the observed ratios in the F₂.

23. For all three pedigrees, let *a* represent the mutant gene and *A* represent its normal allele.

(a) This pedigree is consistent with an X-linked recessive trait because the male would contribute an X chromosome carrying the *a* mutation to the *aa* daughter. The mother would have to be heterozygous *Aa*.

(b) This pedigree is consistent with an X-linked recessive trait because the mother could be *Aa* and transmit her *a* allele to her one son (*a*/Y) and her *A* allele to her other son.

(c) This pedigree is not consistent with an X-linked mode of inheritance because the *aa* mother has an *A*/Y son.

24. (a,b) In looking at the pedigrees, one can see that the condition cannot be dominant because it appears in the offspring (II-3 and II-4) and not the parents in the first two cases. The condition is therefore *recessive*. In the second cross, note that the father is not shaded, yet the daughter (II-4) is. If the condition is recessive, then it must also be *autosomal*.

(c) II-1   = *AA* or *Aa*

II-6   = *AA* or *Aa*

II-9   = *Aa*

25. The test for allelism is made by crossing the various mutant strains. If the resulting offspring are mutant, then the mutations are allelic. If the offspring are wild type, then the mutations are not allelic and complementation is occurring. In Cross 1, all the offspring are wild type indicating that *r1* and *r2* are complementing and therefore not allelic. In Cross 2 all the offspring have tan eyes indicating that the mutations are allelic. Since mutations *r1* and *r3* are in the same gene and *r1* and *r2* are not, the cross *r2* X *r3* should be complemeting, that is, *r2* and *r3* are in different genes.

26. First, look for familiar ratios that will inform you as to the general mode of inheritance. Notice that the last cross (h) gives a 9:4:3 ratio which is typical of epistasis. From this information one can develop a model to account for the results given. Symbolism:

A_B_   = black

A_bb   = golden
aabb   = golden

aaB_   = brown

The combination of *bb* is epistatic to the *A* locus.

(a) *AAB_* X *aaBB* (other configurations possible but each must give all offspring with *A* and *B* dominant alleles)

(b) *AaB_* X *aaBB* (other configurations are possible but both parents cannot be *Bb*)

(c) *AABb* X *aaBb*

(d) *AABB* X *aabb*

(e) *AaBb* X *Aabb*

(f) *AaBb* X *aabb*

(g) *aaBb* X *aaBb*

(h) *AaBb* X *AaBb*

Those genotypes which will breed true will be as follows:

black   = *AABB*

golden = all genotypes which are *bb*

brown = *aaBB*

27. It is important to see that this problem involves multiple alleles, meaning that monohybrid type ratios are expected, and that there is an order of dominance which will allow certain alleles to be "hidden" in various heterozygotes. As with most genetics problems, one must look at the phenotypes of the offspring to assess the genotypes of the parents.

(a)

Phenotypes:

Himalayan   X   Himalayan ⟹albino

Genotypes: $c^h c^a$ $c^h c^a$ $c^a c^a$

The Himalayan parents must both be heterozygous to produce an albino offspring.

Phenotypes:

full color   X   albino ⟹ chinchilla

Genotypes: Cc^{ch} $c^a c^a$ $c^{ch} c^a$

Because of the cc albino parent, the genotype of the chinchilla F_1 must be $c^{ch}c^a$. Also in order to have a chinchilla offspring at all, the full color parent must he heterozygous for chinchilla.

Therefore the cross of albino with chinchilla would be as follows:

$c^a c^a$ X $c^{ch} c^a$

1/2 chinchilla; 1/2 albino

(b)

Phenotypes:

albino   X   chinchilla ⟹ albino

Genotypes: $c^a c^a$ $c^{ch} c^a$ $c^a c^a$

Phenotypes:

full color   X   albino ⟹ full color

Genotypes: $C\_$ $c^a c^a$ Cc^a

It is impossible to determine the complete genotype of the full color parent, but the full color offspring must be as indicated, Cc^a.

Therefore the cross of the albino with full color would be as follows:

$c^a c^a$ X Cc^a

1/2 full color; 1/2 albino

(c)

Phenotypes:

chinchilla   X   albino ⟹ Himalayan

Genotypes: $c^{ch}c^h$ $c^a c^a$ $c^h c^a$

The chinchilla parent must be heterozygous for Himalayan because of the Himalayan offspring.

Phenotypes:

full color   X   albino ⟹ Himalayan

Genotypes: Cc^h $c^a c^a$ $c^h c^a$

Therefore a cross between the two Himalayan types would produce the following offpsring:

$c^h c^a$ X $c^h c^a$

3/4 Himalayan; 1/4 albino

28. (a) This is a case of incomplete dominance in which, as shown in the third cross, the heterozygote (palomino) produces a typical 1:2:1 ratio. Therefore one can set the following symbols:

$C^{ch}C^{ch}$ = chestnut

$C^c C^c$ = cremello

$C^{ch}C^c$ = palomino

(b) The F_1 resulting from matings between cremello and chestnut horses would be expected to be all palomino. The F_2 would be expected to fall in a 1:2:1 ratio as in the third cross in part (a) above.

29. This is a case in which epistasis (from *cc*) results in a "masking" of genes at the *A* locus. In this case there will be modifications of typical 9:3:3:1 and 1:1:1:1 ratios because of gene interactions.

(a) In a cross of

$$AACC \ \ X \ \ \ aacc,$$

the offspring are all *AaCc* (agouti) because the *C* allele allows pigment to be deposited in the hair and when it is it will be agouti. F₂ offspring would have the following "simplified" genotypes with the corresponding phenotypes:

$A\_C\_$ = 9/16 (agouti)

A_cc = 3/16
(colorless because *cc* is epistatic to *A*)

$aaC\_$ = 3/16 (black)

$aacc$ = 1/16
(colorless because *cc* is epistatic to *aa*)

The two colorless classes are phenotyically indistinguishable, therefore the final ratio is 9:3:4.

(b) Results of crosses of female agouti

$$(A\_C\_) \ \ \ X \ \ \ \ aacc \ \text{(males)}$$

are given in three groups:

(1) To produce an even number of agouti and colorless offspring, the female parent must have been *AACc* so that half of the offspring are able to deposit pigment because of *C* and when they do, they are all agouti (having received only *A* from the female parent).

(2) To produce an even number of agouti and black offspring the mother must have been *Aa* and so that no colorless offspring were produced, the female must have been *CC*. Her genotype must have been *AaCC*.

(3) Notice that half of the offspring are colorless, therefore the female must have been *Cc*. Half of the pigmented offspring are black and half are agouti, therefore the female must have been *Aa*. Overall, the *AaCc* genotype is likely.

30. First, make certain that you understand the genetics of all the gene pairs being described in the problem. The ABO system involves multiple alleles, codominance, and dominance. The MN system is codominant. The easiest way to approach these types of problems is to consider those gene pairs that produce a low number of options in the offspring. Notice in cross #1 that there are two options in the offspring for the ABO system (types A and O), but only one option for the MN system (type MN). By looking at the most restrictive classes, one can see that option (c) is the only one that is both MN and O. The remainder of the combinations can be determined using the same logic.

Cross #1 = (c)
Cross #2 = (d)
Cross #3 = (b)
Cross #4 = (e)
Cross #5 = (a)

Given that each parental/offspring grouping can only be used once, there are no other combinations.

31. The clue to the solution comes from the description of the Dexters as not true-breeding and of low fertility. This indicates that Dexters are heterozygous and the Kerry breed is homozygous recessive. The homozygous dominant type is lethal. Polled is caused by an independently assorting dominant allele, while horned is caused by the recessive allele to polled.

32. In cases of extranuclear inheritance, the phenotype is determined by the nuclear (maternal effect) or cytoplasmic (organelle or infectious) condition of the parent that contributes the bulk of the cytoplasm to the offspring. In most cases, the maternal parent provides the basis for the cytoplasmic inheritance.

The pattern of inheritance is more often from one parent to the offspring. One does not see both parents contributing to the characteristics of the offspring as is the case with Mendelian (chromosomal) forms of inheritance. Standard Mendelian ratios (3:1) are usually not present. In general, the results of reciprocal crosses differ. See F4.3.

Female mutant   X   *male wild*

all offspring mutant

Female wild   X   *male mutant*

all offspring wild

In sex-linked inheritance, the pattern is often from grandfather through carrier mother to son. Patterns of extranuclear inheritance are often not influenced by the sex of the individual.

33. The case with *Limnaea* involves a maternal effect in which the *genotype* of the mother influences the *phenotype* of the *immediate* offspring in a non-Mendelian manner. Notice that in the above statement, it is the maternal genotype which determines the phenotype of the offspring, regardless of its own genotype.

Since both of the parents are *Dd*, the parent contributing the eggs must be *Dd*. Therefore, all of the offspring must have the phenotype of the mother's genotype, which is dextral.

34. In a maternal effect, the *genotype* of the mother influences the *phenotype* of her immediate offspring in a non-Mendelian manner. The fact that all of the offspring (F₁) showed a dextral coiling pattern indicates that one of the parents (maternal parent) contains the *D* allele. Taking these offspring and seeing that their progeny (call these F₂) occur in a 1:1 ratio indicates that half of the offspring (F₁) are *dd*. In order to have these results, one of the original parents must have been *Dd* while the other must have been *dd*.

Parents: *Dd*   X   *dd*

Offspring (F1):   1/2 *Dd*,   1/2 *dd*

(all dextral because of the maternal genotype)

Progeny (F₂):

All those from *Dd* parents will be dextral while all those from *dd* parents will be sinistral.

---

35. Developmental phenomena which occur early are more likely to be under maternal influence than those occurring late. Anterior/posterior and dorsal/ventral orientations are among the earliest to be established and in organisms where their study is experimentally and/or genetically approachable, they often show considerable maternal influence. Maternal effect genes produce products which are not carried over for more than one generation as is the case with organelle and infectious heredity. Crosses which illustrate the transient nature of a maternal effect could include the following. However, depending on particular biochemical/developmental parameters, all crosses may not give these types of patterns.

Female *Aa* X male *aa* -----> all offspring of the "A" phenotype.

Take a female "A" phenotype from the above cross and conduct the following mating: *aa* X male *Aa* ----->. All offspring may be of the "a" phenotype because all of the offspring will reflect the *genotype* of the mother, not her *phenotype*. This cross illustrates that maternal effects last only one generation.

36. (a) The presence of *bcd⁻/bcd⁻* males can be explained by the maternal effect: mothers were *bcd⁺/bcd⁻*.

(b) The cross

female *bcd ⁺/bcd ⁻* X male *bcd⁻ /bcd ⁻*

will produce an F_1 with normal embryogenesis because of the maternal effect. In the F_2, any cross having *bcd ⁺/bcd ⁻* mothers will have phenotypically normal embryos. Any cross involving homozygous *bcd ⁻/bcd ⁻* mothers will have problems with embryogenesis.

37. The *mt⁺* strain is the donor of the cpDNA since the inheritance of resistance or sensitivity is dependent on the status of the *mt⁺* gene.

Chapter 5: Sex Determination and Sex Chromosomes

Concept Areas	Corresponding Problems
Sex Chromosomes	1, 3, 7, 8, 9, 12, 13, 26
Life Cycles	2
Sex Determination	4, 5, 6, 7, 9, 10, 12, 13, 14, 17, 22, 25, 29, 30
Sexual Differentiation	3, 4, 11, 22, 23, 24, 27, 28
Dosage Compensation	15, 16, 17, 18, 19, 20, 21, 31, 32, 33

Vocabulary: Organization and Listing of Terms and Concepts

Structures and Substances

Heteromorphic sex chromosomes

   unisexual

   dioecious

   gonochoric

   bisexual

   monoecious

   hermaphroditic

   intersex

   isogamete

   gametophyte

   sporophyte

      stamen (tassels)

   microgametophyte

   pistil

   endosperm nuclei

   oocyte nucleus

Y chromosome

heterogametic sex

homogametic sex

aromatase

testis determining factor (TDF)

pseudoautosomal regions (PARs)

nonrecombining region of the Y (NRY)

male-specific region of the Y (MSY)

amplicon

Cell clone

   X-inactivation center (*Xic*)

   glucose-6-phosphate dehydrogenase deficiency (*G-6-PD*)

   X-inactive specific transcript (*XIST*)

   open reading frame (ORF)

   anhidrotic ectodermal dysplasia

Chapter 5 Sex Determination and Sex Chromosomes

Processes/Methods

Sexual Classification

Sexual Differentiation

    primary

    secondary

    hermaphroditic

Chlamydomonas

    isogametes

Zea mays

    double fertilization

C. elegans

XX/XO *Protenor* mode

XX/XY *Lygaeus* mode

ZZ/ZW

Sex determination (humans)

    XX = female

    XY = male

    Klinefelter syndrome 47, XXY

    48, XXXY

    48, XXYY, etc.

    Turner syndrome 45, X

    mosaics 45X/46XY, 45X/46XX

    47, XXX

    48, XXXX

    49, XXXXX

47, XYY

sexual differentiation

    primordial germ cells

    cortex

    medulla

    human Y chromosome

        pseudoautosomal regions (PARS)

        NRY

        testis determining factor (TDF)

        sex determining region (SRY)

        MSY

            XX males, XY females

            transgenic mice

            SOX9, WT1, SF1

Sex ratio (humans)

    primary, secondary

Dosage compensation

    sex chromatin body (Barr body)

    N-1 rule

    Lyon hypothesis, Lyonization

        G6PD

        red-green color blindness

        anhidrotic ectodermal dysplasia

X-inactivating center (*Xic*)

X-inactive specific transcript (*XIST*)

    open reading frame (ORF)

    epigenetic event

Sex determination (*Drosophila*)

    nondisjunction

        XO = sterile male

        XXY = normal female

ratio (number of X chromosomes to number of haploid sets of autosomes)

    superfemale (metafemale)

    metamale

    intersex

RNA splicing, alternative splicing

Concepts

Sex determination (humans, *Drosophila*)

Environmental factors

Sex differentiation

Dosage compensation

Lyonization

Solutions to Problems and Discussion Questions

1. The term *homomorphic* refers to the situation where both the sex chromosomes have the same form. The term *heteromorphic* refers to the condition in many organisms where there are two different forms (morphs) of chromosomes such as X and Y. In *isogamous* species, there is little visible difference between the haploid vegetative cells that reproduce asexually and the haploid gametes that are involved in sexual reproduction. The two gametes that fuse during mating are morphologically indistinguishable and are called *isogametes*. An organism which is *heterogamous* is one in which there are two morphologically distinct sex chromosomes.

2. Maize (*Zea mays*) is a monoecious seed plant where the sporophyte phase predominates during the life cycle. Both male and female structures are present on the adult plant. The stamens produce diploid microspore mother cells which undergo meiosis to produce four haploid microspores. Each haploid microspore develops into a microgametophyte which contains two sperm nuclei. Female diploid cells, megaspore mother cells, are located in the pistil of the sporophyte. Following meiosis, only one of the four haploid megaspores survives and divides mitotically three times, producing a total of eight haploid nuclei. Two of these nuclei unite to become the endosperm nuclei. At the end of the sac where the sperm enters, three nuclei remain: the oocyte nucleus and two synergids. The other three antipodal nuclei cluster at the opposite end of the embryo sac.

When pollen grains make contact with the stigma and successfully develop, two sperm nuclei enter the embryo sac, one sperm nucleus unites with the haploid oocyte nucleus, and the other sperm nucleus unites with two endosperm nuclei.

In *Caenorhabditis elegans*, there are two sexual phenotypes: males, which have only testes, and hermaphrodites, which contain both testes and ovaries. While in the larval stage of development of hermaphrodites, testes produce sperm, which is stored. Oogenesis does not occur until the adult stage is reached. The eggs are fertilized (self-fertilized) by the stored sperm. The majority of the offspring are hermaphrodites while less than 1 percent of the offspring are males. As adults, males can mate with hermaphrodites, producing about half male and half hermaphrodite offspring.

3. The life cycle of the green alga *Chlamydomonas* exhibits occasional sexual reproduction. Spending most of their life cycle as haploids, they asexually produce daughter cells by mitosis. In unfavorable nutrient conditions, some daughter cells function as gametes forming a diploid zygote after fertilization. When conditions become acceptable, meiosis ensues and haploid vegetative cells are again produced.

Zea mays, like many plants, alternate between the haploid gametophyte stage and the diploid sporophyte stage which are linked together by meiosis and fertilization. It is a monoecious seed plant in which the sporophyte phase predominates the life cycle. Both male and female structures are present in the adult plant. The stamens produce diploid mother cells which undergo meiosis to produce four haploid microspores. Each microspore develops into a mature microgametophyte which contains two sperm nuclei.

Similar female diploid cells, megaspore mother cells, occur in the pistil and following meiosis produce one of the four haploid megaspores which divides mitotically three times, thus producing a total of eight haploid nuclei. Two of these nuclei unite becoming the endosperm nuclei.

Double fertilization results in a diploid zygotic nucleus and the triploid endosperm nucleus. Each ear of corn contains as many as 1000 fertilization products and each kernel may germinate and give rise to a new plant (sporophyte).

The roundworm *Caenorhabditis elegans* consists of only about 1000 cells found in two sexual phenotypes: males, having testes, and hermaphrodites, which have both testes and ovaries. Early in the development of a hermaphrodite, testes form and produce sperm, which is then stored. Ovaries are produced too, but oogenesis occurs in the adult stage. Eggs may be fertilized by the stored sperm from self-fertilization. Most of the offspring are hermaphrodites and less than 1 percent of the offspring are males. Genes located on both the X chromosome and autosomes determine the development of males or hermaphrodites. Hermaphrodites have two X chromosomes while males have only one X chromosome, no Y chromosome is present. As in *Drosophila* the ratio of X chromosomes to the number of sets of autosomes determines the sex of these worms.

4. Sexual differentiation is the response of cells, tissues, and organs to signals provided by the genetic mechanisms of sex determination. In other words, genes are present which signal developmental pathways whereby the sexes are generated. Sexual differentiation is the complex set of responses to those genetic signals.

5. The *Protenor* form of sex determination involves the XX/XO condition while the *Lygaeus* mode involves the XX/XY condition.

6. Calvin Bridges (1916) studied nondisjunctional *Drosophila* which had a variety of sex chromosome complements. He noted that XO produced sterile males while XXY produced fertile females. Other investigators have determined that the Y chromosome is male determining in humans. Individuals with the 47,XXY complement are males while 45,XO produces females.

In *Drosophila* it is the balance between the number of X chromosomes and the number of haploid sets of autosomes which determines sex. In humans there is a small region on the Y chromosome which determines maleness.

7. The Y chromosome is male determining in humans and it is a particular region of the Y chromosome which causes maleness, sex-determining region (SRY). SRY releases a product called the testis-determining factor (TDF) which causes the undifferentiated gonadal tissue to form testes. Individuals with the 47,XXY complement are males while 45,XO produces females. In *Drosophila* it is the balance between the number of X chromosomes and the number of haploid sets of autosomes which determines sex. In contrast to humans, XO *Drosophila* are males and the XXY complement is female.

8. In *primary* nondisjunction half of the gametes contain two X chromosomes while the complementary gametes contain no X chromosomes. Fertilization, by a Y-bearing sperm cell, of those female gametes with two X chromosomes would produce the XXY Klinefelter syndrome. Fertilization of the "no-X" female gamete with a normal X-bearing sperm will produce the Turner syndrome.

9. (a) female $X^{rw}Y$ $\quad$ X $\quad$ male X^+X^+

F_1: females: $\quad$ X^+Y (normal)
$\quad\quad\quad$ males: $\quad$ $X^{rw}X^+$ (normal)

F_2: females: $\quad$ X^+Y (normal)
$\quad\quad\quad\quad\quad\quad$ $X^{rw}Y$ (reduced wing)
$\quad\quad\quad$ males: $\quad$ $X^{rw}X^+$ (normal)
$\quad\quad\quad\quad\quad\quad$ X^+X^+ (normal)

(b) female $X^{rw}X^{rw}$ $\quad$ X $\quad$ male X^+Y

F_1: $\quad$ females: $\quad$ $X^{rw}X^+$ (normal)
$\quad\quad\quad$ males: $\quad$ $X^{rw}Y$ (reduced wing)

F_2: $\quad$ females: $\quad$ $X^{rw}X^+$ (normal)
$\quad\quad\quad\quad\quad\quad$ $X^{rw}X^{rw}$ (reduced wing)
$\quad\quad\quad$ males: $\quad$ X^+Y (normal)
$\quad\quad\quad\quad\quad\quad$ $X^{rw}Y$ (reduced wing)

10. No. Since the Y chromosome cannot be detected in these crosses, there is no way to distinguish the two modes of sex determination.

11. Males and females share a common placenta and therefore hormonal factors carried in blood. Hormones and other molecular species (transcription factors perhaps) triggered by the presence of a Y chromosome lead to a cascade of developmental events which both suppress female organ development and enhance masculinization. Other mammals also exhibit a variety of similar effects depending on the sex of their uterine neighbors during development.

12. Because attached-X chromosomes have a mother-to-daughter inheritance and the father's X is transferred to the son, one would see daughters with the white eye phenotype and sons with the miniature wing phenotype.

13. If the offspring were typical; that is, as if there was no attached-X chromosome to begin with, one would strongly suspect that the X chromosome had become unattached. Specifically, if the male offspring had white eyes and the female offspring were wild type, one might suspect that the attached-X had become unattached.

14. Because synapsis of chromosomes in meiotic tissue is often accompanied by crossing over, it would be detrimental to sex-determining mechanisms to have sex-determining loci on the Y chromosome transferred, through crossing over, to the X chromosome.

15. A *Barr body* is a differentially-staining chromosome seen in some interphase nuclei of mammals with two X chromosomes. There will be one less Barr body than number of X chromosomes. The Barr body is an X chromosome which is considered to be genetically inactive.

16. There is a simple formula for determining the number of Barr bodies in a given cell: N-1, where N is the number of X chromosomes.

Klinefelter syndrome (XXY)	= 1
Turner syndrome (XO)	= 0
47, XYY	= 0
47, XXX	= 2
48, XXXX	= 3

17. The *Lyon hypothesis* states that the inactivation of the X chromosome occurs at random early in embryonic development. Such X chromosomes are in some way "marked" such that all clonally-related cells have the same X chromosome inactivated.

18. Unless other markers, cytological or molecular, are available, one cannot test the Lyon hypothesis with homozygous X-linked genes. The test requires identification of allelic alternatives to see differences in X chromosome activity.

19. Females may display mosaic retinas with patches of defective color perception. Under these conditions, their color vision may be influenced.

20. Refer to the text and notice that the phenotypic mosaicism is dependent on the heterozygous condition of genes on the two X chromosomes. Dosage compensation and the formation of Barr bodies occur only when there are two or more X chromosomes. Males normally have only one X chromosome, therefore such mosaicism cannot occur. Females normally have two X chromosomes. There are cases of male calico cats which are XXY.

21. Many organisms have evolved over millions of years under the fine balance of numerous gene products. Many genes required for normal cellular and organismic function in *both* males and females are located on the X chromosome. These gene products have nothing to do with sex determination or sex differentiation.

22. In mammals, the scheme of sex determination is dependent on the presence of a piece of the Y chromosome. If present, a male is produced. In *Bonellia viridis*, the female proboscis produces some substance which triggers a morphological, physiological, and behavioral developmental pattern which produces males. To elucidate the mechanism, one could attempt to isolate and characterize the active substance by testing different chemical fractions of the proboscis. Mutant analysis usually provides critical approaches into developmental processes. Depending on characteristics of the organism, one could attempt to isolate mutants that lead to changes in male or female development. Third, by using micro-tissue transplantations, one could attempt to determine which anatomical "centers" of the embryo respond to the chemical cues of the female.

23. In general, information about the primary sex ratio in humans is obtained from abortions and miscarriages. In addition, some studies (Barczyk 2001) using "hamster oocyte - human sperm" have been successful in determining some of the causal factors involved in determining the primary sex ratio.

24. There are several possibilities which are discussed in the text. One could account for the significant departures from a 1:1 ratio of males to females by suggesting that at anaphase I of meiosis, the Y chromosome more often goes to the pole that produces the more viable sperm cells. One could also speculate that the Y-bearing sperm has a higher likelihood of surviving in the female reproductive tract, or that the egg surface is more receptive to Y-bearing sperm. At this time the mechanism is unclear.

As Pergament et al. (2002) explain:

"A number of environmental, physiological and genetic factors have been observed to impact on the primary sex ratio: sexual behaviour, variation in hormonal concentrations, natural disasters, environmental pollutants and timing of conception. Nevertheless, no biological mechanism or interaction of factors has suitably explained this phenomenon, or that of the prenatal vulnerability of the male, the suspected higher sex ratio in spontaneous abortion and the male excesses in adult diseases related to the intrauterine environment."

25. Since there is a region of synapsis close to the *Sry*-containing section on the Y chromosome, crossing over in this region would generate XY translocations which would lead to the condition described.

26. Because of the homology between the *red* and *green* genes, there exists the possibility for an irregular synapsis (see the figure below) which, following crossing over, would give a chromosome with only one (*green*) of the duplicated genes. When this X chromosome combines with the normal Y chromosome, the son's phenotype can be explained.

"Normal Synapsis"

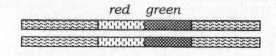

"Oblique Synapsis"

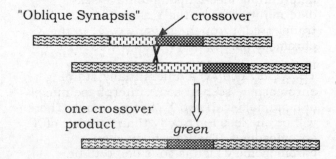

one crossover product

27. The presence of the Y chromosome provides a factor (or factors) which leads to the initial specification of maleness. Subsequent expression of secondary sex characteristics must be dependent on the interaction of the normal X-linked *Tfm* allele with testosterone. Without such interaction, differentiation takes the female path. Since the *Tfm* allele is dominant, one would predict that normal male development would only occur if the mutant *Tfm* allele were deleted and a copy of the normal *Tfm* allele engineered into the genome.

28. (a) Something is missing from the male-determining system of sex determination either at the level of the genes, gene products, or receptors, etc.

(b) The *SOX9* gene or its product is probably involved in male development. Perhaps it is activated by *SRY*.

(c) There is probably some evolutionary relationship between the *SOX9* gene and *SRY*. There is considerable evidence that many other genes and pseudogenes are also homologous to *SRY*.

(d) Normal female sexual development does not require the *SOX9* gene or gene product(s).

29. Since all haploids are male and half of the eggs are unfertilized, 50% of the offspring would be male at the start; adding the X_a/X_a types gives 25% more male, the remainder X_a/X_b would be female. Overall, 75% of the offspring would be male while 25% would be female.

30. In snapping turtles, sex determination is strongly influenced by temperature such that males are favored in the 26-34 °C range. Lizards, on the other hand, appear to have their sex determined by factors other than temperature in the 20-40 °C range.

31. Because of X-chromosome inactivation in mammals, scientists would be interested in determining whether the nucleus taken from Rainbow (donor) would continue to show such inactivation. Would the inactivated X chromosome retain the property of inactivation? See answer #33 below.

32. The white patches of CC are due to an autosomal gene *S* for white spotting which prevents pigment formation in the cell lineages in which it is expressed. Homoygous *SS* cats have more white than heterozygous *Ss* cats and there is no absolute pattern of patches due to the *S* allele. So the distribution of white patches would be expected to be different from Rainbow. In addition, since X chromosome inactivation is random, CC would have a different patch pattern from her genetic mother on the random X inactivation basis alone.

33. Different cells manage X chromosome inactivation in different ways. The absence of orange patches is due to the fact that in gonadal tissue, while oogonia have a single active X chromosome, the inactive X chromosome is reactivated at, or more likely, shortly before, entry into meiotic prophase (Kratzer and Chapman 1981). Thus X chromosome inactivation does not remain in certain ovarian cells as in somatic tissue. However, since the timing of reactivation is variable in different cell lines, there is some uncertainty as to which cell is in which state of inactivation. The actual result was a kitten (CC) with black spots on a white background. With *black* being expressed in the presence of orange, only black shows through in the Carbon Copy's coat. However, if one assumes that the somatic ovarian cell was engaging in X chromosome inactivation, the ovarian somatic cell that Rainbow donated to create CC contained an activated black gene and an inactivated orange gene (from X- inactivation). This would mean that as CC developed, her cells did not change that inactivation pattern. Therefore, unlike Rainbow, CC developed without any cells that specified orange coat color. The result is CC's black and white coat.

Chapter 6: Chromosome Mutations: Variation in Number and Arrangement

Concept Areas	Corresponding Problems
Variation in Chromosome Number	1, 2, 3, 4, 5, 6, 7, 8, 15, 16, 17 18, 19, 20, 24
Nondisjunction	14, 28, 29
Deletions	9
Duplications	9, 12
Inversions	10, 11, 13, 21, 22
Translocations	13, 23, 25, 26, 27, 30

Vocabulary: Organization and Listing of Terms and Concepts

Structures and Substances

Colchicine

Down syndrome critical region (DSCR)

Protoplast

rDNA

Nucleolar organizer (NOR)

Fragile site

Trinucleotide repeat

Processes/ Methods

Chromosome mutations (aberrations)

aneuploidy(F6.1)

nondisjunction

monosomy, trisomy

Klinefelter syndrome

Turner syndrome

partial monosomy

segmental deletions

cri-du-chat syndrome, 46,5p-

trisomy

XXX (*Drosophila*, humans)

pairing configurations

trivalent

Down syndrome (G group)

trisomy 21 (47, +21)

amniocentesis

chorionic villus sampling (CVS)

familial Down syndrome

Chapter 6 Chromosome Mutations: Variation in Number and Arrangement

Patau syndrome (D group)

   trisomy 13 (47, +13)

Edwards syndrome (E group)

   trisomy 18 (47, +18)

   reduced viability

      gametes

      embryos

      spontaneously aborted fetuses

euploidy (F7.1)

   monoploid (n)

   diploid ($2n$)

   polyploid

      triploid ($3n$)

      tetraploid ($4n$)

      pentaploid ($5n$)

   autopolyploidy

      autotriploids ($3n$)

      complete nondisjunction

      dispermic fertilization

         tetraploid X diploid

      autotetraploids ($4n$)

      allopolyploidy

         hybridization

         allotetraploid

         (amphidiploid)

(cotton, *Triticale*)

   Raphanus X *Brassica*

      somatic cell hybrids

      (protoplasts)

   endopolyploidy

      endomitosis

Chromosome structure

   deletions (deficiency)

      terminal, intercalary

      segmental

      loop (deficiency, compensation)

      pseudodominance

   duplications

      evolutionary aspects

         gene families

      gene redundancy

         rDNA

      gene amplification

      nucleolar organizer (NOR)

         micronucleoli

      Bar eye in *Drosophila*

         semidominant

      evolutionary aspects

         gene families

         rearrangements

Chapter 6 Chromosome Mutations: Variation in Number and Arrangement

inversions

    paracentric

    pericentric

      arm ratio

    heterozygotes

    inversion loops

    dicentric chromatids

    acentric chromatids

      dicentric bridges

      evolutionary aspects

    reduction in recovery of recombinants

translocations

    reciprocal

    unorthodox synapsis

    semisterility

    familial Down syndrome

    centric fusion

    Robertsonian fusion

      14/21 or D/G

fragile sites

    X chromosome

    Martin-Bell syndrome (MBS)

    FHIT

    FRA3B

    G-quartets

    genetic anticipation

    cancer

Concepts

Significance of variation in chromosomes

    genomic balance

    sex chromosome balance

    evolution

Gene duplication (evolutionary aspects)

    sequence homology

      nucleic acids

      amino acids

Inversions

    "suppression of crossing over"

    evolutionary consequences

    semisterility

Translocations

Fragile sites

Anticipation

F7.1 Illustration of the chromosomal configurations of diploid and euploid genomes of *Drosophila melanogaster*.

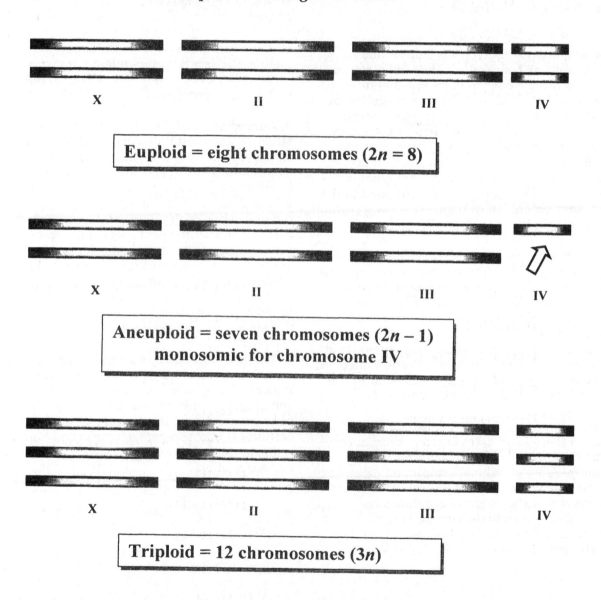

Drosophila melanogaster **female**

Solutions to Problems and Discussion Questions

1. With a diploid chromosome number of 18 ($2n$), a haploid (n) would have nine chromosomes, a triploid ($3n$) would have 27 chromosomes, and a tetraploid ($4n$) would have 36 chromosomes. A trisomic would have one extra chromosome (19) and a monosomic one less than the diploid (17).

2. With frequent exceptions especially in plants, organisms typically inherit one chromosome complement (*haploid* = n = one representative of each chromosome) from each parent. Such organisms are *diploid*, or $2n$. When an organism contains complete multiples of the n complement ($3n$, $4n$, $5n$, etc.) it is said to be *euploid* in contrast to aneuploid in which complete haploid sets do not occur. An example of an aneuploid is *trisomic* where a chromosome is added to the $2n$ complement. In humans, trisomy 21 would be symbolized as $2n+1$ or 47, 21+.

Monosomy is an aneuploid condition in which one member of a chromosome pair is missing, thus producing the chromosomal formula of $2n-1$. Haplo-IV is an example of monosomy in *Drosophila*. *Trisomy* is the chromosomal condition of $2n+1$ where an extra chromosome is present. Down syndrome is an example in humans (47, 21+). See the text and notice that all the chromosomes are present in the diploid state except chromosome #21.

Patau syndrome is a chromosomal condition where there is an extra D group chromosome. Such individuals are 47, 13+ and have multiple congenital malformations. *Edwards syndrome* is a chromosomal condition where there is an extra E group chromosome (47, 18+). Individuals with Edwards syndrome have multiple congenital malformations and reduced life expectancy.

Polyploidy refers to instances where there are more than two haploid sets of chromosomes in an individual cell. *Autopolyploidy* refers to cases of polyploidy where the chromosomes in the individual originate from the same species.

Allopolyploidy involves instances where the chromosomes originate from the hybridization of two different species, usually closely related.

Pericentric inversions have breakpoints which include the centromere while *paracentric* inversions have breakpoints which do not include the centromere.

3. Individuals with Down syndrome, while suffering congenital defects, tendencies toward respiratory disease and leukemia, can live well into adulthood. Individuals with Patau or Edwards syndrome live less than four months on the average. Comparing the different sizes of the involved chromosomes (21, 13, and 18, respectively) in the text for example, suggests that the larger the chromosome, the lower the likelihood of lengthy survival. In addition, it would be expected that certain chromosomes, because of their genetic content, may have different influences on development.

4. The fact that there is a significant maternal age effect associated with Down syndrome indicates that nondisjunction in older females contributes disproportionately to the number of Down syndrome individuals. In addition, certain genetic and cytogenetic marker data indicate the influence of female nondisjunction.

5. While several trisomies (for chromosomes 21, 18, 13, the X and Y) are tolerated, monosomy for the autosomes is not tolerated. Karyotypic analysis of spontaneously aborted fetuses has indicated a relatively large degree of departures from the typical diploid state. The delicate genetic balance produced by millions of years of evolution must be maintained in order for any organism (but especially animals) to develop normally.

Monosomy leads to the exposure of recessive, deleterious genes thus producing developmental abnormalities. Dosage compensation of the sex chromosomes and the relative paucity of Y-linked genes probably contribute to the survival of sex-chromosome aneuploidy. Notice how large the X chromosome is compared with other chromosomes.   At least 20 percent of all conceptions are terminated in natural abortion. Of these, thirty percent show some chromosomal anomaly. Of the chromosomal anomalies that occur, approximately ninety percent are eliminated by spontaneous abortion.

Trisomy for every human chromosome has been observed, however, monosomy, the reciprocal meiotic event of trisomy, is rare. This observation probably results from gamete or early embryonic inviability.

6. Because an allotetraploid has a possibility of producing bivalents at meiosis I, it would be considered the most fertile of the three. Having an even number of chromosomes to match up at the metaphase I plate, autotetraploids would be considered to be more fertile than autotriploids.

7. The sterility of interspecific hybrids is often caused from a high proportion of univalents in meiosis I. As such, viable gametes are rare and the likelihood of two such gametes "meeting" is remote. Even if partial homology of chromosomes allows some pairing, sterility is usually the rule. The horticulturist may attempt to reverse the sterility by treating the sterile hybrid with colchicine. Such a treatment, if sucessful, may double the chromosome number and each chromosome would now have a homologue with which to pair during meiosis.

8. American cultivated cotton has 26 pairs of chromosomes; 13 large, 13 small. Old World cotton has 13 pairs of large chromosomes and American wild cotton has 13 pairs of small chromosomes. It is likely that an interspecific hybridization occurred followed by chromosome doubling. These events probably produced a fertile amphidiploid (allotetraploid). Experiments have been conducted to reconstruct the origin of American cultivated cotton.

9. Basically the synaptic configurations produced by chromosomes bearing a deletion or duplication (on one homologue) are very similar. There will be point-for-point pairing in all sections which are capable of pairing. The section which has no homologue will "loop out" as shown in the text.

10. While there is the appearance that crossing over is suppressed in inversion "heterozygotes" the phenomenon extends from the fact that the crossover chromatids end up being abnormal in genetic content. As such they fail to produce viable (or competitive) gametes or lead to zygotic or embryonic death. Notice in the text the crossover chromatids end up genetically unbalanced.

11. Examine the text and notice that in a paracentric heterozygote, crossing over produces two genetically balanced chromatids (normal and inverted) and two, those resulting from a single crossover in the inversion loop, that are genetically unbalanced and abnormal (dicentric and acentric). The dicentric chromatid will often break, thereby producing genetically unbalanced fragments whereas the acentric fragment is often lost in the meiotic process. Crossing over in the inversion loop of a pericentric heterozygote produces all chromatids with centromeres, but the two chromatids involved in the crossover are genetically unbalanced. The balanced chromatids are of normal or inverted sequence.

12. In a work entitled *Evolution by Gene Duplication*, Ohno suggests that gene duplication has been essential in the origin of new genes. If gene products serve essential functions, mutation, and therefore evolution, would not be possible unless these gene products could be compensated by products of duplicated, normal genes. The duplicated genes, or the original genes themselves, would be able to undergo mutational "experimentation" without necessarily threatening the survival of the organism.

13. It is likely that when certain combinations of genes are of selective advantage in a specific and stable environment, it would be beneficial to the organism to protect that gene combination from disruption through crossing over. By having the genes in an inversion, crossover chromatids are not recovered and therefore are not passed on to future generations.

Translocations offer an opportunity for new gene combinations by associations of genes from nonhomologous chromosomes. Under certain conditions such new combinations may be of selective advantage and meiotic conditions have evolved so that segregation of translocated chromosomes yields a relatively uniform set of gametes.

14. A Turner syndrome female has the sex chromosome composition of XO. If the father had hemophilia it is likely that the Turner syndrome individual inherited the X chromosome from the father and no sex chromosome from the mother. If nondisjunction occurred in the mother, either during meiosis I or meiosis II, an egg with no X chromosome can be the result. See the text for a diagram of primary and secondary nondisjunction.

15. The primrose, *Primula kewensis*, with its 36 chromosomes, is likely to have formed from the hybridization and subsequent chromosome doubling of a cross between the two other species, each with 18 chromosomes. An example of this type of allotetraploidy (amphidiploidy) is seen in the text.

16. Given the basic chromosome set of nine unique chromosomes (a haploid complement) other forms with the "*n* multiples" are forms of autotetraploidy. In the illustration below the *n* basic set is multiplied to various levels as is the autotetraploid in the example.

Basic Set of nine unique chromosomes (*n*)

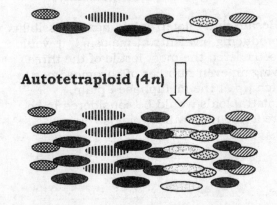

Autotetraploid (4*n*)

Individual organisms with 27 chromosomes are triploids (3*n*) and are more likely to be sterile because there are trivalents at meiosis I which cause a relatively high number of unbalanced gametes to be formed.

17. Set up the cross in the usual manner, realizing that recessive genes in the Haplo-IV individual will be expressed.

Let b = bent bristles; b^+ = normal bristles

(a)

> _/b X b^+/b^+ ⟹
>
> F₁:
>
>   _/b^+ = normal bristles
> b/b^+ = normal bristles
>
> F₂:
>
>   _/b^+ X b/b^+ ⟹
>
>   _/b^+ = normal bristles
>   _/b = bent bristles
> b^+/b^+ = normal bristles
> b/b^+ = normal bristles

(b)

> _/b^+ X b/b ⟹
>
> F₁:
>
>   _/b = bent bristles
> b/b^+ = normal bristles
>
> F₂:
>
>   _/b X b/b^+ ⟹
>
>   _/b^+ = normal bristles
>   _/b = bent bristles
> b^+/b = normal bristles
> b/b = bent bristles

18. The cross would be as follows:

    WWWW   X   *wwww*

(assuming that chromosomes pair at meiosis)

F₁: *WWww*

F₂: 1 *WW*   4 *Ww*   1 *ww*

> 1 *WW*
>
> 4 *Ww*   35 *W _ _ _* and 1 *wwww*
>
> 1 *ww*

19. Given some of the information in the above problem the expression would be as follows:

(35/36 *W_ _ _*:1/36 *wwww*) X
(35/36 *A_ _ _*:1/36 *aaaa*)   ⟹

     $(35/36)^2$ *W_ _ _A_ _ _*

     $35/(36)^2$ *W_ _ _aaaa*

     $35/(36)^2$ *wwwwA_ _ _*

     $1/(36)^2$ *wwwwaaaa*

20. Since two Gl_1 alleles and two ws_3 alleles are present in the triploid, they must have come from the pollen parent. By the wording of the problem, it is implied that the pollen parent contributed an unreduced ($2n$) gamete; however, another explanation, dispermic fertilization is possible. In this case two $Gl_1 ws_3$ gametes could have fertilized the ovule.

21. The rare double crossovers within the boundaries of a paracentric or pericentric inversion heterozygote produce only minor departures from the standard chromosomal arrangement as long as the crossovers involve the same two chromatids. With two-strand double crossovers, the second crossover negates the first. However, three-strand and four-strand double crossovers have consequences which lead to anaphase bridges as well as a high degree of genetically unbalanced gametes.

22. With a crossover within the inversion loop of a paracentric inversion heterozygote, one recombinant chromatid is dicentric (two centromeres) while the other is acentric (lacks a centromere). In a crossover within the inversion loop of a pericentric inversion heterozygote, recombinant chromatids have duplications and deletions, but no acentric or dicentric chromatids are produced.

23. (a) In all probability, crossing over in the inversion loop of an inversion (in the heterozygous state) had produced defective, unbalanced chromatids, thus leading to stillbirths and/or malformed children.

(b) It is probable that a significant proportion (perhaps 50% if there is a high frequency of crossing over in the inversion) of the children of the man will be similarly influenced by the inversion.

(c) Since the karyotypic abnormality is observable, it may be possible to detect some of the abnormal chromosomes of the fetus by amniocentesis or CVS. However, depending on the type of inversion and the ability to detect minor changes in banding patterns, not all abnormal chromosomes may be detected.

24. In plants, gametes with aberrant unbalanced genetic complements usually fail to develop normally, leading to aborted pollen or ovules. Therefore, genetic imbalance is revealed prior to fertilization and inviable seeds result. In animals, aberrant or unbalanced gametes tend to function, but significant embryonic (and subsequent) developmental abnormalities are likely to occur.

25. (a) Reciprocal translocation **(b)**

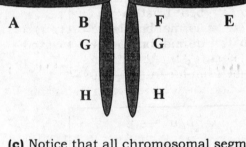

(c) Notice that all chromosomal segments are present and there is no apparent loss of chromosomal material. However, if the breakpoints for the translocation occurred within genes then an abnormal phenotype may be the result. In addition, a gene's function is sometimes influenced by its position; its neighboring genes in other words. If such "position effects" occur then a different phenotype may result.

26. (a, b, c) It is likely that the translocation described above is the cause of the miscarriages. Segregation of the chromosomal elements will produce approximately half unbalanced gametes. The chance of a normal child is approximately one in two, however; half of the normal children will be translocation carriers. Should she abandon her attempts to have a child of her own?

The answer to this question is more one of personal choice than science. It is the task of the scientific community to provide accurate information within the limits of technology. Generally speaking, this information is provided to individuals so that they can make informed decisions. In this case, the woman has been given information that probably fits her circumstance. It is up to her to make such a personal decision.

27. The symbol t(14;21) indicates that part of chromosome 21 is translocated to chromosome 14. When a gamete containing such a chromosome plus a normal chromosome 21 is fertilized by a standard haploid gamete, the individual has 46 chromosomes but effectively has three copies of chromosome 21.

28. (a) The father must have contributed the abnormal X-linked gene.

(b) Since the son is XXY and heterozygous for anhidrotic dysplasia, he must have received both the defective gene and the Y chromosome from his father. Thus nondisjunction must have occurred during meiosis I.

(c) This son's mosaic phenotype is caused by X-chromosome inactivation, a form of dosage compensation in mammals.

29. Notice that a chromosome in this question is defined as having two sisters joined at the centromere. This is the expected chromosome structure at the end of meiosis I.

(a) In light of this information, meiosis I must have produced the abnormal oocytes with more or less than 24 chromosomes, indicating multiple conditions of nondisjunction. More likely, the oocytes consisted of "$22_{1/2}$" chromosomes, those 22 normal dyads and a single monad.

(b) The result will be a monosomic and a normal zygote assuming that the half chromosome (monad) migrates, intact, to one pole or the other.

(c) In all likelihood, premature division of the centromere (at meiosis I) probably causes the single (non-duplicated) chromosome at meiosis II.

(d) We generally consider nondisjunction occurring at meiosis I to consist of intact chromosomes, two sister chromatids, failing to separate appropriately. These data indicate that some forms of aneuploidy result from premature division of the centromere at meiosis I as in the figure on the next page.

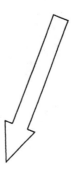

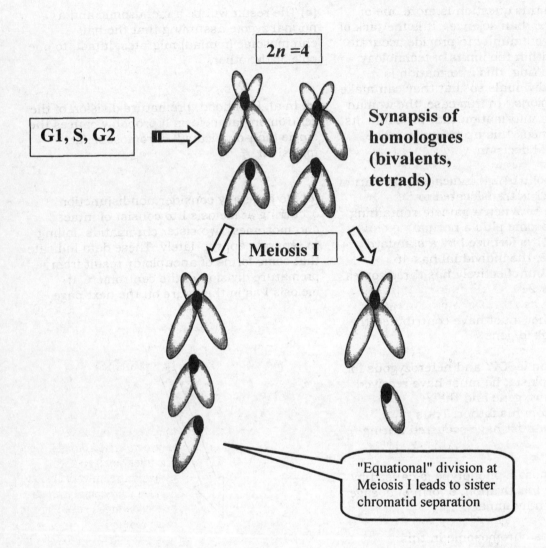

2n =4

G1, S, G2

**Synapsis of
homologues
(bivalents,
tetrads)**

Meiosis I

"Equational" division at
Meiosis I leads to sister
chromatid separation

30. First consider what is meant be a
Robertsonian translocation: breaks at the
short arms of two nonhomologous acrocentric
chromosomes where the small acentric
fragments are lost and the larger
chromosomal segments fuse at or near the
centromeric region, producing a compound,
larger submetacentric or metacentric
chromosome.   Below is a description of
breakage/reunion events which illustrate
such a translocation in relatively small,
similarly sized, chromosomes 19 (metacentric)
and 20 (metacentric/submetacentric). The
case described here is shown occurring before
S phase duplication. The same phenomenon
is shown in the text as occurring after S
phase. Since the likelihood of such a
translocation is fairly small in a general
population, inbreeding played a significant
role in allowing the translocation to "meet
itself."

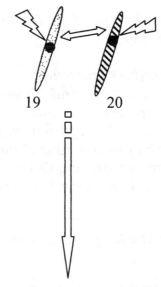

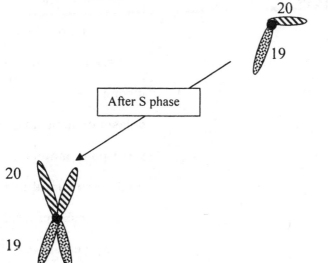

After S phase

20

19

May or may not have a
centromere. Regardless, since
it is often small and/or
contains a significant amount
of heterochromatin, it tends to
be lost during meiosis (fails to
pair properly).

Chapter 7: Linkage and Chromosome Mapping in Eukaryotes

Concept Areas	Corresponding Problems
Linkage vs. Independent Assortment	1, 23, 31, 32
Gene Mapping	3, 4, 5, 6, 7, 8, 9, 10, 11, 12, 13, 24, 25, 26, 31, 32
Mapping to the Centromere	27
Multiple Crossovers and Three-Point Mapping	5, 14, 15, 16, 17, 18, 19
Determining Gene Sequence	15, 16, 17, 20
Interference and Coefficient of Coincidence	6, 15, 16
Crossing Over in the Four-Strand Stage	2, 30
Mechanism of Crossing Over	2, 18, 30
Somatic Cell Hybridization and Human Maps	29
Theory	21, 22, 24, 28

Vocabulary: Organization and Listing of Terms and Concepts

Structures and Substances

Chromosome map

  linkage group

  tetrad

Heterokaryon

Synkaryon

Huntington disease

Cystic fibrosis

Neurofibromatosis

Bromodeoxyuridine (BU*d*R)

Processes/Methods

Linkage

  crossing over

  crossover gametes (recombinant)

recombination

  reciprocal classes

  parental (noncrossover gametes)

incomplete

chiasmata (chiasma)

three-point mapping

product rule (multiple crossovers)

  noncrossovers (NCO)

  single crossovers (SCO)

  double crossovers (DCO)

linkage ratio

Determining gene sequence

  correct heterozygous arrangement

  correct sequence of genes

Chapter 7 Linkage and Chromosome Mapping in Eukaryotes

Cytological evidence (crossing over)

Mechanism of crossing over

Human chromosome maps

    lod score method

Somatic cell hybridization

    random loss of human chromosomes

    synteny testing

Haploid organisms

    tetrad analysis

Mapping to the centromere

    first-division segregation

    second-division segregation

Sister chromatid exchange

    bromodeoxyuridine (BUdR)

Bloom syndrome

Mendel and linkage

    independent assortment

Concepts

Linked genes (linkage groups)

    arrangement (gene sequence)(F7.1)

Chromosome maps

    map unit (% recombination)

    50% maximum

Interference

    coefficient of coincidence

    expected frequency of DCO

    observed frequency of DCO

        positive

        negative

Generation of variation

F7.1 Illustration of critical arrangements of linked genes. Notice that there are two possible arrangements for an *AaBb* double heterozygote. In order to do linkage problems correctly, such arrangements must be understood.

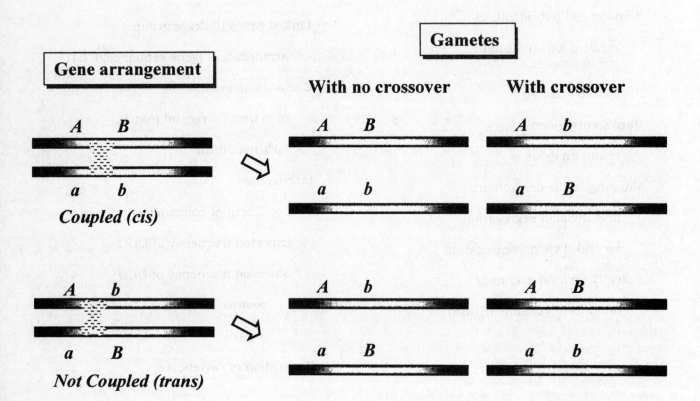

Gene arrangement

Gametes

With no crossover   **With crossover**

A   B

a   b
Coupled (cis)

A   B   *A   b*

a   b   *a   B*

A   b

a   B
Not Coupled (trans)

A   b   *A   B*

a   B   *a   b*

Solutions to Problems and Discussion Questions

1. The biological significance of genetic exchange and recombination appears to be to generate genetic variation in gametes, thereby leading to genetic variation in organisms. By reshuffling genes, new combinations are generated which may then be of evolutionary advantage. In addition, because chromosomal position can influence gene function, variation is created by *position effect*.

2. First, in order for chromosomes to engage in crossing over, they must be in proximity. It is likely that the side-by-side pairing which occurs during synapsis is the earliest time during the cell cycle that chromosomes achieve that necessary proximity. Second, chiasmata are visible during prophase I of meiosis and it is likely that these structures are intimately associated with the genetic event of crossing over.

3. With some qualification, especially around the centromeres and telomeres, one can say that crossing over is somewhat randomly distributed over the length of the chromosome. Two loci which are far apart are more likely to have a crossover between them than two loci that are close together.

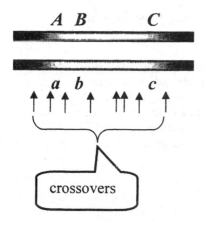

4. Because crossing over occurs at the four-strand stage of the cell cycle (that is, after S phase) notice that each single crossover involves only two of the four chromatids.

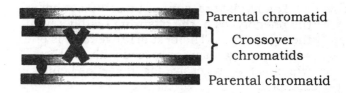

5. As mentioned in an earlier answer (#3) with some qualifications, crossovers occur randomly along the lengths of chromosomes. Within any region, the occurrence of two events is less likely than the occurrence of one event. If the probability of one event is

$$1/X,$$

the probability of two events occurring at the same time will be

$$1/X^2.$$

6. Positive interference occurs when a crossover in one region of a chromosome interferes with crossovers in nearby regions. Such interference ranges from zero (no interference) to 1.0 (complete interference). Interference is often explained by a physical rigidity of chromatids such that they are unlikely to make sufficiently sharp bends to allow crossovers to be close together.

7. Each cross must be setup in such a way as to reveal crossovers because it is on the basis of crossover frequency that genetic maps are developed. It is necessary that genetic heterogeneity exist so that different arrangements of genes, generated by crossing over, can be distinguished.

The organism which is heterozygous must be the sex in which crossing over occurs. In other words, it would be useless to map genes in *Drosophila* if the male parent is the heterozygote since crossing over is not typical in *Drosophila* males.

Lastly, the cross must be setup so that the phenotypes of the offspring readily reveal their genotypes. The best arrangement is one where an organism is crossed with another which is fully recessive for the genes being mapped.

8. Since the distance between *dp* and *ap* is greatest, they must be on the "outside" and *cl* must be in the middle. The genetic map would be as follows:

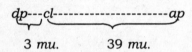

        3 *mu.*   39 *mu.*

9. The initial cross for this problem would be

    AaBb X *aabb.*

(a) If the two loci are on different chromosomes, independent assortment would occur and the following distribution (1:1:1:1) is expected:

    1/4 *AaBb*
    1/4 *Aabb*
    1/4 *aaBb*
    1/4 *aabb*

(b) Even though the two loci are linked and on the same chromosome, the frequency of crossing over is so high that crossovers always occur. Under that condition independent assortment would occur and the following distribution (1:1:1:1) is expected:

    1/4 *AaBb*
    1/4 *Aabb*
    1/4 *aaBb*
    1/4 *aabb*

(c) If crossovers never occur, then all of the gametes from the heterozygous parent are *parental*. If the arrangement is

    AB/ab   X   *ab/ab*

then the two types of offspring will be

    1/2   *AB/ab*

    1/2   *ab/ab.*

Under this condition *AB* are *coupled*. If, however, *A* and *B* are not coupled then the symbolism would be

    Ab/aB   X   *aabb.*

The offspring would occur as follows:

    1/2   *Ab/ab*

    1/2   *aB/ab.*

(d) If the loci are linked with 10 map units between them, then the two recombinant classes must add up to 10% of the total. Assuming that *A* and *B* are coupled, the following distribution would occur:

    45%   *AaBb*   (parental)

    5%   *Aabb*   (crossover)

    5%   *aaBb*   (crossover)

    45%   *aabb*   (parental)

10. In looking at this problem one can immediately conclude that the two loci (kernel color and plant color) are linked because the test cross progeny occur in a ratio other than 1:1:1:1 (and epistasis does not appear because all phenotypes expected are present).

The question is whether the arrangement in the parents is *coupled*

$$RY/ry \quad X \quad ry/ry$$

or *not coupled*

$$Ry/rY \quad X \quad ry/ry$$

Notice that the most frequent phenotypes in the offspring, the parentals, are colored, green (88) and colorless, yellow (92). This indicates that the heterozygous parent in the test cross is coupled

$$RY/ry \quad X \quad ry/ry$$

with the two dominant alleles on one chromosome and the two recessives on the homologue (F6.1). Seeing that there are 20 crossover progeny among the 200, or 20/200, the map distance would be 10 map units (20/200 X 100 to convert to percentages) between the R and Y loci.

11. Start this problem by working through the expected offspring under two models. One with no crossing over and the second with 30% crossing over in the female.

No crossing over.

Female gametes: *Male gametes:*

$1/2\ e\ ca^+$ $1/2\ e\ ca^+$

$1/2\ e^+\ ca$ $1/2\ e^+\ ca$

Offspring:

1/4   "e" phenotype

2/4   wild

1/4   "ca" phenotype

With 30% crossing over.

Female gametes: Male gametes:

35% $e\ ca^+$ $1/2\ e\ ca^+$

35% $e^+\ ca$ $1/2\ e^+\ ca$

15% $e^+\ ca^+$

15% $e\ ca$

Offspring: (obtained by combining gametes and phenotypes)

"e" phenotype   = 17.5% + 7.5%   **= 25%**

wild phenotype = 17.5% + 7.5% + 17.5% + 7.5%
                                                          = 50%

"ca" phenotype = 17.5% + 7.5%   **= 25%**

Notice that the distribution of phenotypes is the same, regardless of the contribution of the crossover classes.

12. Since there is no indication as to the configuration of the P and Z genes (*coupled or not coupled*) in the parent, one must look at the percentages in the offspring. Notice that the most frequent classes are *PZ* and *pz*. These classes represent the parental (non-crossover) groups which indicates that the original parental arrangement in the test cross was

$$PZ/pz \quad X \quad pz/pz$$

Adding the crossover percentages together (6.9 + 7.1) gives 14% which would be the map distance between the two genes.

13. This problem can be approached by looking for the most distant loci (*adp* and *b*) then filling in the intermediate loci. In this case the map for parts **(a)** and **(b)** is the following:

d..........*b*........*pr*..........*vg*........*c*.........*adp*
31   48   54   67   75   83
Map Units

The expected map units between *d* and *c* would be 44, *d* and *vg* would be 36, and *d* and *adp* 52. However, because there is a theoretical maximum of 50 map units possible between two loci in any one cross, that distance would be below the 52 determined by simple subtraction.

14.

	female A:	*female* B:	*Frequency:*
NCO	3, 4	7, 8	first
SCO	1, 2	3, 4	second
SCO	7, 8	5, 6	third
DCO	5, 6	1, 2	fourth

The single crossover classes which represent crossovers between the genes which are closer together (*d-b*) would occur less frequently than the classes of crossovers between more distant genes (*b-c*).

15. For two reasons, it is clear that the genes are in the *coupled* configuration in the F₁ female. First a completely homozygous female was mated to a wild type male and second, the phenotypes of the offspring indicate the following parental classes

$$sc \ s \ v \text{ and } + + +$$

(a)

P₁:

$$sc \ s \ v \ / \ sc \ s \ v \quad X \quad + + +/Y$$

F₁:

$$+ + +/ \ sc \ s \ v \quad X \quad sc \ s \ v/Y$$

(b) Examine the parental classes (most frequent) and compare the arrangement with the double crossover (least frequent) classes. Notice that the *v* gene "switches places" between the two groups (parentals and double crossovers). The gene which switches places is in the middle.

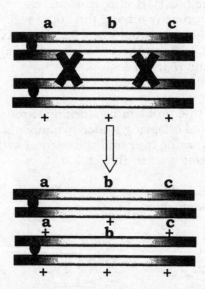

The map distances are determined by first writing the proper arrangement and sequence of genes, then computing the distances between each set of genes.

$$\underline{sc \ v \ s}$$
$$+ + +$$

sc - v = $\dfrac{150 + 156 + 10 + 14}{1000}$ X 100

= 33% (map units)

v - s = $\dfrac{46 + 30 + 10 + 14}{1000}$ X 100

= 10% (map units)

Double crossovers are always added into each crossover group because they represent a crossover in each region.

sc-------v-----s

33   10

(c) The coefficient of coincidence =

$\dfrac{\text{observed freq. double C/O}}{\text{expected freq. double C/O}}$

= $\dfrac{(14 + 10)/1000}{.33 \text{ X } .1}$

= $\dfrac{.024}{.033}$ = .727

which indicates that there were fewer double crossovers than expected, therefore positive chromosomal interference is present.

(d) No, because of dominance, all the genotypic classes would not be apparent.

16. This set-up involves an F_1 in which the fully heterozygous female has the genes y and w in *coupled* and ct *not coupled*. The arrangement for the cross is therefore:

(a) $y w +/+ + ct$ X $y w +/Y$

It is important at this point to determine the gene sequence. Using Methods I or II, examine the parental classes and compare the arrangement with the double crossover (least frequent) classes. Notice that the w gene "switches places" between the two groups (parentals and double crossovers). The gene which switches places is in the middle.

Therefore the arrangement as written above is correct.

(b)

y - w = $\dfrac{9 + 6 + 0 + 0}{1000}$ X 100

= 1.5 map units

w - ct = $\dfrac{90 + 95 + 0 + 0}{1000}$ X 100

= 18.5 map units

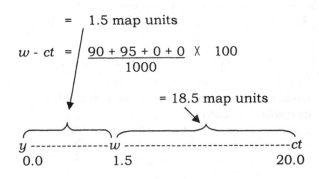

y -------------- w ------------------------------- ct
0.0   1.5   20.0

(c) There were

.185 X .015 X 1000 = 2.775

double crossovers expected.

(d) Because the cross to the F_1 males included the normal (wild type) allele for *cut wings* it would not be possible to unequivocally determine the genotypes from the F_2 phenotypes for all classes.

17. (a) The cross will be as follows. Represent the *Dichaete* gene as an upper-case letter because it is dominant.

P_1: $D + +/ + + +$	X	$+ e p/ \iota e p$
F_1: $D + +/+ e p$	X	$+ e p/+ e p$
F_2: $D + +/+ e p$	Dichaete	
$+ e p /+ e p$	ebony, pink	
$D e +/+ e p$	Dichaete, ebony	
$+ + p/+ e p$	pink	
$D + p/+ e p$	Dichaete, pink	
$+ e +/+ e p$	ebony	
$D e p/+ e p$	Dichaete, ebony, pink	
$+ + +/+ e p$	wild type	

(b) Determine which gene is in the middle by comparing the parental classes with the double crossover classes. Notice that the *pink* gene "switches places" between the two groups (parentals and double crossovers). The gene which switches places is in the middle. So rewriting the sequence of genes with the correct arrangement gives the following:

F₁:

$$D + +/+ p\ e \quad X \quad + p\ e/+ p\ e$$

Distances: remember to add in the double crossover classes

$$D\text{-}p = \frac{12 + 13 + 2 + 3}{1000} \times 100$$

$$= 3.0 \text{ map units}$$

$$p\text{-}e = \frac{84 + 96 + 2 + 3}{1000} \times 100$$

$$= 18.5 \text{ map units}$$

18. The fact that two of the genes are linked and 20 map units apart on the third chromosome, and one is on the second chromosome, the problem is a combination of linkage and independent assortment. First provide the genotypes of the parents in the original cross and the reciprocal. Use a semicolon to indicate that two different chromosome pairs are involved.

P₁:

females: $+/+;\ p\ e/p\ e$

X

males: $dp/dp;\ + +/+ +$

F₁:

females: $+/dp;\ + +/p\ e$

X

males: $dp/dp;\ p\ e/p\ e$

Female gametes: use a modification of the forked-line method for determining the types of gametes to be produced. The *dumpy* locus will give .5 + and .5 *dp* to the gametes because of independent assortment (on a different chromosome) and the other two loci will segregate with 20% (map units) being the recombinants, and 80% being the parentals.

```
               0.4 +   + (parental)    = 0.20 + + +
0.5 +          0.1 +   e (crossover)   = 0.05 + + e
               0.1 p   + (crossover)   = 0.05 + p +
               0.4 p   e (parental)    = 0.20 + p e

               0.4 +   + (parental)    = 0.20 dp + +
               0.1 +   e (crossover)   = 0.05 dp + e
0.5 dp         0.1 p   + (crossover)   = 0.05 dp p +
               0.4 p   e (parental)    = 0.20 dp p e
```

Crossed with *dp p e* from the male gives the following offspring:

0.20 wild type

0.05 ebony

0.05 pink

0.20 pink, ebony

0.20 dumpy

0.05 dumpy, ebony

0.05 dumpy, pink

0.20 dumpy, pink, ebony

92

For the reciprocal cross:

F₁:

males: $+/dp$; $++/p\ e$

X

females: dp/dp; $p\ e/p\ e$

---

there would be no crossover classes.

```
        0.5 +    + (parental) = 0.25 + + +
      /
0.5 + ——— 0.5 p    e (parental) = 0.25 + p e


        0.5 +    + (parental) = 0.25 dp + +
      /
0.5 dp——— 0.5 p   e (parental) = 0.25 dp p e
```

Crossed with *dp p e* from the female gives the following offspring:

.25 wild type

.25 pink, ebony

.25 dumpy

.25 dumpy, pink, ebony

The results would change because of the absence of crossing over in males.

19. Since *Stubble* is a dominant mutation (and homozygous lethal) one can determine whether it is heterozygous (*Sb*/+) or homozygous wild type (+/+). One would use the typical test cross arrangement with the *curled* gene so the male parent arrangement would be

$+\ cu/+\ cu$

20. In typical trihybrid crosses one expects eight kinds of offspring. In this example, only six are listed and one can assume that since the double crossover class is the least frequent, it is the double crossovers which are not listed.

To work this type of problem, examine the list to see which types are not present. In this case, the double crossover classes are the following:

$$+ + c \quad \text{and} \quad a\ b +$$

(a,b) Notice that if you compare the parental classes (most frequent) with the double crossover classes (zero in this case) one can, by using the logic of the methods described in the text, determine that the gene *b* is in the middle and the arrangement is as follows. Note: for consistency the zeros (double crossovers) are included in the calculations.

$$+ b\ c/\ a + +$$

$$a - b \quad = \frac{32 + 38 + 0 + 0}{1000} \times 100$$

$$= 7 \text{ map units}$$

$$b - c \quad = \frac{11 + 9 + 0 + 0}{1000} \times 100$$

$$= 2 \text{ map units}$$

(c) The progeny phenotypes that are missing are $+ + c$ and $a\ b +$, which, of 1000 offspring, 1.4 (.07 X .02 X 1000) would be expected. Perhaps by chance or some other unknown selective factor, they were not observed.

21. Because sister chromatids are genetically identical (with the exception of rare new mutations) crossing over between sisters provides no increase in genetic variability.

22. These observations as well as the results of other experiments indicate that the synaptonemal complex is required for crossing over.

23. (a) There would be $2^n = 8$ genotypic and phenotypic classes and they would occur in a 1:1:1:1:1:1:1:1 ratio.

(b) There would be two classes and they would occur in a 1:1 ratio.

(c) There are 20 map units between the *A* and *B* loci and locus *C* assorts independently from both *A* and *B* loci.

24. Since the genetic map is more accurate when relatively small distances are covered and when large numbers of offspring are scored, this map would probably not be too accurate with such a small sample size.

25. Assign the following symbols for example:

R = Red r = yellow
O = Oval o = long

Progeny A: *Ro/rO* X *rroo* = 10 map units
Progeny B: *RO/ro* X *rroo* = 10 map units

26. The easiest way to approach this problem is to set up fractions representing the proportions of gametes, with the frequency of the recombinant gametes adding up to 25%.

For each, the gamete proportions would be the following:

3/8 *Ab*; 3/8 *aB*; 1/8 *AB*; 1/8 *ab*

Now, combine the gametes from each parent (they are the same) and arrive at the following frequency:

*A_B_* 33/64; *A_bb* 15/64; *aaB_* 15/64; *aabb* 1/64

27. The map distance of a gene to the centromere in *Neurospora* is determined by dividing the percentage of second division asci (tetrads) by two. Patterns other than *BBbb* or *bbBB* are "second division" as discussed in the text and represent a crossover between the gene in question and the centromere. In the data given, the percentage of second division segregation is 20/100 or 20%. Dividing by 2 (because only two of the four chromatids are involved in any single crossover event) gives 10 map units.

28. The purpose of the experiment was to determine whether genetic crossing over involved actual physical exchange of chromosomal material. Other models of the time did not necessarily require an actual physical rearrangement of chromosomal material during recombination. By having microscopically visible markers on the chromosomes, Creighton and McClintock were able to show that homologous chromosomal material physically exchanged segments during crossing over.

29. Look for overlap between chromosome number in given clones and genes expressed. Note that *ENO1* is expressed in clones B,D,E; chromosomes 1 and 5 are common to these clones. However, since *ENO1* is not expressed in clone C which is missing chromosome 1 (and has chromosome 5), *ENO1* must be on chromosome 1.

MDH1: chromosome 2
PEPS: chromosome 4
PMG1: chromosome 1

30. First make a drawing with the genes placed on the homologous chromosomes as follows:

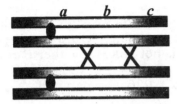

Realize that there are four chromatids in each tetrad and a single crossover involves only two of the four chromatids. Non-involved chromatids must be added to the non-crossover classes. Account for all the crossover classes first, then add up the non-crossover chromatids. For example, in the first crossover class (20 between *a* and *b*) notice that there will be 40 chromatids which were not involved in the crossover. These 40 must be added to the *abc* and +++ classes.

$$
\begin{aligned}
a\,b\,c &= 168 \\
+\,+\,+ &= 168 \\
a\,+\,+ &= 20 \\
+\,b\,c &= 20 \\
+\,+\,c &= 10 \\
a\,b\,+ &= 10 \\
+\,b\,+ &= 2 \\
a\,+\,c &= 2
\end{aligned}
$$

The map distances would be computed as follows:

$$a\text{ - }b \quad \frac{20 + 20 + 2 + 2}{400} \times 100$$

$$= 11 \text{ map units}$$

$$b\text{ - }c \quad = \frac{10 + 10 + 2 + 2}{400} \times 100$$

$$= 6 \text{ map units}$$

31. (a) There are several ways to think through this problem. Remember that there is no crossing over in *Drosophila* males. Therefore any gene on the same chromosome will be completely linked to any other gene on the same chromosome. Since you can get *pink* by itself, *short* cannot be completely linked to it. This leaves linkage to *black* on the second chromosome, the 4th chromosome, or the X chromosome. Since the distribution of phenotypes in males and females is essentially the same, the gene cannot be X-linked.   In addition, the F_1 males were wild and if the *short* gene is on the X, the F_1 males would be short.

It is also reasonable to state that the gene cannot be on the 4th chromosome because there would be eight phenotypic classes (independent assortment of three genes) instead of the four observed. Through these insights, one could conclude that the *short* gene is on chromosome 2 with the *black* gene.

Another way to approach this problem is to make three chromosomal configurations possible in the F_1 male. By producing gametes from this male, the answer becomes obvious.

Case A		Case B		Case C	
p b	*sh*	*p sh*	*b*	*b sh*	*p*
+ +	+	+ +	+	+ +	+

Develop the gametes from <u>Case C</u> and cross them out to the completely recessive triple mutant. You will get the results in the table.

(b) The parental cross is now the following:

Females:	*b sh p*	X	Males:	*b sh p*
	+ + +			*b sh p*

The new gametes resulting from crossing over in the female would be $b +$ and $+ sh$. Since the gene p is assorting independently, it is not important in this discussion. Because 15% of the offspring now contain these recombinant chromatids, the map distance between the two genes must be 15.

32. Notice that in the description of the genotype of the female, no mention is made of the *cis-trans* (coupling-repulsion) arrangement of the genes. The data will supply that information. Begin with a set of symbols as indicated below:

B^+ = wild eye shape
B = Bar eye shape

m^+ = wild wings
m = miniature wings

e^+ = wild body color
e = ebony body color

Superficially, the cross would be as follows:

B^+B m^+m e^+e X $B^+?$ $m?$ $e?$ (The $?$ is used at this point to indicate that we have no information allowing us to decide whether any of the alleles in the male are X-linked.)

Notice from the data that there are approximately as many ebony offspring (282) as those with wild body color (283). Therefore, we can conclude that the *ebony* locus is not linked to B or m. Notice also that the most frequent offspring regarding eye shape and wing size are wild-miniature and Bar-wild. This suggests that the arrangement is "trans" or "repulsion" as indicated below:

B m^+/B^+m; e^+/e

Notice that a semicolon is used to indicate that the *ebony* locus is on a different chromosome.

At this point and without prior knowledge, we still don't know whether any of the genes are X-linked, however, it is of no consequence to the solution of the problem. (In actuality, both B and m loci are X-linked.)

To determine the map distances (again, *ebony* is out of the mapping picture at this point because it is not linked to either B or m):

111 + 115 = 226   = parental

117 + 101 = 218   = parental

26 + 31 = 57   = crossover

29 + 35 = 64   = crossover

Mapping the distance between B and m would be as follows:

$(57 + 64)/ (226 + 218 + 57 + 64)$ X 100 =

121/565 X 100 = 21.4 map units.

We would conclude that the *ebony* locus is either far away from B and m (50 map units or more) or it is on a different chromosome. In fact, *ebony* is on a different chromosome.

Chapter 8: Genetic Analysis and Mapping in Bacteria and Bacteriophages

Concept Areas	Corresponding Problems
Genetic Recombination in Bacteria	1
Conjugation	2, 3, 4, 5, 6, 7, 25, 28, 29, 30
Transformation	8, 9, 10, 26, 27
Bacteriophages	11, 12, 13, 14, 15, 16, 17, 23, 24
Transduction	18, 19, 20
Mutation and Recombination in Viruses	21, 22

Vocabulary: Organization and Listing of Terms and Concepts

Structures and Substances

Bacteria

Bacteriophage

Spontaneous mutations

Growth conditions

    minimal medium

    liquid culture

    prototroph

    auxotroph

Donor strain

    E. coli K12

    F sex pilus

    fertility factor, F factor

    RecA, RecBCD proteins

    rec genes

lysozyme

Hfr, circular chromosome

F', merozygotes

    partial diploid

Plasmids

    F factors

    R plasmids

        resistance transfer factor (RTF)

        r-determinants

        antibiotic resistance

    Col plasmids

        ColE1

            colicins

            colicinogenic

Chapter 8: Genetic Analysis and Mapping in Bacteria and Bacteriophages

Protein capsid

Lysozyme

Plaque

Episome

Prophage P22

Processes/Methods

Sensitive

Resistant

    lag, log, stationary phases

Bacterial recombination

    conjugation

        F⁺, F⁻

        physical contact

        unidirectional

        donor, "male"

        recipient, "female"

        high frequency recombination, Hfr

            oriented transfer

            interrupted mating technique

            circular map

F' state

    merozygotes

Transformation

    competence

    heteroduplex

linkage

    cotransformation

Transduction

    phage life cycle

        plaque (plaque assay)

            lysis

        lysogeny

            temperate phage

            symbiotic relationship

            prophage

            lysogenic bacterium

        U-tube experiment

            filterable agent (FA)

            P22

        generalized transduction (F8.1)

            abortive transduction

            complete transduction

        cotransduction

        mapping

Mutations (viral)

    rapid lysis, host range

    mixed infection experiments

Concepts

Adaptation hypothesis

Dilution

Bacterial recombination - all forms

    relationship to *rec* genes

Fine structure analysis

    complementation

    cistron

    recombinational analysis

    deletion testing

F8.1 Simple illustration comparing *abortive* and *complete* transduction.

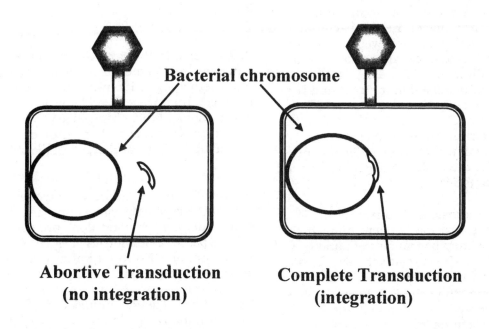

Solutions to Problems and Discussion Questions

1. Three modes of recombination in bacteria are *conjugation*, *transformation*, and *transduction*. Conjugation is dependent on the F factor which, by a variety of mechanisms, can direct genetic exchange between two bacterial cells. Transformation is the uptake of exogenous DNA by cells. Transduction is the exchange of genetic material using a bacteriophage.

2. (a) The requirement for physical contact between bacterial cells during conjugation was established by placing a filter in a U-tube such that the medium can be exchanged but the bacteria cannot come in contact. Under this condition, conjugation does not occur.

(b) By treating cells with streptomycin, an antibiotic, it was shown that recombination would not occur if one of the two bacterial strains was inactivated. However, if the other was similarly treated, recombination would occur. Thus, directionality was suggested, with one strain being a donor strain and the other being the recipient.

(c) An F⁺ bacterium contains a circular, double-stranded, structurally independent, DNA molecule, the F⁺ factor plasmid, that can direct recombination.

3. In an F⁺ X F⁻ cross, the transfer of the F factor produces a recipient bacterium which is F⁺. Any gene may be transferred, and the frequency of transfer is relatively low. Crosses which are Hfr X F⁻ produce recombinants at a higher frequency than the F⁺ X F⁻ cross. The transfer is oriented (nonrandom) and the recipient cell remains F⁻.

4. Bacteria which are F⁺ possess the F factor, while those that are F⁻ lack the F factor. In Hfr cells the F factor is integrated into the bacterial chromosome and in F' bacteria, the F factor is free of the bacterial chromosome yet possesses a piece of the bacterial chromosome.

5. Mapping the chromosome in an Hfr X F⁻ cross takes advantage of the oriented transfer of the bacterial chromosome through the conjugation tube. For each F type, the point of insertion and the direction of transfer are fixed, therefore breaking the conjugation tube at different times produces partial diploids with corresponding portions of the donor chromosome being transferred. The length of the chromosome being transferred is contingent on the duration of conjugation, thus mapping of genes is based on time.

6. In an Hfr X F⁻ cross, the F factor is directing the transfer of the donor chromosome. It takes approximately 90 minutes to transfer the entire chromosome. Because the F factor is the last element to be transferred and the conjugation tube is fragile, the likelihood for complete transfer is low.

7. As shown in the text, the F⁺ element can enter the host bacterial chromosome and upon returning to its independent state, it may pick up a piece of a bacterial chromosome. When transferred to a bacterium with a complete chromosome, a partial diploid, or merozygote, is formed.

8. Transformation requires *competence* on the part of the recipient bacterium, meaning that only under certain conditions are bacterial cells capable of being transformed. Transforming DNA must initially be *double-stranded* to begin with yet is converted to a single-stranded structure upon insertion into the host cell. The most efficient length of the transforming DNA is about 1/200 of the size of the host chromosome. Transformation is an energy-requiring process and the number of sites on the bacterial cell surface is limited.

9. In the first data set, the transformation of each locus, a^+ or b^+, occurs at a frequency of .031 and .012 respectively. To determine if there is linkage, one would determine whether the frequency of double transformants a^+b^+ is greater than that expected by a multiplication of the two independent events. Multiplying .031 X .012 gives .00037 or approximately 0.04%. From this information, one would consider no linkage between these two loci. Notice that this frequency is approximately the same as the frequency in the second experiment, where the loci are transformed independently.

10. Notice that the incorporation of loci a^+ or b^+ occurs much more frequently than the incorporation of b^+ and c^+ together (210 to 1) and the incorporation of all three genes $a^+b^+c^+$ occurs relatively infrequently. If a and b loci are close together and both are far from locus c then fewer crossovers would be required to incorporate the two linked loci compared to all three loci (see diagram). If all three loci were close together, then the frequency of incorporation of all three would be similar to the frequency of incorporation of any two contiguous loci, which is not the case.

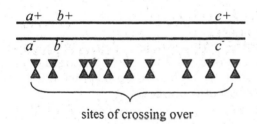

sites of crossing over

11. Not only does the phage lack genes for ribosomal construction, it contains no ribosomes. Upon infection, phage genes are transcribed and the transcripts are translated using bacterial ribosomes.

12. Depending on the particular phage, the life cycle is generally initiated when the virus binds by adsorption to the bacterial host cell. Contraction of the tail sheath causes the central core to cross the cell wall. The DNA in the head is injected through the cell membrane into the bacterium. Bacterial DNA, RNA, and protein synthesis is inhibited, and synthesis of viral RNAs begins using bacterial machinery. Degradation of the host DNA is initiated. Phage DNA replication occurs, leading to a pool of viral DNA molecules. The components of the head, tail, and tail fibers are then synthesized. Three sequential pathways occur to assemble the progeny phage:

(1) DNA packaging as the viral heads are assembled,

(2) tail assembly, and

(3) tail fiber asssembly.

After DNA is packaged into the head, it combines with the tail components, and the tail fibers are added.

13. A single plaque originates from the replicative activity of a single bacteriophage.

14. A single plaque is a clearing of bacteria resulting from the lytic action of millions of bacteriophage.

15. Notice that each of the serial dilutions is hundred-fold and three dilutions were made. This leads to a final 10^{-2} X 10^{-2} X 10^{-2} = 10^{-6} dilution. Assuming the typical introduction of 0.1ml to the bacterial solution, since 17 plaques were formed, the initial density of bacteriophage suspension would be calculated as follows:

170phage/ml X 10^6 = 1.7 X 10^8 phage/ml

16. A lytic cycle occurs as bacteriophages enter a bacterial host and form progeny phages after a relatively short period of time. There is no extensive latent period in that progeny may be produced within an hour or two. *Lysogeny* is a complex process whereby certain temperate phage can enter a bacterial cell and instead of following a lytic developmental path, integrate their DNA into the bacterial chromosome. In doing so, the bacterial cell becomes lysogenic. The latent, integrated phage chromosome is called a *prophage*.

17. A prophage is the latent, non-infective state of the bacteriophage chromosome when it is incorporated into the host, bacterial chromosome.

18. In their experiment a filter was placed between the two auxotrophic strains which would not allow contact. F-mediated conjugation requires contact and without that contact, such conjugation cannot occur. The treatment with DNase showed that the filterable agent was not naked DNA.

19. In *generalized transduction* virtually any genetic element from a host strain may be included in the phage coat and thereby be transduced. If the transduced bacterial chromosomal fragment does not integrate and thus replicate with the host bacterial chromosome, transduction is said to be *abortive*. If the introduced bacterial DNA recombines with a homologous region of the host bacterial chromosome, all daughter cells will inherit the introduced element and transduction is termed *complete*. See F8.1 in this book.

20. Cotransduction of genes in generalized transduction allows linkage relationships to be determined because the closer two genes are to each other, the higher the likelihood that they will be physically "linked" together in a single DNA strand during transduction.

21. The first problem to be solved is the gene order. Clearly, the parental types are

$$a^+b^+c^+ \text{ and } a^-b^-c^-$$

because they are the most frequent. The double crossover types are the least frequent,

$$a^-b^-c^+ \text{ and } a^+b^+c^-.$$

Because it is the gene in the middle which switches places when one compares the parental and double crossover classes, the *c* gene must be in the middle. The map distances are as follows:

a to c = (740 + 670 + 90 + 110)/10,000

= 16.1 map units

c to b = (160 + 140 + 90 + 110)/10,000

= 5 map units

22. Viral recombination occurs when there is a sufficiently high number of infecting viruses so that there is a high likelihood that more than one type of phage will infect a given bacterium. Under this condition phage chromosomes can recombine by crossing over.

23. Starting with a single bacteriophage, one lytic cycle produces 200 progeny phages, three more lytic cycles would produce $(200)^4$ or 1,600,000,000 phages.

24. (a) Remembering that 0.1ml is typically used in the plaque assay, the initial concentration of phage per ml is greater than 10^5.

(b) Remembering that 0.1ml is typically used in the plaque assay, the initial concentration of phage per ml is around 140×10^5 or 1.4×10^7.

(c) Remembering that 0.1ml is typically used in the plaque assay, the initial concentration of phage is less than 10^7. Coupling this information with the calculations in part (b) above, it would appear that the initial concentration of phage is around 1×10^7 and the failure to obtain plaques in this portion of the experiment is expected and due to sampling error.

25. One can approach this problem by lining up the data from the various crosses in the following order:

Hfr Strain	*Order*
1	T C H R O
2	H R O M B
3	<<C H R O M
4	M B A K T>>
5	< <B A K T C

Overall:

$$\boxed{\text{T C H R O M B A K}}$$

Notice that all of the genes can be linked together to give a consistent map and that the ends overlap, indicating that the map is circular. The order is reversed in two of the crosses indicating the orientation of transfer is reversed.

26. Because the frequency of double transformants is quite high (compare the *trp⁺tyr⁺* transformants in A and B experiments) one may conclude that the genes are quite closely linked together.

27. Part B in the experiment gives one the frequencies of transformations of the individual genes and the frequency of transformants receiving two pieces of DNA (2 in the data table). One must know these numbers in order to estimate the actual number of *trp⁺tyr⁺* cotransformations. Since the number of *trp⁺tyr⁺* cotransformants is much lower in part B than part A, the two genes must be linked.

28. (a) Rifampicin eliminates the donor strain which is *rif*ˢ.

(b)

b *a*			*c*	F

(c) To determine the location of the *rif* gene one could use a donor strain which was *rif*ʳ but sensitive to another antibiotic (ampicillin for example). The interrupted mating experiment is conducted as usual on an ampicillin-containing medium but the recombinants must be replated on a rifampicin medium to determine which ones are sensitive.

29. The basis for answering this question rests in the fact that it is easier to transform two genes which are close together (that is, cotransform) than if the same two genes are far apart. If two genes are cotransforming at a relatively high rate they are said to be "linked" in a sense that they are closer together than two genes which do not cotransform. The data indicate that *a* and *d* are linked, *b* and *c* are linked and since *f* cotransforms with *b*, *b*,*c*, and *f* are likely to be linked. However if the arrangement is *c b f* or the reverse, there is a possibility that whereas both *c* and *f* are "linked" to *b*, *c* and *f* may not be strongly enough linked to cotransform. Gene *e* does not cotransform with any gene so it must be more distant from the other linkage groups.

30. Since *g* cotransforms with *f* it is likely to be in the *c b f* "linkage group" and would be expected to cotransform with each. One would not expect transformation with *a, d* or *e*.

31. (a) Some strains, *E. fergusonii* for example, undergo relatively low transfer as a donor strain, while others, *E. chrysanthemi*, undergo relatively frequent transfer as a donor strain. Within-species transfer is not necessarily more frequent than between-species transfer. The direction of transfer (which is the donor and recipient strain) in some cases influences the frequency of transfer; for example, notice the frequencies of transfer when *E. chrysanthemi* is the donor and *E. coli* is the recipient (-1.7), compared to when *E. coli* is the donor and *E. chrysanthemi* is the recipient (-3.7).

(b) *E. chrysanthemi* (-2.4); *E. coli-E. chrysanthemi* (-1.7).

(c) Conjugative plasmids can share genes when bacteria are in proximity and since such plasmids may contain either pathological genes or genes that compromise the use of antibiotics, any harmful variant which develops in one species may be spread to others. While a particular gene may be harmless in one bacterium, it may confer pathogenicity or drug resistance to a different species.

32. (a) No, all functional groups do not impact similarly on conjugative transfer of R27. Regions 1, 2, and 4 appear to be least influenced by mutation because transfer is at 100%.

(b) Regions 3, 5, 6, 8, 9, 10, 12, 13, and 14 appear to have the most impact on conjugation because when mutant, conjugation is abolished.

(c) Regions 7 and 11, when mutant, only partially abolish conjugation, therefore they probably have less impact on conjugation than those listed in part (b).

(d) The data in this problem provide some insight into the complexity of the genetic processes involved in bacterial conjugation. The regions which have the most impact on conjugation fall into three different functional groups. In addition, notice that regions 1, 2, 4, 7, and 11, those which appear to have little if any impact on conjugation, are functionally related as indicated by their shading.

Chapter 9: DNA Structure and Analysis

Concept Areas	Corresponding Problems
Central Dogma	1, 2, 8, 9, 19
Transformation	3, 4
Differential Labeling of Macromolecules	5, 6, 7
Genetic Variation	24, 33, 34
Model Building	15, 16, 28, 31, 35, 36
Nucleic Acid Structure	10, 11, 12, 13, 14, 17, 18, 20, 23, 27, 28, 29, 30, 32
Genomic Complexity	24
Analytical Methods	20, 21, 22, 24, 25, 26, 27, 30, 36, 37

Vocabulary: Organization and Listing of Terms and Concepts

Historical

Miescher (1868- nuclein)

   proteins

   nucleic acids

      tetranucleotide hypothesis

      base ratios, Erwin Chargaff

      transforming principle

         Avery et al. (1944)

         deoxycholate

         T2 bacteriophage (phage)

            Hershey and Chase (1952)

               ^{32}P, ^{35}S

Watson and Crick (1953)

Franklin

Wilkins

Structures and Substances

Messenger RNA (mRNA)

Transfer RNA (tRNA)

Ribosomal RNA (rRNA)

Ribonuclease

Deoxyribonuclease

Lysozyme

   Diplococcus

Protoplasts (spheroplasts)

Ultraviolet light action spectrum

   260nm, 280nm

RNA core

Coat protein

Qβ

Retrovirus

Reverse transcriptase

Nucleic acids

   nucleotides

      nitrogenous base

         purines

            adenine

            guanine

         pyrimidines

            cytosine

            thymine

            uracil

      pentose sugar

         ribose

         deoxyribose

      phosphoric acid

   nucleoside

      monophosphate

      diphosphate

      triphosphate

         adenosine triphosphate

         guanosine triphosphate

phosphodiester bond (5'-3')

inorganic phosphate

      hydrolysis

polynucleotide

base composition

      A=T, G=C

      (A+G) = (C+T)

      (A+T)/(C+G) = variable

X-ray diffraction

antiparallel

0.34 nm (stacked bases) (3.4 Å)

3.4 nm (complete turn)

10 bases per turn

      10.4 bases per turn

2.0nm diameter (20 Å)

hydrogen bonds

      (A to T, G to C)

complementarity

major and minor grooves

hydrophobic bases

hydrophilic backbone

A-DNA

B-DNA

C-DNA

D-DNA

E-DNA

Z-DNA

P- DNA

RNA

    ribosomal RNA (rRNA)

        ribosomes

    messenger RNA (mRNA)

        primary transcripts

    transfer RNA (tRNA)

    small nuclear RNA (snRNA)

    telomerase RNA

    antisense RNA

repetitive DNA

polyacrylamide gel

agarose gel

Processes/Methods

Replication (9.1)

Storage of information (F10.1)

Expression (F9.1)

    transcription

    translation

        central dogma

Transformation

    Diplococcus pneumoniae

        Streptococcus pneumoniae

        virulent

        avirulent

        serotypes (II, III)

        smooth, rough

    heat-killed IIIS

        ribonuclease

        proteolytic enzymes

        deoxyribonuclease

recombinant DNA research

transgenic mice

RNA as genetic material

    TMV (tobacco mosaic virus)

    Qβ phage

    retroviruses

        reverse transcription

Bonding

    sugar to purine

    sugar to pyrimidine

    nucleotide to nucleotide

Single crystal X-ray analysis

    Svedberg coefficient (S)

    Absorption of ultraviolet light (UV)

        260 nm (OD_{260})

Denaturation (melting)

    heat, chemical treatment

Spectrophotometry

Melting profile

Melting temperature (T_m)

Renaturation (hybridization)

DNA/DNA

DNA/RNA

in situ hybridization

autoradiography

fluorescent label

FISH

kinetics

C_0t

$C_0t_{1/2}$

sequence complexity

electrophoresis

polyacrylamide

agarose

Concepts

Central dogma

Characteristics of genetic material

Tetranucleotide hypothesis

Transformation

Differential labeling of macromolecules

Indirect evidence

DNA content (n, $2n$)

mutagenesis

action spectrum

absorption spectrum

260 nm, 280 nm

Direct evidence

recombinant DNA technology

Model building

DNA double helix

storage of genetic information

information flow

mutation

Genomic complexity

reassociation kinetics

Separation strageties

Labeling strategies

F9.1 Illustration of relationships between DNA, its functions and related products.

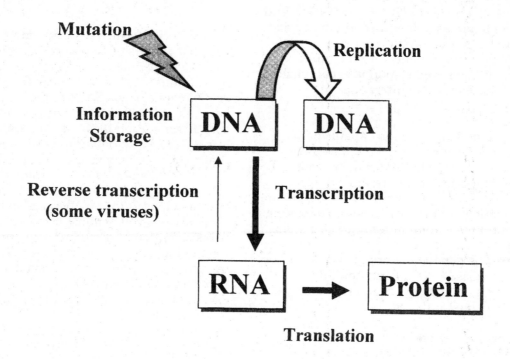

Solutions to Problems and Discussion Questions

1. *Replication* is that process which leads to the production of identical copies of the existing genetic information. Since daughter cells contain essentially exact copies (with some exceptions) of genetic information of the parent cell, and through the production and union of gametes, offspring contain copies (with variation) of parental genetic information, the genetic material must copy (replicate) itself. Replication is accomplished during the S phase of interphase in eukaryotes.

The genetic material is capable of *expression* through the production of a phenotype. Through transcription and translation, proteins are produced which contribute to the phenotype of the organism. The genetic material must be stable enough to maintain information in "*storage*" from one cell to the next and one organism to the next. Because the genetic material is not "used up" in the processes of transcription and translation, genetic information can be stored and used constantly.

Above, it was stated that the genetic material must be stable enough to store genetic information; however, variation through *mutation* provides the raw material for evolution. The genetic material is capable of a variety of changes, both at the chromosomal and nucleotide levels. See F10.1.

2. Prior to 1940 most of the interest in genetics centered on the transmission of similarity and variation from parents to offspring (transmission genetics). While some experiments examined the possible nature of the hereditary material, abundant knowledge of the structural and enzymatic properties of proteins generated a bias which worked to favor proteins as the hereditary substance.

In addition, proteins were composed of as many as twenty different subunits (amino acids) thereby providing ample structural and functional variation for the multiple tasks which must be accomplished by the genetic material. The tetranucleotide hypothesis (about DNA structure) provided insufficient variability to account for the diverse roles of the genetic material.

3. Griffith performed experiments with different strains of *Diplococcus pneumoniae* in which a heat-killed pathogen, when injected into a mouse with a live nonpathogenic strain, eventually led to the mouse's death. A summary of this experiment is provided in the text. Examination of the dead mouse revealed living pathogenic bacteria. Griffith suggested that the heat-killed virulent (pathogenic) bacteria transformed the avirulent (non-pathogenic) strain into a virulent strain. Alloway showed that a chemical extract of the virulent cells was sufficient to cause transformation of avirulent cells, further reinforcing the hypothesis that the transforming factor has a chemical basis. Avery and coworkers systematically searched for the transforming principle originating from the heat-killed pathogenic strain and determined it to be DNA. Others showed that transformed bacteria are capable of serving as donors of transforming DNA indicating that the process of transformation involves a stable alteration in the genetic material (DNA).

4. Transformation is dependent on a macromolecule (DNA) which can be extracted and purified from bacteria. During such purification however, other macromolecular species may contaminate the DNA. Specific degradative enzymes, proteases, RNase, and DNase were used to selectively eliminate components of the extract and, if transformation is concomitantly eliminated, then the eliminated fraction is the transforming principle. DNase eliminates DNA and transformation, therefore it must be the transforming principle.

110

5. Nucleic acids contain large amounts of phosphorus and no sulfur whereas proteins contain sulfur and no phosphorus. Therefore the radioisotopes ^{32}P and ^{35}S will selectively label nucleic acids and proteins, respectively.

The Hershey and Chase experiment is based on the premise that the substance injected into the bacterium is the substance responsible for producing the progeny phages and therefore must be the hereditary material. The experiment demonstrated that most of the ^{32}P -labeled material (DNA) was injected while the phage ghosts (protein coats) remained outside the bacterium. Therefore the nucleic acid must be the genetic material.

6. Actually phosphorus is found in approximately equal amounts in DNA and RNA. Therefore labeling with ^{32}P would "tag" both RNA and DNA. However, the T2 phage, in its mature state, contains very little if any RNA, therefore DNA would be interpreted as being the genetic material in T2 phage.

7. In theory, the general design would be appropriate in that some substance, if labeled, would show up in the progeny of transformed bacteria. However, since the amount of transforming DNA is extremely small compared to the genomic DNA of the recipient bacterium and its progeny, it would be technically difficult to assay for the labeled nucleic acid. In addition, it would be necessary to know that the small stretch of DNA which caused the genetic transformation was actually labeled. This in itself would be relatively easy using present-day recombinant DNA techniques; however, in earlier times, such specific labeling would have been difficult.

8. The early evidence would be considered indirect in that at no time was there an experiment, like transformation in bacteria, in which genetic information in one organism was transferred to another using DNA. Rather, by comparing DNA content in various cell types (sperm and somatic cells) and observing that the *action* and *absorption* spectra of ultraviolet light were correlated, DNA was considered to be the genetic material. This suggestion was supported by the fact that DNA was shown to be the genetic material in bacteria and some phage. Direct evidence for DNA being the genetic material comes from a variety of observations including gene transfer which has been facilitated by recombinant DNA techniques.

9. Some viruses contain a genetic material composed of RNA. The tobacco mosaic virus is composed of an RNA core and a protein coat. "Crosses" can be made in which the protein coat and RNA of TMV are interchanged with another strain (Holmes ribgrass). The source of the RNA determines the type of lesion, thus, RNA is the genetic material in these viruses. Retroviruses contain RNA as the genetic material and use an enzyme known as *reverse transcriptase* to produce DNA which can be integrated into the host chromosome. See F9.1. Note: the term "organism" generally refers to membrane-bound, nonviral, living systems. Therefore, technically all organisms have DNA as their genetic material.

10. The structure of deoxyadenylic acid is given below and in the text. Linkages among the three components require the removal of water (H_2O).

11. The numbering of the carbons on the sugar is especially important (see diagram below). Examine the text for the numbers on the carbons and nitrogens of the bases:

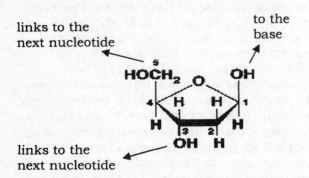

links to the next nucleotide

to the base

links to the next nucleotide

12. Examine the structures of the bases in the text. The other bases would be named as follows:

Guanine: 2-amino-6-oxypurine

Cytosine: 2-oxy-4-aminopyrimidine

Thymine: 2,4-dioxy-5-methylpyrimidine

Uracil: 2,4-dioxypyrimidine

13. Examine the text for the format for this drawing. Note that the complementary strand must be drawn in the antiparallel orientation.

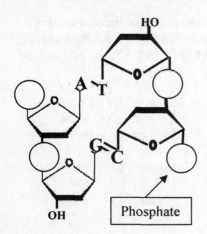

HO

A—T

G—C

OH

Phosphate

14. The following are characteristics of the Watson-Crick double-helix model for DNA:

The base composition is such that A=T, G=C and (A+G) = (C+T). Bases are stacked, 0.34 nm (3.4 Angstoms) apart, in a plectonic, antiparallel manner. There is one complete turn for each 3.4 nm which constitutes 10 bases per turn. Hydrogen bonds hold the two polynucleotide chains together, each being formed by phosphodiester linkages between the five-carbon sugars and the phosphates. There are two hydrogen bonds forming the A to T pair and three forming the G to C pair. The double helix exists as a twisted structure, approximately 20 Angstroms in diameter, with a topography of major and minor grooves. The hydrophobic bases are located in the center of the molecule while the hydrophilic phosphodiester backbone is on the outside.

15. In addition to creative "genius" and perseverance, model building skills, and the conviction that the structure would turn out to be "simple" and have a natural beauty in its simplicity, Watson and Crick employed the X-ray diffraction information of Franklin and Wilkins, and the base ratio information of Chargaff and the knowledge of the nucleotide structures.

16. Because in double-stranded DNA, A=T and G=C (within limits of experimental error), the data presented would have indicated a lack of pairing of these bases in favor of a single-stranded structure or some other nonhydrogen-bonded structure.

Alternatively, from the data it would appear that A=C and T=G, which would negate the chance for typical hydrogen bonding since opposite charge relationships do not exist. Therefore, it is quite unlikely that a tight helical structure would form at all.

17. A covalent bond is a relatively strong bond which involves the sharing of electrons between two or more atoms. Hydrogen bonds, much weaker than covalent bonds, are formed as a result of

"electrostatic attraction between a covalently bonded hydrogen atom and an atom with an unshared electron pair. The hydrogen atom assumes a partial positive charge, while the unshared electron pair-characteristic of covalently bonded oxygen and nitrogen atoms- assumes a partial negative charge. These opposite charges are responsible for the weak chemical attraction."(Klug, Cummings and Spencer)

Complementarity, responsible for the chemical attraction between adenine and thymine (uracil in RNA) and guanine and cytosine, is responsible for DNA and RNA assuming its double-stranded character. Complementarity is based on hydrogen bonding.

18. Three main differences between RNA and DNA are the following:

(1) uracil in RNA replaces thymine in DNA,

(2) ribose in RNA replaces deoxyribose in DNA, and

(3) RNA often occurs as both single- and partially double-stranded forms whereas DNA most often occurs in a double-stranded form.

19. While there are many types of RNA, the three main types described in this section are presented below:

ribosomal RNA: rRNA combines with proteins to form ribosomes which function to align mRNA and charged tRNA molecules during translation.

transfer RNA: tRNAs are involved in protein synthesis in that they represent a "link" between the sequences in DNA (as reflected in mRNA) and the ordering of amino acids in proteins. Transfer RNAs are specific in that each species is attached to only one type of amino acid.

messenger RNA: the coding sequences in DNA is transferred to the site of protein synthesis by a relatively short-lived molecule called messenger RNA. In eukaryotes, mRNA carries genetic information from the nucleus to the cytoplasm. It is the sequence of bases in mRNA which specifies the order of amino acids in proteins.

20. The nitrogenous bases of nucleic acids (nucleosides, nucleotides, and single- and double-stranded polynucleotides), absorb UV light maximally at wavelengths 254 to 260 nm. Using this phenomenon, one can often determine the presence and concentration of nucleic acids in a mixture. Since proteins absorb UV light maximally at 280 nm, this is a relatively simple way of dealing with mixtures of biologically important molecules.

UV absorption is greater in single-stranded molecules (hyperchromic shift) as compared to double-stranded structures. Therefore, one can easily determine, by applying denaturing conditions, whether a nucleic acid is in the single- or double-stranded form. In addition, A-T rich DNA denatures more readily than G-C rich DNA. Therefore one can estimate base content by denaturation kinetics.

21. Various treatments, such as heat, or certain chemical environments cause separation of the hydrogen bonds which hold together the complementary strands of DNA. Under these conditions, double-stranded DNA is changed to single-stranded DNA.

22. *A hyperchromic effect* is the increased absorption of UV light as double-stranded DNA (or RNA for that matter) is converted to single-stranded DNA. As illustrated in the text, the change in absorption is quite significant, with a structure of higher G-C content *melting* at a higher temperature than an A-T rich nucleic acid. If one monitors the UV absorption with a spectrophotometer during the melting process the hyperchromic shift can be observed. The T_m is the point on the profile (temperature) at which half (50%) of the sample is denatured.

23. Because G-C base pairs are formed with three hydrogen bonds while A-T base pairs by two such bonds, it takes more energy (higher temperature) to separate G-C pairs.

24. Carefully examine the text. First understand the concept of molecular hybridization, then see that as the degree of strand uniqueness increases, the time required for reassociation increases. Repetitive sequences renature relatively quickly because the likelihood of complementary strands interacting increases.

For curve A in the problem, there is evidence for a rapidly renaturing species (repetitive) and a slowly renaturing species (unique). The fraction which reassociates faster than the *E. coli* DNA is highly repetitive and the last fraction (with the highest $Cot_{1/2}$ value) contains primarily unique sequences. Fraction B contains mostly unique, relatively complex DNA.

25. The reassociation of separate complementary strands of a nucleic acid, either DNA or RNA, is based on hydrogen bonds forming between A-T (or U) and G-C.

26. In one sentence of their first *Nature* paper, Watson and Crick state,

"It has not escaped our notice that the specific pairing we have postulated immediately suggests a possible copying mechanism for the genetic material."

The model itself indicates that unwinding of the helix and separation of the double-stranded structure into two single strands immediately exposes the specific hydrogen bonds through which new bases are brought into place.

27.

(1) As shown, the extra phosphate is not normally expected.

(2) In the adenine ring, a nitrogen is at position 8 rather than position 9.

(3) The bond from the C-1' to the sugar should form with the N at position 9 (N-9) of the adenine.

(4) The dinucleotide is a "deoxy" form, therefore each C-2' should not have a hydroxyl group. Notice the hydroxyl group at C-2' on the sugar of the adenylic acid.

(5) At the C-5 position on the thymine residue, there should be a methyl group.

(6) There are too many bonds at the N-3 position on the thymine.

(7) There are too few bonds at the C-5 of thymine.

28. As provided in the text, a direct proportionality between $C_0t_{1/2}$ and the number of base pairs exists under certain conditions.

The ratios for MS-2 would be as follows:

$0.5/10^5 = 0.001/X$

or

$X/0.001 = 10^5/0.5$

$X = (0.001)(10^5)/0.5$

$X = 200$ base pairs

The ratios for *E. coli* would be as follows:

$0.5/10^5 = 10.0/X$ or

$X/10.0 = 10^5/0.5$

$X = (10.0)(10^5)/0.5$

$X = 2 \times 10^6$ base pairs

29.

(a) The X-ray diffraction studies would indicate a helical structure, for it is on the basis of such data that a helical pattern is suggested. The fact that it is irregular may indicate different diameters (base pairings), additional strands in the helix, kinking, or bending.

(b) The hyperchromic shift would indicate considerable hydrogen bonding, possibly caused by base pairing.

(c) Such data may suggest irregular base pairing in which purines bind purines (all the bases presented are purines), thus giving the atypical dimensions.

(d) Because of the presence of ribose, the molecule may show more flexibility, kinking, and/or folding.

While there are several situations possible for this model, the phosphates are still likely to be far apart (on the outside) because of their strong like charges. Hydrogen bonding probably exists on the inside of the molecule and there is probably considerable flexibility, kinking, and/or bending.

30. Left side (a) = right, right side (b) = left.

31. Since cytosine pairs with guanine and uracil pairs with adenine, the result would be a base substitution of G:C to A:T after rounds of replication.

32. Under this condition, the hydrolyzed 5-methyl cytosine becomes thymine.

33. Without knowing the exact bonding characteristics of hypoxanthine or xanthine it may be difficult to predict the likelihood of each pairing type. It is likely that both are of the same class (purine or pyrimidine) because the names of the molecules indicate a similarity. In addition, the diameter of the structure is constant which, under the model to follow, would be expected. In fact, hypoxanthine and xanthine are both purines.

Because there are equal amounts of A, T, and H, one could suggest that they are hydrogen bonded to each other; the same may be said for C, G, and X. Given the molar equivalence of erythrose and phosphate, an alternating sugar-phosphate-sugar backbone as in "earth-type" DNA would be acceptable. A model of a triple helix would be acceptable, since the diameter is constant. Given the chemical similarities to "earth-type" DNA, it is probable that the unique creature's DNA follows the same structural plan.

34. (a) Heat application would yield a hyperchromic shift if the DNA is double-stranded. One could also get a rough estimation of the GC content from the kinetics of denaturation and the degree of sequence complexity from comparative renaturation studies.

(b) Determination of base content by hydrolysis and chromatography could be used for comparative purposes and could also provide evidence as to the strandedness of the DNA.

(c) Antibodies for Z-DNA could be used to determine the degree of left-handed structures, if present.

(d) Sequencing the DNA from both viruses would indicate sequence homology. In addition, through various electronic searches readily available on the Internet (Web site: *ncbi.nlm.nih.gov*, for example) one could determine whether similar sequences exist in other viruses or in other organisms.

35. The way the question is stated suggests that DNA which is separated electrophoretically is of the same shape (long rod). In fact, DNA can exist in a variety of shapes as seen in supercoiled plasmids, relaxed (nicked) plasmids, and linear molecules. Size comparisons with DNA must be such that linear molecules are compared with linear molecules and supercoiled with supercoiled, etc. In comparing DNA migration to RNA, even though RNA molecules have the same charge-to-mass ratios, they also exist in a variety of shapes. Complementary intra-strand base pairing can make more compact structures compared to the more relaxed, open conformation. For electrophoretic size comparisons, RNA molecules must be denatured to eliminate secondary structural variables.

Chapter 10: DNA Replication and Synthesis

Concept Areas	Corresponding Problems
Replication	1, 2, 3, 4, 5, 14, 15, 16, 17, 20 26, 28, 29, 32
In vitro Experiments	6, 7, 8, 9, 10
Eukaryotic Replication	18, 25, 30
Base Composition	19
Enzymology	8, 10, 11,12, 13, 16, 23, 27, 31
Telomerase	24
Conditional Mutations	21
Gene Conversion	22

Vocabulary: Organization and Listing of Terms and Concepts

Structures and Substances

DNA polymerase I

5'-nucleotides (F10.1)

3'-nucleotides (F10.1)

Phage φX174

DNA ligase (polynucleotide joining enzyme)

DNA polymerase II

DNA polymerase III

   primer

   exonuclease

   holoenzyme

   subunits

   γ complex

   replisome

DNA polymerases IV, V

Helicases, *dna*A, *dna*B, *dna*C

Single-stranded DNA binding proteins

DNA gyrase (topoisomerase)

RNA primer

   primase

    free 3' hydroxyl group

DNA ligase

   ligase deficient mutant

ori C

   9mer, 13mer

   β-subunit clamp

Eukaryotic DNA polymerases

   six forms

   multiple replicons

117

Chapter 10 DNA Replication and Synthesis

Antonomously replicating sequence (ARS)

Origin replication complex (ORC)

Pre-replication complex

Nucleosome

Telomerase

    Tetrahymena

    5'-TTGGGG-3'

    hairpin loop

    ribonucleoprotein

Endonuclease

Heteroduplex DNA molecules

    Holliday structures

    chi form

    recombinant duplexes

    *rec*A, *rec*B, *rec*C, *rec*D

Processes/Methods

Replication of DNA

    semiconservative

    conservative

    dispersive

Meselson and Stahl - 1958

    E. coli

        equilibrium centrifugation

        $^{15}NH_4Cl$, $^{14}NH_4Cl$

Taylor, Woods, and Hughes - 1957

    Vicia faba

    ^{3}H-thymidine

    autoradiography

    colchicine

    sister chromatid exchanges

bidirectional (*vs.* unidirectional)

    origin of replication, *ori*

    replicon

    replication fork

    continuous, discontinuous

        leading strand

        lagging strand

        Okazaki fragments

Synthesis of DNA *in vitro*

    Kornberg - 1957

    reaction mixture

    chain elongation

        fidelity

    base comparisons (template/product)

    biologically active DNA

        infection of *E. coli*

    faithful copying

    processivity

Polymerase switching

Exonuclease proofreading

Conditional mutation

    temperature sensitive

Genetic recombination

    homologous recombination

    single-stranded nick

    endonuclease and ligation

Gene conversion

    Neurospora

    nonreciprocal

Concepts

Replication

    semiconservative

    antiparallel

    continuous, discontinuous

    conservative (F10.3)

    dispersive (F10.3)

Biological activity

Repair

Proofreading

Eukaryotic DNA replication

Telomere replication

Conditional mutants (F10.2)

Genetic recombination

Gene conversion

F10.1 Shorthand structures for 3' and 5' nucleotides.

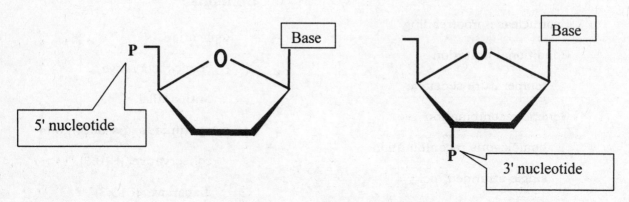

F10.2 Illustration of the influence of a conditional mutation on protein structure and function.

Changes in the environment of the protein may cause conformational changes in the protein to alter function of that protein.

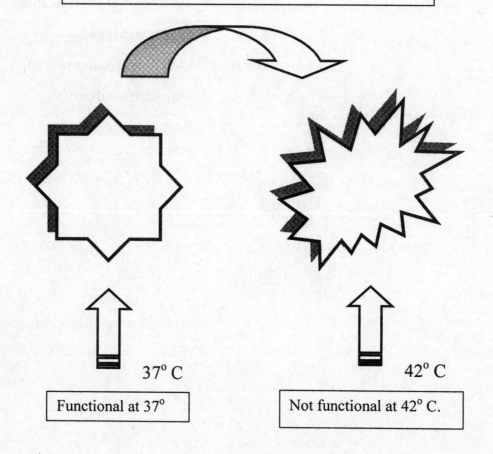

37° C

Functional at 37°

42° C

Not functional at 42° C.

F10.3 Figure relating to question #4 in the problems section depicts labeling pattern under *Conservative* and *Dispersive* replication patterns.

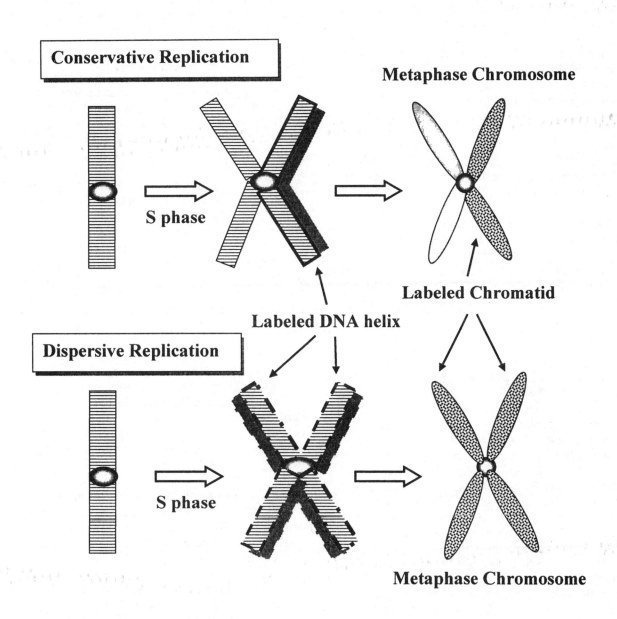

Solutions to Problems and Discussion Questions

1. The differences among the three models of DNA replication relate to the manner in which the new strands of DNA are oriented as daughter DNA molecules are produced.

Conservative: In the conservative scheme, the original double helix remains as a complete unit and the new DNA double helix is produced as a single unit. The old DNA is completely conserved.

Semiconservative: Each daughter strand is composed of one old DNA strand and one new DNA strand. Separation of hydrogen bonds is required.

Dispersive: In the dispersive scheme, the original DNA strand is broken into pieces and the new DNA in the daughter strand is interspersed among the old pieces. Separation of the individual covalent, phosphodiester bonds is required for this mode of replication.

2. The Meselson and Stahl experiment has the following components. By labeling the pool of nitrogenous bases of the DNA of *E. coli* with a heavy isotope ^{15}N, it would be possible to "follow" the "old" DNA. This is accomplished by growing the cells for many generations in medium containing ^{15}N. Cells were transferred to ^{14}N medium so that "new" DNA could be detected. A comparison of the density of DNA samples at various times in the experiment (initial ^{15}N culture, and subsequent cultures grown in the ^{14}N medium) showed that after one round of replication in the ^{14}N medium, the DNA was half as dense (intermediate) as the DNA from bacteria grown only in the ^{15}N medium. In a sample taken after two rounds of replication in the ^{14}N medium, half of the DNA was of the intermediate density and the other half was as dense as DNA containing only ^{14}N DNA.

3. Under a conservative scheme the first round of replication in ^{14}N medium produces one dense double helix and one "light" double helix in contrast to the intermediate density of the DNA in the semiconservative mode. Therefore, after one round or replication in the ^{14}N medium, the conservative scheme can be ruled out.

After one round of replication in ^{14}N under a dispersive model, the DNA is of intermediate density, just as it is in the semiconservative model. However, in the next round of replication in ^{14}N medium, the density of the DNA is between the intermediate and "light" densities.

4. Refer to the text for an illustration of the labeling of *Vicia* chromosomes under a Taylor, Woods, and Hughes experimental design. Notice that only those cells which pass through the S phase in the presence of the ^{3}H-thymidine are labeled and that each double helix (per chromatid) is "half-labeled." See Figure F10.3 in this book for a graphic description of the conservative and dispersive replication patterns.

(a) Under a conservative scheme, all of the newly labeled DNA will go to one sister chromatid, while the other sister chromatid will remain unlabeled. In contrast to a semiconservative scheme, the first replicative round would produce one sister chromatid which has label on both strands of the double helix. (See F10.3 above)

(b) Under a dispersive scheme, all of the newly labeled DNA will be interspersed with unlabeled DNA. Because these preparations (metaphase chromosomes) are highly coiled and condensed structures derived from the "spread out" form at interphase (which includes the S phase), it is impossible to detect the areas where label is not found. Rather, both sister chromatids would appear as evenly labeled structures. (See F10.3 above)

5. Because the semiconservative scheme predicts that *half* of the DNA in each daughter double helix is labeled, it would be difficult to envision a scheme where three strands are replicated in such a semiconservative manner. It would seem that either the conservative or dispersive scheme would fit more appropriately. To examine the nature of replication, one could devise an experiment similar to that of Meselson and Stahl or Taylor, Woods, and Hughes.

6. The *in vitro* replication requires a DNA template, a primer to give a double stranded portion, a divalent cation (Mg⁺⁺), and all four of the deoxyribonucleoside triphosphates: dATP, dCTP, dTTP, and dGTP. The lower case "d" refers to the deoxyribose sugar.

7. Prior to the development of highly efficient methods of enzyme isolation, large cultures, containing large numbers of bacterial cells, were needed to yield even small quantities of enzymes.

8. Several analytical approaches showed that the products of DNA polymerase I were probably copies of the template DNA. *Base composition* was used initially to compare both templates and products.   Within experimental error, those data strongly suggested that the DNA replicated faithfully.

9. The *in vitro* rate of DNA synthesis using DNA polymerase I is slow, being more effective at replicating single-stranded DNA than double-stranded DNA. In addition, it is capable of degrading as well as synthesizing DNA. Such degradation suggested that it functioned as a repair enzyme. In addition, DeLucia and Cairns discovered a strain of *E. coli* (*pol*A1) which still replicated its DNA but was deficient in DNA polymerase I activity.

10. As stated in the text, *biologically active* DNA implies that the DNA is capable of supporting typical metabolic activities of the cell or organism and is capable of faithful reproduction.

11. The *pol*AI mutation was instrumental in demonstrating that DNA polymerase I activity was not necessary for the *in vivo* replication of the *E. coli* chromosome. Such an observation opened the door for the discovery of other enzymes involved in DNA replication.

12. All three enzymes share several common properties. First, none can *initiate* DNA synthesis on a template but all can *elongate* an existing DNA strand assuming there is a template strand as shown in the figure below. Polymerization of nucleotides occurs in the 5' to 3' direction where each 5' phosphate is added to the 3' end of the growing polynucleotide.

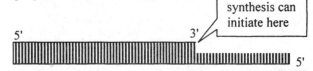

All three enzymes are large complex proteins with a molecular weight in excess of 100,000 daltons and each has 3' to 5' exonuclease activity. Refer to the text.

DNA polymerase I:
    polymerization
    3'-5' exonuclease activity
    5'-3' exonuclease activity
    present in large amounts
    relatively stable
    removal of RNA primer
DNA polymerase II:
    polymerization
    3'-5' exonuclease activity
    possibly involved in repair function
DNA polymerase III:
    polymerization
    3'-5' exonuclease activity
    essential for replication
    complex molecule

13. Refer to the text for a listing of the components of DNA polymerase III. The active form of the enzyme is called the holoenzyme. The region responsible for actual polymerization is called the "core" portion.

14. Given a stretch of double-stranded DNA, one could initiate synthesis at a given point and either replicate strands in one direction only (unidirectional) or in both directions (bidirectional) as shown below. Notice that in the text the synthesis of complementary strands occurs in a *continuous* 5'>3' mode on the leading strand in the direction of the replication fork, and in a *discontinuous* 5'>3' mode on the lagging strand opposite the direction of the replication fork. Such discontinuous replication forms Okazaki fragments.

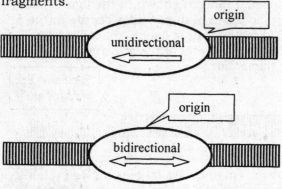

15. *Helicase, dnaA* and *single-stranded DNA binding proteins* initially unwind, open, and stabilize DNA at the initiation point. *DNA gyrase*, a DNA topoisomerase, relieves supercoiling generated by helix unwinding. This process involves breaking both strands of the DNA helix.

16. *Okazaki fragments* are relatively short (1000 to 2000 bases in prokaryotes) DNA fragments which are synthesized in a discontinuous fashion on the lagging strand during DNA replication. Such fragments appear to be necessary because template DNA is not available for 5'>3' synthesis until some degree of continuous DNA synthesis occurs on the leading strand in the direction of the replication fork. The isolation of such fragments provides support for the scheme of replication shown in the text. DNA *ligase* is required to form phosphodiester linkages in gaps which are generated when DNA polymerase I removes RNA primer and meets newly synthesized DNA ahead of it.

Notice in the text the discontinuous DNA strands are ligated together into a single continuous strand. *Primer* RNA is formed by RNA primase to serve as an initiation point for the production of DNA strands on a DNA template. None of the DNA polymerases are capable of initiating synthesis without a free 3' hydroxyl group. The primer RNA provides that group and thus can be used by DNA polymerase III.

17. The synthesis of DNA is thought to follow the pattern described in the text. The model involves opening and stabilization of the DNA helix, priming DNA with synthesis with RNA primer, movement of replication forks in both directions which includes elongation of RNA primers in continuous and discontinuous 5'>3' modes and their removal by the exonucleolytic activity of DNA polymerase I. Okazaki fragments generated in the replicative process are joined together with DNA ligase. DNA gyrase relieves supercoils generated by DNA unwinding.

18. Eukaryotic DNA is replicated in a manner which is very similar to that of *E. coli.* Synthesis is bidirectional, continuous on one strand and discontinuous on the other, and the requirements of synthesis (four deoxyribonucleoside triphosphates, divalent cation, template, and primer) are the same. Okazaki fragments of eukaryotes are about one-tenth the size of those in bacteria.

Because there is a much greater amount of DNA to be replicated and DNA replication is slower, there are multiple initiation sites for replication in eukaryotes (and increased DNA polymerase per cell) in contrast to the single replication origin in prokaryotes. Replication occurs at different sites during different intervals of the S phase. The proposed functions of four DNA polymerases are described in the text. Because most eukaryotic chromosomes are linear, enzymes such as telomerase are needed to replicate the telomeres, or ends of chromosomes.

19. Even though the base composition between two species may be *similar*, sequences can vary considerably.

20. (a) In *E. coli*, 100kb are added to each growing chain per minute. Therefore the chain should be about 4,000,000bp.

(b) Given (4×10^6 bp) $\times$ 0.34nm/bp =

1.36×10^6nm or 1.3mm

21. (a) No repair from DNA polymerase I and/or DNA polymerase III.

(b) No DNA ligase activity.

(c) No primase activity.

(d) Only DNA polymerase I activity.

(e) No DNA gyrase activity.

22. *Gene conversion* is likely to be a consequence of genetic recombination in which nonreciprocal recombination makes it appear that one allele is "converted" to another. Gene conversion is now considered a result of heteroduplex formation which is accompanied by mismatched bases. Some of the ways in which these mismatches can be corrected, result in the "conversion."

23. (a) Because DNA polymerase III is essential for DNA chain elongation, it is necessary for replication of the *E. coli* chromosome. Thus strains which are mutant for this enzyme must contain conditional mutations or may rely on DNA polymerase I and replicate their DNA more slowly. **(b)** The 3' - 5' exonuclease activity is involved in proofreading. Thus proofreading would be hampered in such mutant strains and a higher than expected mutation rate would occur.

24. Telomerase activity is present in germ linc tissue to maintain telomere length from one generation to the next. In other words, telomeres can not shorten indefinitely without eventually eroding genetic information.

25. Since synthesis is bidirectional, one can multiply the rate of synthesis by two to come up with a figure of 18,000 bases replicated per five minutes (30bases/second $\times$ 300 seconds). Dividing 1.6×10^8 by 1.8×10^4 gives 0.88×10^4 or about 8,800 replication sites.

26. If replication is conservative, the first autoradiograms (see metaphase I in the text) would have label distributed only on one side (chromatid) of the metaphase chromosome as shown below.

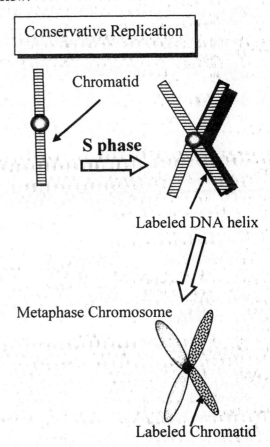

Conservative Replication

Chromatid

S phase

Labeled DNA helix

Metaphase Chromosome

Labeled Chromatid

27.

(a) DNA polymerase would catalyze a bond between the 5' end of the last nucleotide added and the 3' end of the incoming nucleotide. In this reaction, the energy would be provided by the cleavage of the gamma- and beta- phosphates of the last nucleotide added to the chain rather than of the incoming nucleotide.

(b) If DNA polymerase removed a base, it would not be able to add any more bases to the chain because the penultimate base would have a monophosphate rather than a triphosphate and there would be no source of energy for the polymerization reaction.

28. If the DNA contained parallel strands in the double helix and the polymerase would be able to accommodate such parallel strands, there would be continuous synthesis and no Okazaki fragments. The telomere problem would only be at one end. Several other possibilities exist. If the DNA strands were replicated as complete single strands, the synthesis could begin at the opposite free ends. In addition, if the DNA existed only as a single strand, the same results would occur.

29. (a) 5'ACCUAAGU **(b)** U

30. Conservative replication can be eliminated. This is because under a conservative mode of replication, both of the original DNA strands remain together in one chromatid and the two new strands form a single double helix in the other chromatid. Such is not the case in this figure.

31. (a) DNA, since one of the nitrogenous bases is T; also, notice the lack of a OH group at the 2' carbon. **(b)** 3' **(c)** Since spleen diesterase cuts between the 5' carbon and the phosphate, the original 5' phosphate is transferred to the 3' carbon of the 5' neighbor.

Therefore deoxyadenosine would obtain the phosphate at its 3' position.

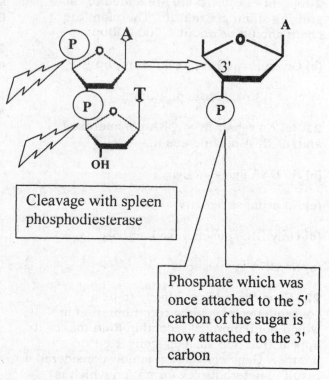

Cleavage with spleen phosphodiesterase

Phosphate which was once attached to the 5' carbon of the sugar is now attached to the 3' carbon

32. First, given that label is distributed on both ends of the structure, replication must be bidirectional. Second, since both upper and lower portions contain label, no restrictions to synthesis are apparent. The distribution of low density grains in the center would indicate that replication begins in the middle and proceeds to the outward areas in both directions rather evenly.

Chapter 11: Chromosome Structure and DNA Sequence Organization

Concept Areas	Corresponding Problems
Viral and Bacterial Chromosomes	1, 2, 18, 19, 26
Mitochondrial and Chloroplast DNA	3, 4, 5, 6
Specialized Chromosomes	7, 8, 9, 11
Organization of DNA in Chromatin	12, 13, 14, 15, 17, 20, 23, 24, 25
Organization of the Eukaryotic Genome	10, 16, 21, 22, 27, 28, 29, 30

Vocabulary: Organization and Listing of Terms and Concepts

Structures and Substances

Viral chromosomes

  DNA, RNA

    double-stranded

    single-stranded

    often circular

  protein coat

  φX174

  polyoma

  lambda (λ)

Bacterial chromosomes

  DNA

  double-stranded

  nucleoid

  E. coli

    circular

DNA-binding proteins

  HU, H

  topoisomer

  topoisomerase

Mitochondrial DNA (mtDNA)

  plant

  animal

  coding (mtDNA)

    rRNAs

    tRNAs

    respiratory components

  coding (nuclear)

    imported products

Chapter 11 Chromosome Structure and DNA Sequence Organization

Chloroplast DNA (cpDNA)

   circular

   double-stranded

   different than nuclear DNA

   coding (cpDNA)

      rRNAs

      tRNAs

   ribulose-1-5-bisphosphate carboxylase

Eukaryotic chromosomes

   chromatin

   mitotic chromosomes

      condensed chromatin

         folded fiber

Chromatin

   nucleoprotein

   histones

      amino acid composition

      tetramers

         nucleosome core particle

   nonhistones

   micrococcal nuclease

      nucleosomes

      linker DNA

         histone H1

   solenoid

Heterochromatin, euchromatin

   telomere

   kinetochore

   satellite and repetitive DNA

   GP island

   pseudogene

Processes/Methods

Semiconservative replication

Importing of nuclear-coded gene products

Autoradiography

Folded-fiber (eukaryotic chromosome)

   coiling-twisting-condensing

Chromatin remodeling

   methylation, phosphorylation

Heterochromatin

   few genes

   late replicating

   position effect

Repetitive DNA

   non-coding sequences

      satellite DNA

      highly repetitive DNA

   centromeric DNA (CEN)

      alphoid family

   telomeric DNA sequences

telomeric-associated sequences

telomerase

moderately repetitive DNA

short interspersed elements (SINES)

   Alu family

long interspersed elements (LINES)

variable number tandem repeats (VNTR)

DNA fingerprinting

minisatellites

microsatellites

repetitive transposed sequences

moderately repetitive multicopy genes

pseudogene formation

Concepts

Variety of DNA conformations

Evolution of cellular organelles

   endosymbiont theory

Heterochromatin/euchromatin

Chromatin remodeling

Centromeric/telomeric structure

Repetitive DNA

Pseudogene formation

Solutions to Problems and Discussion Questions

1. Bacteriophage λ has a linear, double-stranded DNA while in the phage coat and upon infection closes to form a circular chromosome with a size of about 50kb. T2 phage also has a linear, double-stranded DNA chromosome; less than 200kb. *E. coli* has a circular, double-stranded DNA chromosome of about 4.2×10^3kb. Both intact phages are about 1/150 the size of *E.coli*. Since phages are obligate parasites of bacteria, they are dependent on their hosts for the manufacture of materials for their replication. Bacteria contain all genetic information for metabolism, replication, and *de novo* synthesis of numerous life-supporting materials. Phages, on the other hand, contain relatively few genes; namely, those needed to adsorb, inject, and produce progeny using primarily bacterial materials.

2. By having a circular chromosome, no free ends present the problem of linear chromosomes, namely complete replication of terminal sequences.

3. Mitochondrial DNA and chloroplast DNA exist as double-stranded closed circles which replicate semiconservatively. They are both free of chromosomal proteins which are characteristic of eukaryotic chromosomes. Lengths of mtDNA, but cpDNA vary and multiple copies of each DNA may occur in each organelle. Few, if any, introns or repetitive sequences occur in mtDNA, however, cpDNA does contain duplications and long noncoding regions.

4. Mitochondrial DNA varies in size from 16kb in humans to over 350kb in some plants and codes for ribosomal, transfer and messenger RNAs. The protein-synthesizing apparatus and many components of cellular respiration are jointly formed from nuclear and mitochondrial genes. Chloroplast DNA codes for ribosomal RNAs, as well as tRNAs and mRNAs for ribosomal proteins and photosynthesis. Nuclear genes also contribute to the pool of functional proteins in chloroplasts.

5. Mitochondria import nuclear-coded gene products for DNA and RNA synthesis (polymerases) as well as initiation and elongation factors essential for translation, ribosomal proteins, aminoacyl tRNA synthetases, and several tRNA species. Such imported components are distinct from those used in the host cells, often making them susceptible to antibiotics specific for bacteria. Likewise, chloroplasts import vital protein components from nuclear genes including the small subunit of RuBP, one of the most abundant proteins on earth.

6. Mitochondria and chloroplasts contain proteins more similar to bacterial forms than those found in eukaryotes. This finding supports the endosymbiont hypothesis for the origin of such organelles from bacteria.

7. Polytene chromosomes are formed from numerous DNA replications, pairing of homologues, and absence of strand separation or cytoplasmic division. Each chromosome contains about 1000-5000 DNA strands in parallel register. They appear in specific tissues, such as salivary glands, of many dipterans like *Drosophila*. They appear as comparatively long, wide, fibers with sharp light and dark sections (bands) along their length. Such bands (chromomeres) are useful in chromosome identification, and detection of chromosomal rearrangements.

8. Since eukaryotic chromosomes are "multirepliconic" in that there are multiple replication forks along their lengths, one would expect to see multiple clusters of radioactivity.

9. Puffs represent active genes as evidenced by staining and uptake of labeled RNA precursors as assayed by autoradiography.

10. Long interspersed elements (LINEs) are repetitive transposable DNA sequences in humans. Members of the most prominent family, designated **L1**, have a length of about 6.4kb each and are represented about 100,000 times. LINEs are often referred to as retrotransposons because their mechanism of transposition resembles that used by retroviruses.

11. Lampbrush chromosomes are typically present in vertebrate oocytes and are so named because of their similar appearance to brushes used to clean kerosene lamp chimneys in the 19th century. They are also found in spermatocytes of some insects. They are found as diplotene stage structures and are active uncoiled versions of condensed meiotic chromosomes. Lampbrush chromosomes are typically viewed using light and electron microscopy.

12. While greater DNA content per cell is associated with eukaryotes, one cannot universally equate genomic size with an increase in organismic complexity. There are numerous examples where DNA content per cell varies considerably among closely related species. Because of the diverse cell types of multicellular eukaryotes, a variety of gene products is required, which may be related to the increase in DNA content per cell. In addition, the advantage of diploidy automatically increases DNA content per cell. However, seeing the question in another way, it is likely that a much higher *percentage* of the genome of a prokaryote is actually involved in phenotype production than in a eukaryote.

Eukaryotes have evolved the capacity to obtain and maintain what appear to be large amounts of "extra," perhaps "junk," DNA. This concept will be examined in subsequent chapters of the text. Prokaryotes on the other hand, with their relatively short life cycle, are extremely efficient in their accumulation and use of their genome.

Given the larger amount of DNA per cell and the requirement that the DNA be partitioned in an orderly fashion to daughter cells during cell division, certain mechanisms and structures (mitosis, nucleosomes, centromeres, etc.) have evolved for packaging and distributing the DNA. In addition, the genome is divided into separate entities (chromosomes) to perhaps facilitate the partitioning process in mitosis and meiosis.

13. Digestion of chromatin with endonucleases, such as micrococcal nuclease, gives DNA fragments of approximately 200 base pairs or multiples of such segments. X-ray diffraction data indicated a regular spacing of DNA in chromatin. Regularly spaced bead-like structures (nucleosomes) were identified by electron microscopy.

14. Nucleosomes are octomeric structures of two molecules of each histone (H2A, H2B, H3, and H4) except H1. On the surface of the nucleosomes and complexed with linker DNA is histone H1. A 146-base pair sequence of DNA wraps around the nucleosome.

15. As chromosome condensation occurs, a 300Å fiber is formed. It appears to be composed of 5 or 6 nucleosomes coiled together. Such a structure is called a solenoid. These fibers form a series of loops that further condense into the chromatin fiber which are then coiled into chromosome arms making up each chromatid.

16. *Heterochromatin* is chromosomal material which stains deeply and remains condensed when other parts of chromosomes, euchromatin, are otherwise pale and less condensed. Heterochromatic regions replicate late in S phase and are relatively inactive in a genetic sense because there are few genes present or if they are present, they are repressed. Telomeres and the areas adjacent to centromeres are composed of heterochromatin.

17. (a) Since there are 200 base pairs per nucleosome (as defined in this problem) and 10^9 base pairs, there would be 5 X 10^6 nucleosomes.

(b) Since there are 5×10^6 nucleosomes and nine histones (including H1) per nucleosome, there must be $9(5 \times 10^6)$ histone molecules: 4.5×10^7. **(c)** Since there are 10^9 base pairs present and each base pair is 3.4 Å, the overall length of the DNA is 3.4×10^9 Å. Dividing this value by the packing ratio (50) gives 6.8×10^7 Å.

18. The first step of this solution is to convert all of the given values to cubic Å remembering that 1 mm = 10,000 Å. Using the formula πr^2 for the area of a circle and $4/3 \, \pi r^3$ for the volume of a sphere, the following calculations apply:

Volume of DNA: 3.14×10 Å $\times 10$ Å $\times (50 \times 10^4$ Å$) = 1.57 \times 10^8$ Å^3

Volume of capsid: $4/3 \, (3.14 \times 400$ Å $\times 400$ Å $\times 400$ Å$) = 2.67 \times 10^8$ Å^3

Because the capsid head has a greater volume than the volume of DNA, the DNA will fit into the capsid.

19. One base pair occupies 0.34nm, therefore the equation would be as follows:

$52\mu m/(0.34nm/bp) \times 1000nm/mm =$

152,941 base pairs

20. Volume of the nucleus = $4/3 \, \pi r^3$

$= 4/3 \times 3.14 \times (5 \times 10^3 nm)^3$

$= 5.23 \times 10^{11} nm^3$

Volume of the chromosome = $\pi r^2 \times$ length

$= 3.14 \times 5.5nm \times 5.5nm \times (2 \times 10^9 nm)$

$= 1.9 \times 10^{11} nm^3$

Therefore, the percentage of the volume of the nucleus occupied by the chromatin is

$= 1.9 \times 10^{11} nm^3 / 5.23 \times 10^{11} nm^3 \times 100$
$=$ about 36.3%

21. Data by Sun *et al.* support the general observation that heterochromatic genes are less active than euchromatic genes and, more specifically, the possibility that heterochromatin may contain genes which are repressed. Heterochromatin is located in eukaryotic chromosomes as differentially staining compared with euchromatin. It is relatively inactive genetically either because of a lack of genes or the presence of repressed genes. Heterochromatin replicates later in S phase than euchromatic segments. Centromeric and telomeric regions of chromosomes are typically heterochromatic.

22. Chromosomes are not randomly distributed within nuclei. Homologous chromosomes tend to distribute themselves opposite each other and in an antiparallel manner, meaning that their positions are in reverse order on opposite sides of the nucleus. Assuming that such patterns are maintained throughout the entire cell cycle, it is possible that chromosomal positions may influence gene function and/or chromosomal behavior during mitosis and/or meiosis. If gene function is influenced not only by gene position in a chromosome but also by gene position in a nucleus, then an alternative explanation for position effect exists.

23. The intimate relationships among histones, nucleosomes, and DNA in chromatin clearly account for structural remodeling of chromosomes as the cell cycle proceeds from interphase to metaphase. That nucleosomes are associated with chromatin during periods of gene activity raises the question as to the possible roles they play in influencing not only chromosome structure but also gene function. The findings that natural chemical modification of nucleosomal components, as indicated in the question, increases gene activity suggests that changes in the binding of nucleosomes to DNA enables genes to be more accessible to factors which promote gene function.

In addition, the finding that heterochromatin, containing fewer genes and more repressed genes, is undermethylated, further supports the suggestion that histone modification is functionally related to changes in gene activity.

24. DNA replicates in a *semiconservative* fashion with each daughter DNA double helix containing one new and one original single strand. Nucleosomes follow a *dispersive* pattern with each daughter chromatid containing a mixture of old and original nucleosomes. One could test the distribution of nucleosomes by conducting an autoradiographic experiment similar to Taylor-Woods-Hughes, but instead of labeling the DNA with ^{3}H-thymidine, one would label some or all the histones H2A, H2B, H3, and H4 in nucleosomes.

25. Dividing 3×10^9 base pairs by 10^6 gives an average of 3000 base pairs or 3kb between *Alu* sequences.

26. Bacteriophage lambda is composed of a double-stranded, linear DNA molecule of about 48,000 base pairs. It is capable of forming a closed, double-stranded circular molecule because of a 12-base pair, single-stranded, complementary "overhanging" sequence at the 5' end of each single strand.

27. The distribution of microsatellites varies in a taxon-related manner. Microsatellites are more common within genes of yeast and fungi and quite infrequent in genes of mammals. There appears to be a general decrease in within-gene microsatellites in more recently evolved taxa.

28. The general frequency and pattern of various trinucleotide repeat motifs are similar in all taxonomic groups. Within-gene trinucleotide repeats are the most frequent repeat motif in all taxonomic groups followed by hexanucleotide repeats. One explanation might be that various microsatellite types (mono-, di-, tri-, etc.) are generated at different rates in different genomic regions (within and between genes). A second possibility is that selection acts differentially depending on the type and location of a repeat. The correlation between the high frequency of tri- and hexanucleotide repeats within genes and a triplet code specifying particular amino acids within genes may not be coincidental. Specifically, insertion or deletion of a tri- or hexanucleotide sequence within a coding sequence may not result in a frameshift mutation, while insertion or deletion of other sequence lengths always does.

29. (a) The microsatellite motif is imperfect and can be represented as (GTCPy)$_n$.

(b) The sequence of the nonmicrosatellite region is TCGATATAGC(PuPy)AT. It is not perfectly conserved in that there is one base difference among strains of *D. nigrodunni* and among strains of *D. dunni*.

30. If microsatellites in general are flanked by a conserved sequence, those conserved sequences may be involved in the generation and/or maintenance of the microsatellite. Alternatively, the microsatellite may generate the nonmicrosatellite region. Any hypothesis presented is in need of additional investigation before definitive statements can be made.

Chapter 12: The Genetic Code and Transcription

Concept Areas	Corresponding Problems
Genetic Code	1, 5, 9, 10, 12, 13, 15, 17
Deciphering the Code	3, 4, 6, 7, 8, 11
Characteristics of the Code	2, 14, 16, 26
Information Flow	18, 19, 20, 21, 22, 23, 24, 25, 27
RNA Structure	14, 16

Vocabulary: Organization and Listing of Terms and Concepts

Structures and Substances

Codon

    triplet

Messenger RNA

Phage T4

Polynucleotide phosphorylase

    random assembly of nucleotides

Homopolymer codes

    RNA homopolymers

    RNA heteropolymers

      anticodon

N-formylmethionine (fmet)

Ribosome

RNA polymerase

    holoenzyme

    $(\alpha_2, \beta, \beta', \sigma)$

    consensus sequences

Pribnow box (-10) TATA

  -35 region

termination factor

RNA polymerase (eukaryotic)

  heterogeneous nuclear RNA (hnRNA)

  heterogeneous nuclear

    ribonucleoprotein (hnRNP)

  promoters (promoter sequences)

Consensus sequences

  adenine and thymine richness

cis-acting elements

Goldberg-Hogness (-30, TATA box)

CCAAT sequence

enhancers

trans-acting factors

transcription factors

TATA-factor (TFIIA, B, D)

TATA-binding protein (TBP)

134

pre-mRNAs

split genes (intervening sequences)

   introns

   exons

poly-A

cap (7mG)

   5' to 5'

ADAR (adenosine deaminase acting on RNA)

Processes/Methods

Transcription, translation

Frameshifts

Cell-free protein-synthesizing system

   ribosomes, tRNAs, amino acids, etc.

   artificial mRNAs

Triplet binding assay

Transcription

   RNA polymerase II

      cleft, clamp

   template binding

      template strand, partner strand

   denaturation (unwinding)

   DNA footprinting

   initiation

   chain elongation (5' to 3')

chain termination

gene amplification

RNA processing

   split genes

   post-transcriptional changes

      poly-A (3'), cap (5')

   mechanisms

      rRNA self-excision (ribozyme)

      spliceosome

         snRNAs, snurps (snRNP)

      branch point

      alternative splicing

         isoform

RNA editing

   substitution

   insertion/deletion

   guide RNA (gRNA)

Concepts

Genetic code

   triplet codon

      frameshift mutations (r_{II})

         nonsense triplets

      codon assignments

         artificial mRNAs

         triplet binding assay

Chapter 12 The Genetic Code and Transcription

repeating copolymers

ordered codons

confirmation of codon assignments

MS2

unambiguous

degenerate, wobble

support for degenerate code

punctuation

start, AUG

stop, UAA, UAG, UGA

nonoverlapping

support for nonoverlapping code

universal, exceptions

ordered

overlapping genes

Hypotheses

messenger RNA

wobble hypothesis

pattern of degeneracy

Information flow (F12.1)

transcription

primary transcript

intermediate molecule

RNA polymerases

translation (F12.2)

gene amplification

RNA splicing

beta-globin gene

ovalbumin gene

pro-α-2(I) collagen

mechanisms

Alternative splicing, RNA editing

Comparisons (eukaryotic, prokaryotic)

F12.1 Illustration of the processes, transcription and translation, involved in protein synthesis. Such relationships are often called the Central Dogma.

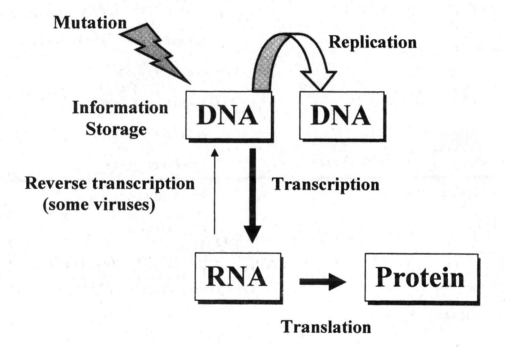

F12.2 Illustration of transcription in prokaryotes coupled with translation. Transcription involves production of RNA from a DNA template.

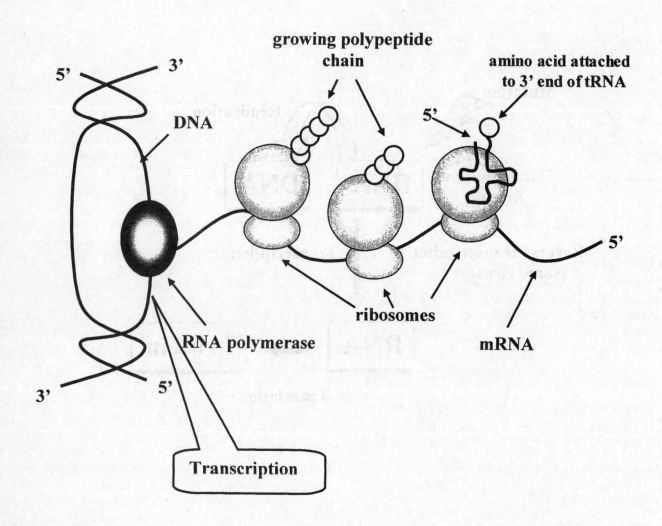

Solutions to Problems and Discussion Questions

1. In eukaryotes, protein synthesis occurs primarily in the cytoplasm, far from the location of DNA and the encoded information. In addition, while some of the basic amino acids would be able to associate directly with DNA, the acidic amino acids would be unable to do so. Thus some sort of "adaptor" system was needed for DNA to direct amino acid assembly.

2. (a) The reason that (+++) or (- - -) restored the reading frame is because the code is triplet. By having the (+++) or (- - -), the translation system is "out of phase" until the third "+" or "-" is encountered. If the code contained six nucleotides (a sextuplet code), then the translation system is "out of phase" until the sixth "+" or "-" is encountered. In this case, the "out of phase" region would probably be more extensive and likely cause more amino acid alterations, but the reading frame would eventually be established. **(b)** Given a sextuplet code, restoration of the reading frames would only occur with the addition or loss of 6 nucleotides. Lay out a sequence such as

CATDOGPIGOWLCATDOGPIGOWLCAT...

and test parts "a" and "b" in the problem.

3. (a) The way to determine the fraction which each triplet will occur with a random incorporation system is to determine the likelihood that each base will occur in each position of the codon (first, second, third), then multiply the individual probabilities (fractions) for a final probability (fraction).

GGG = $3/4 \times 3/4 \times 3/4$ = 27/64

GGC = $3/4 \times 3/4 \times 1/4$ = 9/64

GCG = $3/4 \times 1/4 \times 3/4$ = 9/64

CGG = $1/4 \times 3/4 \times 3/4$ = 9/64

CCG = $1/4 \times 1/4 \times 3/4$ = 3/64

CGC = $1/4 \times 3/4 \times 1/4$ = 3/64

GCC = $3/4 \times 1/4 \times 1/4$ = 3/64

CCC = $1/4 \times 1/4 \times 1/4$ = 1/64

(b) Glycine:

GGG and one G_2C (adds up to 36/64)

Alanine:

one G_2C and one C_2G (adds up to 12/64)

Arginine:

one G_2C and one C_2G (adds up to 12/64)

Proline:

one C_2G and CCC (adds up to 4/64)

(c) With the wobble hypothesis, variation can occur in the third position of each codon.

Glycine: GGG, GGC

Alanine: CGG, GCC, CGC, GCG

Arginine: GCG, GCC, CGC, CGG

Proline: CCC, CCG

4. Assume that you have introduced a copolymer (ACACACAC. . .) to a cell free protein synthesizing system. There are two possibilities for establishing the reading frames: ACA, if one starts at the first base and CAC if one starts at the second base. These would code for two different amino acids (ACA = threonine; CAC = histidine) and would produce repeating polypeptides which would alternate *thr-his-thr-his.* . . or *his-thr-his-thr.* . .

Because of a triplet code, a trinucleotide sequence will, once initiated, remain in the same reading frame and produce the same code all along the sequence regardless of the initiation site.

Given the sequence CUACUACUACUA, notice the different reading frames producing three different sequences each containing the same amino acid.

Codons: CUA   CUA   CUA   CUA. . .

Amino Acids: leu   leu   leu   leu. . .

           UAC   UAC   UAC   UAC. . .
           tyr   tyr   tyr   tyr. . .

           ACU   ACU   ACU   ACU. . .
           thr   thr   thr   thr. . .

If a tetranucleotide is used, such as ACGUACGUACGU...

Codons: ACG   UAC   GUA   CGU   ACG

Amino Acids: thr   tyr   val   arg   thr

        CGU   ACG   UAC   GUA   CGU

        arg   thr   tyr   val   arg

        GUA   CGU   ACG   UAC   GUA

        val   arg   thr   tyr   val

        UAC   GUA   CGU   ACG   UAC

        tyr   val   arg   thr   tyr

Notice that the sequences are the same except that the starting amino acid changes.

5. The UUACUUACUUAC tetranucleotide sequence will produce the following triplets depending on the initiation point: UUA = leu; UAC = tyr; ACU = thr; CUU = leu. Notice that because of the degenerate code, two codons correspond to the amino acid leucine.

The UAUCUAUCUAUC tetranucleotide sequence will produce the following triplets depending on the initiation point: UAU = tyr; AUC = ile; UCU = ser; CUA = leu. Notice that in this case, degeneracy is not revealed and all the codons produce unique amino acids.

6. From the repeating polymer ACACA. . . one can say that threonine is either CAC or ACA. From the polymer CAACAA. . . with ACACA. . . , ACA is the only codon in common. Therefore, threonine would have the codon ACA.

7. As in the previous problem the procedure is to find those sequences which are the same for the first two bases but which vary in the third base. Given that AGG = arg, then information from the AG copolymer indicates that AGA also codes for arg and GAG must therefore code for glu.

Coupling this information with that of the AAG copolymer, GAA must also code for glu, and AAG must code for lys.

8. The basis of the technique is that if a trinucleotide contains bases (a codon) which are complementary to the anticodon of a charged tRNA, a relatively large complex is formed which contains the ribosome, the tRNA, and the trinucleotide. This complex is trapped in the filter whereas the components by themselves are not trapped. If the amino acid on a charged, trapped tRNA is radioactive, then the filter becomes radioactive.

9. List the substitutions, then from the code table, apply the codons to the original amino acids. Select codons which provide single base changes.

Original		**Substitutions**
threonine	----->	*alanine*
<u>AC</u>(U,C,A, or G)		<u>GC</u>(U,C,A, or G)
glycine	----->	*serine*
<u>GG</u>(U or C)		<u>AG</u>(U or C)
isoleucine	----->	*valine*
<u>AU</u>(U, C or A)		<u>GU</u>(U, C or A)

10. Apply the most conservative pathway of change.

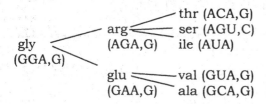

gly
(GGA,G)

thr (ACA,G)
arg ser (AGU,C)
(AGA,G) ile (AUA)

glu val (GUA,G)
(GAA,G) ala (GCA,G)

11. The enzyme generally functions in the degradation of RNA, however in an *in vitro* environment, with high concentrations of the ribonucleoside diphosphates, the direction of the reaction can be forced toward polymerization. *In vivo*, the concentration of ribonucleoside diphosphates is low and the degradative process is favored.

12. Because Poly U is complementary to Poly A, double-stranded structures will be formed. In order for an RNA to serve as a messenger RNA it must be single-stranded, thereby exposing the bases for interaction with ribosomal subunits and tRNAs.

13. Applying the coding dictionary, the following sequences are "decoded"

Sequence 1: met-pro-asp-tyr-ser-(term)

Sequence 2: met-pro-asp-(term)

The 12th base (a uracil) is deleted from Sequence #1 thereby causing a frameshift mutation which introduced a terminating triplet UAA.

14. (a)

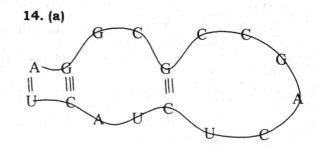

(b) 3'-TCCGCGGCTGAGATGA-5' (use complementary bases, substituting T for U)

(c) 3'-GCU-5'

(d) Assuming that the AGG. . . is the first codon in the reading frame of the mRNA, then the sequence would be

arg-arg-arg-leu-tyr

15. Given the sequence GGA, by changing each of the bases to the remaining three bases, then checking the code table, one can determine whether amino acid substitutions will occur.

G G A gly		G G U gly	
U G A **term**		G G C gly	
C G A **arg**		G G A gly	
A G A **arg**		G G G gly	
G U A **val**		U G U **cys**	
G C A **ala**		C G U **arg**	
G A A **glu**		A G U **ser**	
G G U gly		G U U **val**	
G G C gly		G C U **ala**	
G G A gly		G A U **asp**	

141

16. (a) Starting from the 5' end and locating the AUG triplets, one finds two initiation sites leading to the following two sequences:

met-his-thr-tyr-glu-thr-leu-gly

met-arg-pro-leu-asp (or glu)

(b) In the shorter of the two reading sequences (the one using the internal AUG triplet), a UGA triplet was introduced at the second codon. While not in the reading frames of the longer polypeptide (using the first AUG codon) the UGA triplet terminates the product starting at the second initiation codon.

17. By examining the coding dictionary one will notice that the number of codons for each particular amino acid (synonyms) is directly related to the frequency of amino acid incorporation stated in the problem.

18. The central dogma of molecular genetics and to some extent, all of biology, states that DNA produces, through transcription, RNA, much of which (mRNA) is "decoded" (during translation) to produce proteins. See F12.2 for a graphic description.

19. Several observations indicated that a "messenger" molecule exists. First, DNA, the genetic material, is located in the nucleus of a eukaryotic cell whereas protein synthesis occurs in the cytoplasm. DNA, therefore, does not directly participate in protein synthesis. Second, RNA, which is chemically similar to DNA, is synthesized in the nucleus of eukaryotic cells. Much of the RNA migrates to the cytoplasm, the site of protein synthesis. Third, there is generally a direct correlation between the amounts of RNA and protein in a cell. More direct support was derived from experiments showing that an RNA other than that found in ribosomes was involved in protein synthesis, and that shortly after phage infection, an RNA species is produced which is complementary to phage DNA.

20. RNA polymerase from *E. coli* is a complex, large (almost 500,000 daltons) molecule composed of subunits (α,β,β',σ) in the proportion $\alpha2$,β,β', σ for the holoenzyme. The β subunit provides catalytic function while the sigma (σ) subunit is involved in recognition of specific promoters. The core enzyme is the protein without the sigma.

21. Ribonucleoside triphosphates and a DNA template in the presence of RNA polymerase and a divalent cation (Mg^{++}) produce a ribonucleoside monophosphate polymer, DNA, and pyrophospate (diphosphate). Equimolar amounts of precursor ribonucleoside triphosphates, and product ribonucleoside monophosphates and pyrophosphates (disphosphates) are formed. In *E. coli* transcription and translation can occur simultaneously. Ribosomes attach to the 5' end of the nascent mRNA and progress to the 3' end during translation. While transcription/ translation can be "visualized" in *E. coli* (F12.2), the predominant components "visualized" are the strings of ribosomes (polysomes).

22. While some folding (from complementary base pairing) may occur with mRNA molecules, they generally exist as single-stranded structures which are quite labile. Eukaryotic mRNAs are generally processed such that the 5' end is "capped" and the 3' end has a considerable string of adenine bases. It is thought that these features protect the mRNAs from degradation. Such stability of eukaryotic mRNAs probably evolved with the differentiation of nuclear and cytoplasmic functions. Because prokaryotic cells exist in a more unstable environment (nutritionally and physically, for example) than many cells of multicellular organisms, rapid genetic response to environmental change is likely to be adaptive. To accomplish such rapid responses, a labile gene product (mRNA) is advantageous. A pancreatic cell, which is developmentally stable and existing in a relatively stable environment, could produce more insulin on stable mRNAs for a given transcriptional rate.

23. Apply complementary bases, substituting U for T:

(a)

Sequence 1: 3'-GAAAAAACGGUA-5'

Sequence 2: 3'-UGUAGUUAUUGA-5'

Sequence 3: 3'-AUGUUCCCAAGA-5'

(b)

Sequence 1: *met-ala-lys-lys*

Sequence 2: *ser-tyr-[ter]*

Sequence 3: *arg-thr-leu-val*

(c) Apply complementary bases:

3'-GAAAAAACGGTA-5'

24. First, compute the frequency (percentages would be easiest to compare) for each of the random codons.

For 4/5 C: 1/5 A:

CCC= 4/5 X 4/5 X 4/5 = 64/125 (51.2%)

C_2A = 3(4/5 X 4/5 X 1/5) = 48/125 (38.4%)

CA_2 = 3(4/5 X 1/5 X 1/5) = 12/125 (9.6%)

AAA = 1/5 X 1/5 X 1/5 = 1/125 (0.8%)

For 4/5 A: 1/5 C:

AAA = 4/5 X 4/5 X 4/5 = 64/125 (51.2%)

A_2C = 3(4/5 X 4/5 X 1/5) = 48/125 (38.4%)

AC_2 = 3(4/5 X 1/5 X 1/5) = 12/125 (9.6%)

CCC = 1/5 X 1/5 X 1/5 = 1/125 (0.8%)

Proline: C_3, and one of the C_2A triplets

Histidine: one of the C_2A triplets

Threonine: one C_2A triplet,

             and one A_2C triplet

Glutamine: one of the A_2C triplets

Asparagine: one of the A_2C triplets

Lysine: A_3

25.

(a) #1: *nonsense mutation*
#2: *missense mutation*
#3: *frameshift mutation*

(b) #1: mutation in third position to A or G
#2: change U to C in third triplet
#3: removal of a G in the UGG triplet (trp)

(c) termination

(d) All of the amino acids can be assigned specific triplets including the third base of each triplet. Compare the sequences for the wild type and mutant #2. After removal of a G in the UUG triplet of tryptophan, the frameshift mutation shifts the first base of the following triplet to the third (often ambiguous) base of the previous triplet. The only tricky solution is with serine which has six triplet possibilities, but it can still be resolved.

AUG UGG UAU CGU GGU AGU CCA ACA

(e) The mutation may be in a promoter or enhancer, although many posttranscriptional alterations are possible.

26. (a,b) Use the code table to determine the number of triplets which code each amino acid, then construct a graph and plot such as this one below:

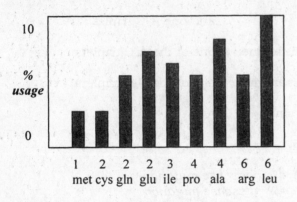

codons

(c) There appears to be a weak correlation between the relative frequency of amino acid usage and the number of triplets for each.

(d) To continue to investigate this issue, one might examine additional amino acids in a similar manner.   In addition, different phylogenetic groups use code synonyms differently. It may be possible to find situations in which the relationships are more extreme. One might also examine more proteins to determine whether such a weak correlation is stronger with different proteins.

27. Consider the following diagram representing the possibility described in the problem. If the promoter is not transcribed, as is the case of typical protein-coding genes, retrotransposition would produce a "daughter" *Alu* void of a promoter. Such an *Alu* would be a "dead-end" because it would not be capable of giving rise to its own *Alu* sequences. Perhaps an *Alu* sequence inserted 3' to a promoter would produce daughters, but this would likely be rare.

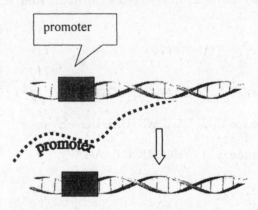

28. (a, b, c) Both nucleic acids include the expected bases; A, T, G, C for DNA and A, U, G, C for RNA. The DNA sample is compatible with a double stranded structure because the purine/pyrimidine ratio for DNA is 1.0 and is therefore consistent with a Watson-Crick model for DNA. The purine/pyrimidine ratio is not 1.0 for RNA, so the RNA must not be double stranded.

(d) If all the DNA is transcribed as stated in the problem, the $(A+U)/(C+G)$ ratio in RNA should equal the $(A+T)/(C+G)$ ratio in DNA and it does (1.2). To show that it doesn't matter if one or two strands are copied, draw out a double stranded DNA with a 1.2 ratio of $(A+T)/(C+G)$. Make RNA copies from one or both strands to see the resulting $(A+U)/(C+G)$ RNA ratios. Notice that if both strands are copied, the purine/pyrimidine ratio $(A+G)/(U+C)$ should be 1.0 and it is not. Therefore, it is likely that only one of the two strands is copied and the strand that is copied is richer in Ts and/or Cs compared with As and/or Gs. This would produce more As and Gs in the numerator of the equation thereby giving the ratio of 1.3. Consider this explanation in light of the *template* strand given below:

ATTAAATTTTATCCGGGCCGCC

29.
(a)

gucccaaccaugcccaccgaucuuccgccugcuucugaa
gAUGCGGGCCCAG

(b)

5' gtc cca acc **atg** ccc acc gat ctt ccg cct gct tct
gaa gAT GCG GGC CCA G

(c)

5' gtcccaaccatgcccaccgatcttccgcctgcttctgaag
ATG CGG GCC CAG

The two initiator codons are not in the same
reading frame.

(d)

5' gtc cca acc **atg** ccc acc gat ctt ccg cct gct tct
gaa gAT GCG GGC CCA G

```
                    met pro thr  asp leu pro  pro ala
ser glu  asp   ala   gly       pro
```

5' gtcccaaccatgcccaccgatcttccgcctgcttctgaag
ATG CGG GCC CAG

```
  met   arg   ala   gln
```

The amino acid sequences in the region of
overlap are not the same.

(e) One might argue for the conservation of
DNA by having the same region code for a
multiple of products, and that might be the
case in viruses and prokaryotes where
genomic efficiency is more of an issue.
However, eukaryotes appear to be much less
likely to evolve strategies which conserve DNA
sequences *per se*. However, if functionally
and/or structurally related products can be
conveniently regulated by such an
arrangement, then perhaps an evolutionary
advantage exists. The most obvious
disadvantage is that if a mutation occurs in

the common region, then two gene products
are altered instead of one.

30. The advantage would be that if sequence
homologies can be identified for a variety of
HIV isolates, then perhaps a single or a few
vaccines could be developed for the multitude
of subtypes which infect various parts of the
world. In other words, the wider the match of
a vaccine to circulating infectives, the more
likely the efficacy. On the other hand, the
more finely aligned a vaccine is to the target,
the more likely it is that new or previously
undiscovered variants will escape vaccination
attempts.

31.
(a)

(b)

(c) Since the antisense strand is relatively
short, under physiological conditions, non-
specific binding of the antisense strand to
other RNAs in the cell may cause the
degradation of non-targeted RNAs.

(d) Since the exact behavior of antisense DNA
in a cell is not completely known, the answer
to this question is elusive. However, given the
complexity of intracellular events, it is likely
that reduction of expression of a repressor
gene group may induce other genes by
eliminating such repressors.

(e) One of the major drawbacks to antisense therapy is the lack of specificity described here and the relative unknown behavior of DNA oligodeoxynucleotides in living cells.

32. Alternative splicing occurs when pre-mRNAs are spliced in more than one way to yield various combinations of exons in the final mRNA product. Upon translation of a group of alternatively spliced mRNAs, a series of related proteins, called isoforms, are produced. It is likely that alternative splicing evolved to provide a variety of functionally related proteins in a particular tissue from one original source. In other words, varieties of similar proteins can be produced by alternative splicing rather than independent evolution.

Some tissues might be more prone to develop alternative splicing if they depend on a number of related protein functions. In addition, if genes found in certain tissues have more exons in their active genes, alternative splicing would be expected. While some information is available concerning the mechanisms of alternative splicing, at this time little is known about the underlying forces which drove the evolution of tissue-specific alternative splicing. The use of alternative splicing to generate varieties of products is also known to exist at different developmental stages. In such cases, as development occurs, different splicing mechanisms occur.

Chapter 13: Translation and Proteins

<u>Concept Areas</u>	<u>Corresponding Problems</u>
Translation	1, 4, 21, 22, 26, 28
RNAs	2, 3, 6, 7, 28, 35
Information Flow	5, 8, 9, 10
One-gene: One-enzyme	14
Pathways	11, 12, 13, 27, 29, 30, 32
Proteins	15, 16, 17, 18, 19, 20, 23, 24, 25, 31, 32
Antibiotic Resistance	33, 34
Antisense Therapy	35

Vocabulary: Organization and Listing of Terms and Concepts

Structures and Substances

Polypeptide, protein

Signal sequence

Chaperone

Ribosome

   monosome

rRNA

   5S, 16S, 23S RNA (single transcript)

     proteins

   5.8S, 18S, 28S RNA (single transcript)

     5S

     proteins

     tandem repeats and spacer DNA

     clustered on chromosomes:
      13, 14, 15, 21, 22

ribosomal proteins

Ribosome complex

   peptidyl (P site)

   aminoacyl (A site)

   exit (E site)

   tunnel

   peptidyl transferase

Transfer RNAs - tRNA

   75-90 nucleotides

   unusual bases

   cloverleaf model

   cognate amino acid

     anticodon, codon

     ...pCpCpA (3')

     ...pG (5')

aminoacyl tRNA synthetases

    charging

    activated form

        (aminoacyladenylic acid)

    isoaccepting tRNAs

Initiation factors

    initiation complex

    Shine-Delgarno sequence

Formylmethionine (N-formylmethionine)

    tRNA^{fmet}

Elongation factors

GTP-dependent release factors

    termination (nonsense)

    stop codons UAA, UAG, UGA

Polyribosomes (polysomes)

mRNA

Heterogeneous RNA (hnRNA)

    poly-A

    cap (7mG)

        5' to 5'

    Kozak sequences

    5'-ACCAUGG

Inborn Errors of Metabolism

alkaptonuria

    homogentisic acid

        (alkapton 2,5-dihydrophenylacetic acid)

phenylketonuria

    phenylalanine hydroxylase

Neurospora

arginine

citrulline

ornithine

sickle-cell anemia (trait)

    HbA, HbS, HbA$_2$

    heme group

    globin portion

Amino acid

carboxyl group

amino group

R (radical) group

central carbon

hydrophobic

polar (hydrophilic)

    negative, positive

Peptide bond

Primary structure

Secondary structure

Chapter 13 Translation and Proteins

α-helix

β-pleated sheet

Tertiary structure

Quaternary structure

  collagen

  keratin

  actin, myosin

  immunoglobin

  transport proteins

    hemoglobin, myoglobin

  enzyme (active site)

  hormone, receptor

    anabolic, catabolic

      energy of activation

    protein domain

    LDL receptor protein

    epidermal growth factor

Processes/Methods

Transcription, translation

RNA processing

  post-transcriptional modification

Translation

  codon, anticodon

  tRNA charging

aminoacyl tRNA synthetases

  chain initiation

  chain elongation

  translocation

  chain termination, UAG, UAA, UGA

Simultaneous transcription and translation (Prokaryotes, F13.1)

  wobble hypothesis

Starch gel electrophoresis

Exon shuffling

Posttranslational modification

    protein targeting

    modification, trimming

Concepts

Information flow

Transcription, translation (F13.1)

Comparisons (eukaryotic, prokaryotic)

One-gene: One-enzyme hypothesis

One-gene: One-protein

One-gene: One-polypeptide chain

Pathway analysis

Protein structure

Posttranslational modification

Structure/function relationships

F13.1 Polarity constraints associated with simultaneous transcription and translation in prokaryotes. The RNA polymerase is moving downward (arrow) in this sketch.

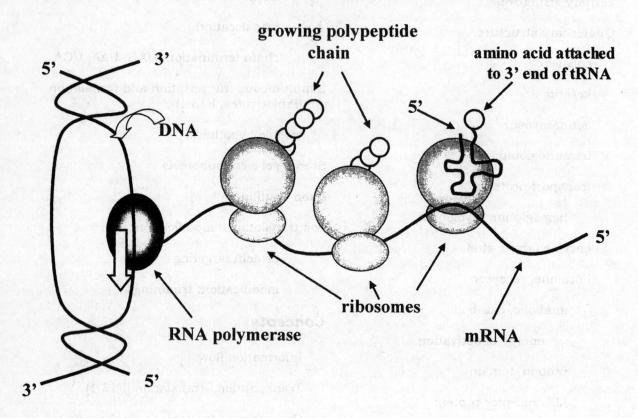

Solutions to Problems and Discussion Questions

1. A functional polyribosome will contain the following components: mRNA, charged tRNA, large and small ribosomal subunits, elongation and perhaps initiation factors, peptidyl transferase, GTP, Mg^{++}, nascent proteins, and possibly GTP-dependent release factors.

2. Transfer RNAs are "adaptor" molecules in that they provide a way for amino acids to interact with sequences of bases in nucleic acids. Amino acids are specifically and individually attached to the 3' end of tRNAs which possess a three-base sequence (the anticodon) to base-pair with three bases of mRNA. Messenger RNA, on the other hand, contains a copy of the triplet codes which are stored in DNA. The sequences of bases in mRNA interact, three at a time, with the anticodons of tRNAs.

Enzymes involved in transcription include the following: RNA polymerase (*E. coli*), and RNA polymerase I, II, III (eukaryotes). Those involved in translation include the following: aminoacyl tRNA synthetases, peptidyl and transferase.

3. It was reasoned that there would not be sufficient affinity between amino acids and nucleic acids to account for protein synthesis. For example, acidic amino acids would not be attracted to nucleic acids. With an adaptor molecule, specific hydrogen bonding could occur between nucleic acids, and specific covalent bonding could occur between an amino acid and a nucleic acid tRNA.

4. The sequence of base triplets in mRNA constitutes the sequence of codons. A three-base portion of the tRNA constitutes the anticodon.

5. Since there are three nucleotides which code for each amino acid, there would be 423 code letters (nucleotides), 426 including a termination codon. This assumes that other features, such as the polyA tail, the 5'cap, promoter, and 5' and 3' untranslated sequences are omitted.

6. The steps involved in tRNA charging are outlined in the text. An amino acid in the presence of ATP, Mg^{++}, and a specific aminoacyl synthetase produces an amino acid-AMP enzyme complex (+ PP$_i$). This complex interacts with a specific tRNA to produce the aminoacyl tRNA.

7. The four sites in tRNA which provide for specific recognition are the following: attachment of the specific amino acid, interaction with the aminoacyl tRNA synthetase, interaction with the ribosome, and interaction with the codon (anticodon).

8. Phenylalanine is an amino acid which, like other amino acids, is required for protein synthesis. While too much phenylalanine and its derivatives cause PKU in phenylketonurics, too little will restrict protein synthesis.

9. Both phenylalanine and tyrosine can be obtained from the diet. Even though individuals with PKU cannot convert phenylalanine to tyrosine, it is obtained from the diet.

10. Tyrosine is a precursor to melanin, skin pigment. Individuals with PKU fail to convert phenylalanine to tyrosine and even though tyrosine is obtained from the diet, at the population level, individuals with PKU have a tendency for less skin pigmentation.

11. (a) In this cross, two gene pairs are operating because the F₂ ratio is a modification of a 9:3:3:1 ratio, which is typical of a dihybrid cross. If one assumes that homozygosity for either or both of the two loci gives white, then let strain A be *aaBB* and strain B, *AAbb*. The F₁ is *AaBb* and pigmented (purple). The typical F₂ ratio would be as follows:

   9/16   *A_B_*   Purple

   3/16   *aaB_*   white

   3/16   *A_bb*   white

   1/16   *aabb*   white

If a pathway exists which has the following structure, then the genetic and biochemical data are explained.

(b) For this condition, with the pink phenotype present, leave the symbols the same, however, change the Y compound such that when accumulated, a pink phenotype is produced:

   9/16   *A_B_*   Purple

   3/16   *aaB_*   white

   3/16   *A_bb*   **pink**

   1/16   *aabb*   white

12. The best way to approach these types of problems, especially when the data are organized in the form given, is to realize that the substance (supplement) which "repairs" a strain, as indicated by a (+), is *after* the metabolic block for that strain. In addition, and most important, is that the substance which "repairs" the highest number of strains is either *the end product* or is *closest to the end product*.

Looking at the table, notice that the supplement tryptophan "repairs" all the strains. Therefore it must be at the end of the pathway or at least after all the metabolic blocks (defined by each mutation). Indole "repairs" the next highest number of strains (3) therefore it must be second from the end. Indole glycerol phosphate "repairs" two of the four strains so it is third from the end. Anthranilic acid "repairs" the least number of strains, so it must be early (first) in the pathway.

Minimal medium is void of supplements and mutant strains involving this pathway would not be expected to grow (or be "repaired'). The pathway therefore would be as follows:

To assign the various mutations to the pathway, keep in mind that if a supplement "repairs" a given mutant, the supplement must be after the metabolic block. Applying this rationale to the above pathway, the metabolic blocks are created at the following locations.

13. In general, the rationale for working with a branched chain pathway is similar to that stated in the previous problem. Since thiamine "repairs" each of the mutant strains, it must, as stated in the problem, be the final synthetic product.

Remembering the "one-gene:one-enzyme" statement, each metabolic block should only occur in one place, so even though pyrimidine and thiazole supplements each "repair" only one strain, they will not occupy the same step; rather a branched pathway is suggested. Consider that pyrimidine and thiazole are products of distinct pathways and that both are needed to produce the end product, thiamine, as indicated below:

thi-2

Precursor ⟹ **pyrimidine**
　　　　　　　　　　　thi-3
　　　　　　　　⟹　⟹ **thiamine**
Precursor ⟹ **thiazole**

thi-1

14. The fact that enzymes are a subclass of the general term *protein*, a *one-gene:one-protein* statement might seem to be more appropriate. However, some proteins are made up of subunits, each different type of subunit (polypeptide chain) being under the control of a different gene. Under this circumstance, the *one-gene:one polypeptide* might be more reasonable.

It turns out that many functions of cells and organisms are controlled by stretches of DNA which either produce no protein product (operator and promoter regions, for example) or have more than one function as in the case of overlapping genes and alternative mRNA splicing. A simple statement regarding the relationship of a stretch of DNA to its physical product is difficult to justify.

15. The electrophoretic mobility of a protein is based on a variety of factors, primarily the net charge of the protein and to some extent, the conformation in the electrophoretic environment. Both are based on the type and sequence (primary structure) of the component amino acids of a protein.

The interactions (hydrogen bonds) of the components of the peptide bonds, hydrophobic, hydrophilic, and covalent interactions (as well as others) are all dependent on the original sequence of amino acids and take part in determining the final conformation of a protein. A change in the electrophoretic mobility of a protein would therefore indicate that the amino acid sequence had been changed.

16. The following types of normal hemoglobin are presented in the text:

Hemoglobin	Polypeptide chains
HbA	$2\alpha 2\beta$ (alpha, beta)
HbA$_2$	$2\alpha 2\delta$ (alpha, delta)
HbF	$2\alpha 2\gamma$ (alpha, gamma)
Gower 1	$2\zeta 2\varepsilon$ (zeta, epsilon)

The *alpha* and *beta* chains contain 141 and 146 amino acids, respectively. The *zeta* chain is similar to the alpha chain while the other chains are like the beta chain. Each chain represents a primary structure of amino acids connected by covalent peptide bonds. Secondary structures are determined by hydrogen bonding between components of the peptide bonds. Alpha helices and pleated sheets result. Tertiary structures are formed from interactions of the amino acid side chains while the quaternary level results from the associations of chains shown above.

17. Sickle-cell anemia is coined a *molecular* disease because it is well understood at the molecular level; at the level of a base change in DNA which leads to an amino acid change in the β chain of hemoglobin. It is a *genetic* disease in that it is inherited from one generation to the next. It is not contagious as might be the case of a disease caused by a microorganism. Diseases caused by microorganisms may not necessarily follow family blood lines whereas genetic diseases do.

18. In the late 1940s, Pauling demonstrated a difference in the electrophoretic mobility of HbA and HbS (sickle-cell hemoglobin) and concluded that the difference had a chemical basis. Ingram determined that the chemical change occurs in the primary structure of the globin portion of the molecule using the fingerprinting technique. He found a change in the 6th amino acid in the β chain.

19. It is possible for an amino acid to change without changing the electrophoretic mobility of a protein under standard conditions. If the amino acid is substituted with an amino acid of like charge and similar structure there is a chance that factors which influence electrophoretic mobility (primarily net charge) will not be altered. Other techniques such as chromatography of digested peptides may detect subtle amino acid differences.

20. Dividing 20 by 0.34 gives the number of nucleotides (about 59) occupied by a ribosome. Dividing 59 by three gives the approximate number of triplet codes, approximately 20.

21. "Fine-mapping" meaning precise mapping of mutations *within* a gene, is possible in some phage systems because many recombinants can often be generated relatively easily. Having the precise intragenic location of mutations as well as the ability to isolate the products, especially mutant products, allows scientists to compare the locations of lesions within genes.

Mutations occurring nearer to the initiation site in a gene will produce proteins with defects near the N-terminus. In this problem, the lesions cause chain termination, therefore the nearer the mutations are to the 5' end of the mRNA, the shorter will be the polypeptide product. Relating the position of the mutation with the length of the product establishes the colinear relationship.

22. As stated in the text, the four levels of protein structure are the following:

Primary: the linear arrangement or sequence of amino acids. This sequence determines the higher level structures.

Secondary: α-helix and β-pleated sheet structures generated by hydrogen bonds between components of the peptide bond.

Tertiary: folding which occurs as a result of interactions of the amino acid side chains. These interactions include, but are not limited to the following: covalent disulfide bonds between cysteine residues; interactions of hydrophilic side chains with water; interactions of hydrophobic side chains with each other.

Quaternary: the association of two (dimer) or more polypeptide chains. Called *oligomeric,* such a protein is made up of more than one protein.

Since all higher levels are dependent on the sequence of amino acids (primary structure) it is the primary structure which is most influential in determining protein structure and function.

23. There are probably as many different types of proteins as there are different types of structures and functions in living systems. Some examples are given below:

Oxygen transport: hemoglobin, myoglobin
Structural: collagen, keratin, histones
Contractile: actin, myosin
Immune system: immunoglobins
Cross-membrane transport: a variety of proteins in and around membranes, such as receptor proteins
Regulatory: hormones, perhaps histones

24. Enzymes function to regulate catabolic and anabolic activities of cells. They influence (lower) the *energy of activation,* thus allowing chemical reactions to occur under conditions which are compatible with living systems. Enzymes possess active sites and/or other domains which are sensitive to the environment. The active site is considered to be a crevice, or pit, which binds reactants, thus enhancing their interaction. The other domains mentioned above may influence the conformation and therefore function of the active site.

25. All of the substitutions involve one base change.

26. When an expectant mother returns to consumption of phenylalanine in her diet, she subjects her baby to higher than normal levels of phenylalanine throughout its development. Since increased phenylalanine is toxic, many (approximately 90%) newborns are severely and irreversibly retarded at birth. Expectant mothers (who are genetically phenylketonurics) should return to a low phenylalanine intake during pregnancy.

27. One can conclude that the amino acid is not involved in recognition of the codon.

28. Even though three gene pairs are involved, notice that because of the pattern of mutations, each cross may be treated as monohybrid **(a)** or dihybrid **(b,c)**.

(a) F_1:   *AABbCC* = speckled
    F_2: 3   *AAB_CC* = speckled
        1   *AAbbCC* = yellow

(b) F_1:   *AABbCc* = speckled
    F_2: 9   *AAB_C_* = speckled
        3   *AAB_cc* = green
        3   *AAbbC_* = yellow ⎫ 4
        1   *AAbbcc* = yellow ⎭

(c) F_1:   *AaBBCc* = speckled
    F_2: 9   *A_BBC_* = speckled
        3   *A_BBcc* = green
        3   *aaBBC_* = colorless ⎫ 4
        1   *aaBBcc* = colorless ⎭

29. Because cross **(a, b)** is essentially a monohybrid cross, there would be no difference in the results if crossing over occurred (or did not occur) between the *a* and *b* loci.

30. With the codes for valine being GUU, GUC, GUA, and GUG, single base changes from glutamic acid's GAA and GAG can cause the glu>>>val switch. The normal glutamic acid is a negatively charged amino acid whereas valine carries no net charge and lysine is positively charged. Given these significant charge changes, one would predict some, if not considerable, influence on protein structure and function. Such changes could stem from internal changes in folding or interactions with other molecules in the RBC, especially other hemoglobin molecules.

31. Because of a change in the net charge of the polypeptide, one would expect individuals with HbC to suffer some altered hemoglobin function and perhaps be resistant to malaria as well. In fact, HbC homozygotes suffer mild hemolytic anemia (a benign hemoglobinopathy). The HbC gene is distributed particularly in malarial-infested areas suggesting that some resistance to malaria is conferred. Recent studies indicate that HbC may be protective against severe forms of malaria, but not to more uncomplicated forms.

32. A cross of the following nature would satisfy the data:

AABBCC   X   aabbcc

Offspring in the F$_2$:

27   A_B_C_   = purple
9   A_B_cc   = pink
9   A_bbC_   = rose
9   aaB_C_   = orange
3   A_bbcc   = pink
3   aaB_cc   = pink
3   aabbC_   = rose
1   aabbcc   = pink

pink-**c**-> rose -**b**-> orange -**a**-> purple

The above hypothesis could be tested by conducting a backcross as given below:

AaBbCc   X   aabbcc

The cross should give a

4(pink):2(rose):1(orange):1(purple) ratio

33.

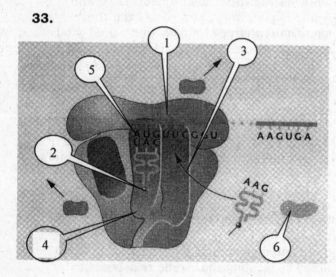

34.

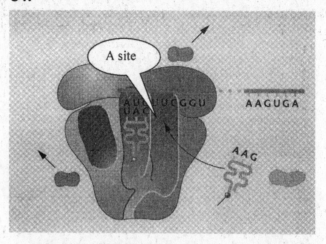

35. (a) Since protein synthesis is dependent on the passage of mRNA from DNA to ribosomes, any circumstance which compromises that flow will cause a reduction in protein synthesis. The more specific the binding of the antisense oligonucleotide to the target mRNA, the more specific the influence on protein synthesis. The ideal situation would be where a particular species of antisense oligonucleotide impacted on one and only one protein population.

(b) Clearly, a length of around 15-16 nucleotides is most effective in causing RNA degradation.

(c) A number of factors, including length of the oligonucleotide, are probably important for the ability of the antisense oligonucleotide to target a specific RNA *in vivo*. It is likely that stability of the oligonucleotide is dependent on its base composition and length. The oligonucleotide must be small enough to diffuse effectively throughout the cell in order to "locate" the targeted mRNA and it must not assume a folded conformation which blocks opportunities for base pairing. Since the oligonucleotide is so much smaller than the target mRNA, it is also likely that the actual location of binding to the target is important in mRNA degradation. One of the main problems of antisense therapy is the introduction of the oligonucleotide into the interior of target cells.

Chapter 14: Gene Mutation, DNA Repair, and Transposition

Concept Areas	Corresponding Problems
Random and Adaptive Mutations	3
Classes of Mutations	4, 5, 6, 7, 31
Detection of Mutations	2, 13, 17, 18, 22, 28
Spontaneous Mutation Rates	7, 22, 25
Induced Mutations	8, 9, 10, 11
Molecular Basis of Mutation	4, 14, 15, 16, 25, 27, 30
Case Studies	1, 26, 29, 31
Repair of DNA	12, 13
UV Radiation and Skin Cancer	16, 32
High-Energy Radiation	10, 13
Transposable Elements	19, 20, 21

Vocabulary: Organization and Listing of Terms and Concepts

Structures and Substances

Somatic cells

Gamete forming cells

   germ line

   gametes

   missense

5-Bromouracil

2-Amino purine

Acridine dyes

Acridine orange

Proflavin

Mustard gas

Ethylmethane sulfonate

6-Methylguanine

Apurinic site

ABO antigens

   H substance

   glycosyltransferase

Dystrophin

Pyrimidine dimers

FMR-1

uvr gene product

DNA polymerase I (*polA*1)

AP endonuclease

DNA glycosylases

XPA, XPF, XPG

TFIIH

*rec*A

*lex*A

Photoreactivation enzyme

Adenine methylase

Heterokaryon

Transposable elements

    insertion sequence

    copia, P

Transposon, transposase

Processes/Methods

Variation by mutation

       replication

       repair errors

       background radiation

          cosmic sources

          mineral sources

          ultraviolet light

      rates

    induced

    X-rays

    gametic, germ-line

      autosomal dominant

      X-linked recessive

      autosomal recessive

loss-of-function

gain-of-function

null mutations

somatic

Detection

    Drosophila

      attached X

    humans

      pedigree analysis

      cell culture (*in vitro*)

      molecular basis

        direct sequencing of DNA

ABO antigens

H substance modification

muscular dystrophy

    Duchenne muscular dystrophy

    Becker muscular dystrophy

      dystrophin

      trinucleotide

fragile-X syndrome

    repeats

MDPK
(serine-threonine protein kinase)

Huntington disease

Ames test

    Salmonella typhimurium

Molecular basis

    base substitution or point mutations

        transition

        transversion

        frameshift

    tautomeric shifts (forms)

    base analogues

        5-bromouracil

        2-amino purine

    reverse mutation

        alkylation

        mustard gases

        ethylmethane sulfonate

    frameshift mutations

        acridine dyes (acridines)

            acridine orange

        proflavin

        apurinic sites

            deamination

    oxygen radicals

        H_2O_2

        OH^- (hydroxyl radical)

        superoxide (O_2^-)

ultraviolet light

pyrimidine dimers

    T-T

    recA, lexA, uvr

SOS response

high-energy radiation

    ionizing radiation

    X-rays

    gamma radiation

    cosmic radiation

Repair

    ultraviolet radiation (260nm)

        pyrimidine dimers

        T-T, C-C, T-C

        photoreactivation

            photoreactivation enzyme (PRE)

        excision repair

            base excision repair (BER)

            nucleotide excision repair (NER)

            uvr gene product

            DNA polymerase I

            DNA ligase

            AP endonuclease

            DNA glycosylases

proofreading and mismatch repair

strand discrimination

DNA methylation

GATC sequence

mut H, L, S

postreplication repair

homologous recombinational repair

xeroderma pigmentosum (XP)

unscheduled DNA synthesis

photoreactivation enzyme

heterokaryon

somatic cell genetics

Transposable genetic elements

insertion sequence (IS)

terminal repeats

transposon (Tn) elements

AC-DS system

transposable controlling elements

open reading frames (ORFs)

transposase

other systems

copia (*Drosophila*)

direct terminal repeat (DTR)

inverted terminal repeat (ITR)

P elements (*Drosophila*)

hybrid dysgenesis P

Alu (humans)

SINES, LINES

Concepts

Mutation

basis of organismic diversity (F14.1)

somatic, germ line (F14.2)

autosomal dominant

X-linked, autosomal recessive

morphological

nutritional or biochemical

behavioral

regulatory

lethal

conditional, temperature-sensitive

Sources

exogenous (environmental)

endogenous

spontaneous

Detection of mutations

Molecular diversity of mutations

Repair

Transposable elements

Complementation

F14.1 Graphic representation of the relationship between mutation and Darwinian evolutionary theory. Mutation provides the original source of variation on which natural selection operates.

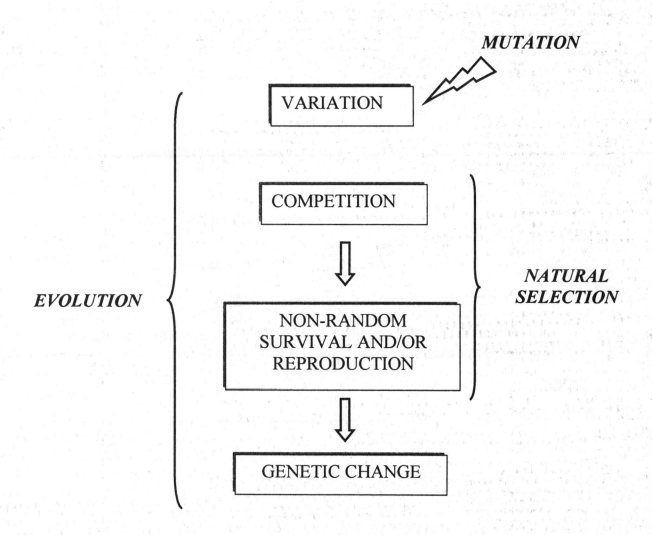

F14.2 Illustration of the difference between somatic and germ-line mutations. Somatic mutations are not passed to the next generation, whereas those in the germ line may be passed to offspring.

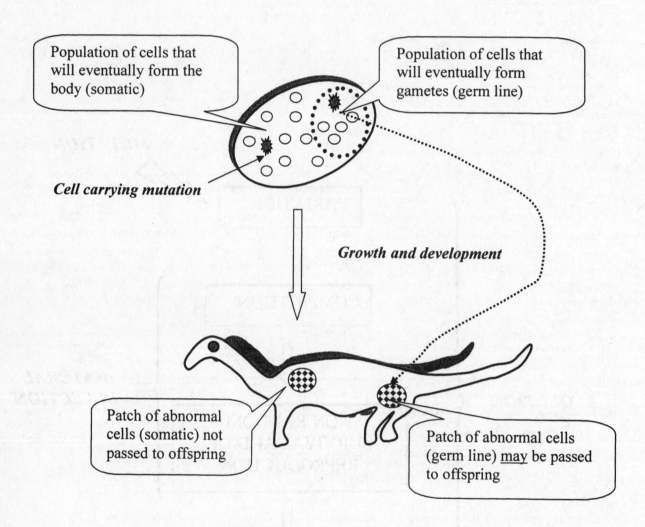

Solutions to Problems and Discussion Questions

1. Mutations are the "windows" through which geneticists look at the normal function of genes, cells, and organisms. When a mutation occurs, it allows the investigator to formulate questions as to the function of the normal allele of that mutation. For example, hemophilia is an inherited blood-clotting disease. Because there are three different inherited forms of the disease, two X-linked and one autosomal, all determined by non-allelic genes, one can say that there are at least three different proteins involved in blood clotting. At a different level, mutations provide "markers" with which biologists can study the genetics and dynamics of populations.

2. When conducting genetic screens, one assumes that all the cells of an organism are genetically identical. Therefore, the organism responds to the screen enabling detection of the mutation. If a somatic cell of a multicellular organism is mutated, it is highly unlikely that the organism will be sufficiently altered to respond to a screen. That's not to say that somatic mutations can't influence the organism. Cancer cells generally originate from a single altered cell and can have a profound influence on the fate of an organism.

3. It is true that *most* mutations are thought to be deleterious to an organism. A gene is a product of perhaps a billion or so years of evolution and it is only natural to suspect that random changes will probably yield negative results. However, *all* mutations may not be deleterious. Those few, rare variations that are beneficial will provide a basis for possible differential propagation of the variation. Such changes in gene frequency represent the basis of the evolutionary process. See F14.1 in this book.

4. As stated in the previous question, a functional sequence of nucleotides, a gene, is likely to be the product of perhaps a billion or so years of evolution. Each gene and its product function in an environment that has also evolved, or co-evolved. A coordinated output of each gene product is required for life. Deviations from the norm, caused by mutation, are likely to be disruptive because of the complex and interactive environment in which each gene product must function. However, on occasion a beneficial variation occurs.

5. A diploid organism possesses at least two copies of each gene (except for "hemizygous" genes) and in most cases, the amount of product from one gene of each pair is sufficient for production of a normal phenotype. Recall that the condition of "recessive" is defined by the phenotype of the heterozygote. If output from one normal (non-mutant) gene in a heterozygote gives the same phenotype as in the normal homozygote, where there are two normal genes, the normal allele is considered "dominant."

Phenotype, if mutant is:

Genotypes	recessive	dominant
wild/wild	wild	wild
wild/mutant	wild	mutant
mutant/mutant	mutant	mutant

6. A *conditional* mutation is one that produces a wild type phenotype under one environmental condition and a mutant phenotype under a different condition. A conditional *lethal* is a gene that under one environmental condition, leads to premature death of the organism.

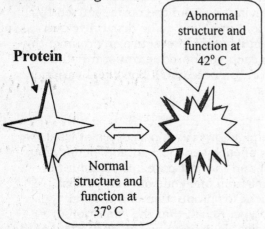

Protein

Abnormal structure and function at 42° C

Normal structure and function at 37° C

7. Watson and Crick recognized that various tautomeric forms, caused by single proton shifts, could exist for the nitrogenous bases of DNA. Such shifts could result in mutations by allowing hydrogen bonding of normally noncomplementary bases so that incorrect nucleotide bases may be added during DNA replication. As stated in the text, important tautomers involve keto-enol pairs for thymine and guanine, and amino-imino pairs for cytosine and adenine.

8. All three of the agents are mutagenic because they cause base substitutions. Deaminating agents oxidatively deaminate bases such that cytosine is converted to uracil and adenine is converted to hypoxanthine. Uracil pairs with adenine and hypoxanthine pairs with cytosine. Alkylating agents donate an alkyl group to the amino or keto groups of nucleotides, thus altering base-pairing affinities. 6-ethyl guanine acts like adenine, thus pairing with thymine. Base analogs such as 5-bromouracil and 2-amino purine are incorporated as thymine and adenine, respectively, yet they basepair with guanine and cytosine, respectively.

9. Frameshift mutations are likely to change more than one amino acid in a protein product because as the reading frame is shifted, a different set of codons is generated. In addition, there is the possibility that a nonsense triplet could be introduced, thus causing premature chain termination. If a single pyrimidine or purine has been substituted, then only one amino acid is influenced.

10. X-rays are of higher energy and shorter wavelength than UV light. They have greater penetrating ability and can create more disruption of DNA.

11. In contrast to UV light, X-rays penetrate beyond surface layers of cells and thus can affect gamete-forming tissues in multicellular organisms. In addition, X-rays break chromosomes and a variety of chromosomal aberrations can result. Ions and free radicals are formed in the paths of X-rays and these interact with components of DNA to cause mutations. UV light generates pyrimidine dimers, primarily thymines, which distort the normal conformation of DNA and inhibit normal function.

12. *Photoreactivation* can lead to repair of UV-induced damage. An enzyme, photoreactivation enzyme, will absorb a photon of light to cleave thymine dimers. *Excision repair* involves the products of several genes, DNA polymerase I and DNA ligase, to clip out the UV-induced dimer, fill in, and join the phosphodiester backbone in the resulting gap. The excision repair process can be activated by damage that distorts the DNA helix. *Recombinational repair* is a system that responds to DNA that has escaped other repair mechanisms at the time of replication. If a gap is created on one of the newly synthesized strands, a "rescue operation or SOS response" allows the gap to be filled. Many different gene products are involved in this repair process: *rec*A and *lex*A. In SOS repair, the proofreading by DNA polymerase III is suppressed and this therefore is called an "error-prone system."

13. Because mammography involves the use of X-rays and X-rays are known to be mutagenic, it has been suggested that frequent mammograms may do harm. This subject is presently under considerable debate. At the 2002 World Health Organization conference in Barcelona, Spain, the conclusion was that "mammograms can prevent breast cancer deaths in one in 500 women ages 50 to 69."

14. Each involves a ballooning of trinucleotide repeats. See the text for a detailed description of the role of trinucleotide repeats in a variety of human diseases. Genetic anticipation is the occurrence of an earlier age of onset of a genetic disease in successive generations.

15. In the *Ames assay,* the compound to be tested is incubated with a mammalian liver extract to simulate an *in vivo* environment. This solution is then placed on culture plates with an indicator microorganism, *Salmonella typhimurium,* which is defective in its normal repair processes. The frequency of mutations in the tester strains is an indication of the mutagenicity of the compound. Because cancer results from the mutation of genes in somatic cells, mutagenic chemicals are considered to be potentially carcinogenic.

16. *Xeroderma pigmentosum* is a form of human skin cancer caused by perhaps several rare autosomal genes, which interfere with the repair of damaged DNA. Studies with heterokaryons provided evidence for complementation, indicating that there may be as many as seven different genes involved. The enzymes responsible for nucleotide excision repair appear to be involved. Since cancer is caused by mutations in several types of genes, interfering with DNA repair can enhance the occurrence of these types of mutations.

17. Given that the cells were treated, then allowed to complete one round of replication, the final computation of the mutation rate should be divided by two (two cells are plated for each cell treated). The general expression for the mutation rate is the number of mutant cells divided by the total number of cells. In this case the equation would be as follows:

$$\frac{18 \times 10^1}{6 \times 10^7}$$

or 3×10^{-6}

Now dividing by two (as stated above) gives

1.5×10^{-6}

18. Each organism mentioned in the problem possesses a variety of transposable elements. Bacteria possess insertion sequences (about 800 to 1500 base pairs in length) as well as transposons, which are larger. Both are mobile in bacterial, viral, and plasmid DNAs and both have repeated base sequences at their ends. Barbara McClintock described the genetic behavior of mobile elements (*Ds* and *Ac*) in maize. *Ds* can move if *Ac* is present, thus *transposable controlling elements* exist. An *Ac* element is 4563 base pairs long and similar in structure to some bacterial transposons. Transposons often code for transposase enzymes, which are essential for transposition. *Copia* elements in *Drosophila* may be present in numerous copies in the genome and contain direct and inverted terminal repeats. *P* elements, also in *Drosophila,* are responsible for a phenomenon called hybrid dysgenesis.

Humans possess a variety of transposable elements including the *Alu* family of short interspersed elements (SINES), which are between 200 and 300 base pairs long and may exist in 300,000 copies per genome. Long interspersed elements (LINES) also occur in the human genome and seem to be capable of movement. Such elements share common structural features, are often mobile, and may influence gene activity.

19. It is probable that the IS occupied or interrupted normal function of a controlling region related to the *galactose* genes, which are in an operon with one controlling upstream element.

20. It is likely that the reverse transcriptase, in making DNA, provides a DNA segment that is capable of integrating into the yeast chromosome as other types of DNA are known to do.

21. First, while less likely, one might suggest that transposons, for one reason or another, are more likely to insert in noncoding regions of the genome. One might also suggest that they are more stable in such regions. Second, and more likely, it is possible that transposons insert rather randomly and that selection eliminates those that have interrupted coding regions of the genome. Since such regions are more likely to influence the phenotype, selection is more likely to influence such regions.

22. It is possible that through the reduction of certain environmental agents that cause mutations, mutation rates might be reduced. On the other hand, certain industrial and medical activities actually concentrate mutagens (radioactive agents and hazardous chemicals). Unless human populations are protected from such agents, mutation rates might actually increase. If one asks about the accumulation of mutations (not rates) in human populations as a result of improved living conditions and medical care, then it is likely that as the environment becomes less harsh (through improvements), more mutations will be tolerated as selection pressure decreases. In addition, as individuals live longer and have children at a later age, some studies indicate that older males accumulate more gametic mutations.

23. Any agent that inhibits DNA replication, either directly or indirectly, through mutation and/or DNA crosslinking, will suppress the cell cycle and may be useful in cancer therapy. Since guanine alkylation often leads to mismatched bases, they can often be repaired by a variety of mismatched repair mechanisms. However, DNA crosslinking can be repaired by recombinational mechanisms; thus, for such agents to be successful in cancer therapy, suppressors of DNA repair systems are often used in conjunction with certain cancer drugs. See: Wang, Z. et al. 2001. J Nat'l Cancer Inst. 93(19):1434-6.

24. Both major forms of muscular dystrophy include muscular wasting of differing severity and age of onset. Both forms are caused by mutations in the *dystrophin* gene, which is very large, composed of 97 exons and is 2.6Mb in length. Given the size of this gene and the number of exons/introns, many opportunities exist for mutational upset. Interestingly, the severity of the phenotype is not always connected with the size of a deleted segment. What seems to be quite important in determining expression is whether a frameshift is introduced. See: http://compbio.berkeley.edu/people/ed/rust/Dystrophin.html.

25. Replication slippage is a process that generates small deletions and insertions during DNA replication. While it can occur anywhere in the genome, it is most prevalent in regions already containing repeated sequences. Thus, repeated sequences are hypermutable.

26. There are several ways in which an unexpected mutant gene may enter a pedigree. If a gene is incompletely penetrant, it may be present in a population and only express itself under certain conditions. It is unlikely that the gene for hemophilia behaved in this manner. If a gene's expression is suppressed by another mutation in an individual, it is possible that offspring may inherit a given gene and not inherit its suppressor. Such offspring would have hemophilia. Since all genetic variations must arise at some point, it is possible that the mutation in Queen Victoria's family was new, arising in one of her parents. Lastly, it is possible that her mother was heterozygous and by chance, no other individuals in her family were unlucky enough to receive the mutant allele.

27. Unscheduled DNA synthesis represents DNA repair. One can determine complementation groupings by placing each heterokaryon giving a "-" into one group and those giving a "+" into a separate group. For instance, *XP1* and *XP2* are placed into the same group because they do not complement each other. However, *XP1* and *XP5* do complement ("+") therefore they are in different groups. Completing such pairings allows one to determine the following groupings:

XP1	*XP4*	*XP5*
XP2		*XP6*
XP3		*XP7*

The groupings (complementation groups) indicate that there are at least three "genes" that form products necessary for unscheduled DNA synthesis. All of the cell lines that are in the same complementation group are defective in the same product.

28. Your study should include examination of the following short-term aspects: immediate assessment of radiation amounts distributed in a matrix of the bomb sites as well as a control area not receiving bomb-induced radiation, radiation exposure as measured by radiation sickness and evidence of radiation poisoning from tissue samples, abortion rates, birthing rates, and chromosomal studies.

Long-term assessment should include: sex-ratio distortion (males being more influenced by X-linked recessive lethals than females), chromosomal studies, birth and abortion rates, cancer frequency and type, and genetic disorders. In each case, data should be compared with a suitable control site to see if changes are bomb-related. In addition, to attempt to determine cause-effect, it is often helpful to show a dose response. Thus, by comparing the location of individuals at the time of exposure with the matrix of radiation amounts, one may be able to determine whether those most exposed to radiation suffer the most physiologically and genetically. If a positive correlation is observed, then statistically significant conclusions may be possible.

29. The cystic fibrosis gene produces a complex membrane transport protein that contains several major domains: a highly conserved ATP binding domain, two hydrophobic domains, and a large cytoplasmic domain, which probably serves in a regulatory capacity. The protein is like many ATP-dependent transport systems, some of which have been well studied. When a mutation causes clinical symptoms, fluid secretion is decreased and dehydrated mucus accumulates in the lungs and air passages. Mutations that radically alter the structure of the protein (frameshift, splicing, nonsense, deletions, duplications, etc.) would probably have more influence on protein function than those which cause relatively minor amino acid substitutions, although this generalization does not always hold true. A protein with multiple functional domains would be expected to react to mutational insult in a variety of ways.

30. (a) For those organisms that generate energy by aerobic respiration, a process occurs that involves the reduction of molecular oxygen. Partially reduced species are produced as intermediates and by-products of such molecular action: O_2^-, H_2O_2, and OH^-. These species are potent electrophilic oxidants that escape mitochondria and attack numerous cellular components. Collectively, these are called reactive oxygen species (ROS).

(b)

Guanine

Cytosine — Guanine

When casually examining the structures in the above diagrams, it is not immediately obvious that oxoG:A pairs should occur. However, hydrogen bonding can occur to any other base, including self pairs. Homopurine (A:A, G:G) and heteropurine (A:G) pairs represent anomalous base pairing possibilities even with nonaltered bases. While G:C is undoubtedly the most stable, several mispairs are actually stronger than the A-T pair.

Base pairing is complicated by the fact that the purines possess two H-bonding faces; the Watson-Crick face, involving ring positions 1 and 6 for adenine and, 1, 2, and 6 for guanine, and the Hoogsteen face involving ring positions 6 and 7. The typical pairing mode is indicated as *wc* where pairing occurs on the Watson-Crick face in the normal orientation, even for the mispair A:G. Alteration of pairing and favoring of the Hoogsteen face can be favored with the alteration generated by oxoGuanine. Indeed, triple helix configurations commonly involve the Hoogsteen face.

(c) If not repaired (see below), the first round of replication involves the pairing of oxoG to adenine (see above), while in the next round of replication, adenine pairs with its normal thymine. Therefore, if one starts with a G:C pair, one ends up with an A:T pair.

(d) It turns out that G:G>T:A transversions are quite commonly found in human cancers and are especially prevalent in the tumor suppressor gene *p53*. Thus, the cellular defense system has been extensively studied. One component is a triphosphatase that cleanses the nucleotide precursor pool by removing the two outermost phosphates from oxo-dGTP. Another involves a DNA glycosylase that initiates repair of misreplicated oxoG:A by hydrolyzing the glycosidic bond linking the adenine base to the sugar. Another is a DNA gycosylase/lyase system that recognizes oxoG opposite cytosine. Of the three systems, the DNA glycosylases are probably the most effective.

31. Since Betazoids have a 4-letter genetic code and the gene is 3,332 nucleotides long, the protein involved must be 833 amino acids in length.

(mr-1) Codon 829 specifies an amino that is very close to the end (carboxyl) of the gene. While a nonsense mutation would terminate translation prematurely, the protein would only be shortened by five amino acids. Thus, the protein's ability to fold and perform its cellular function must not be seriously altered. Because of the direction of translation (5' to 3' on the mRNA) the carboxyl terminal amino acids in a protein are the last to be included in folding priorities and are sometimes (often) less significant in determining protein function.

(mr-2) Since the phenotype is mild, this amino acid change does not completely inactivate the protein, but it does change its activity to some extent. Perhaps the substitution causes the protein to fold in a slightly aberrant manner, allowing it to have some residual function but preventing it from functioning entirely normally. Additionally, even if the protein folds similar to the wild type protein, charge or structural differences in the protein's active site may be only mildly influenced.

(mr-3) This deletion contains a total of 68 nucleotides, which account for 17 amino acids. Since Betazoids' codons contain four nucleotides, the mRNA reading frames are maintained subsequent to the deletion. Protein function significantly depends on the relative positions of secondary levels of structure: α-helices and β-sheets. If the deleted section is a "benign" linker between more significant protein domains, then perhaps the protein can tolerate the loss of some amino acids in a part of the protein without completely losing its function.

(mr-4) Amino acid specified by codon 192 must be critical to the function of the protein. Altering this amino acid must disrupt a critical region of the protein, thus causing it to lose most or all of its activity. If the protein is an enzyme, this amino acid could be located in its active site and be critical for the ability of the enzyme to bind and/or influence its substrate. One might expect that the amino acid alteration is rather radical such as one sees in the generation of sickle cell anemia. HbS is caused by the substitution of a valine (no net charge) for glutamic acid (negatively charged).

(mr-5) A deletion of 11 base pairs, a number that is not divisible by four, will shift the reading frames subsequent to its location. Even though this deletion is smaller than the deletion discussed above (83--150) and is located in the same region, it causes a reading frame shift and some or all of the amino acids that are added downstream from the mutation may be different from those in the normal protein. The reason that all will not likely change is because of synonyms in the code. There is also the possibility that a nonsense triplet may be introduced in the "out-of-phase" region, thus causing premature chain termination. Because this mutation occurs early in the gene, most of the protein will be affected. This may well explain the severe insensitive phenotype.

32. Individuals with xeroderma pigmentosum (XP) are much more likely to contract skin cancer in youth than non-XP individuals. By age 20, approximately 80% of the XP population has skin cancer compared with approximately 4% in the non-XP group. XP individuals lack one or more functional genes involved in DNA repair.

Chapter 15: Regulation of Gene Expression

Concept Areas	Corresponding Problems
Overview	1, 2, 3, 13, 14, 15, 16, 17, 20, 23
Lactose Metabolism in E. coli	4, 5, 6, 7, 8, 9, 10
Positive and Negative Control	2, 3, 17, 14, 15, 16, 17, 18, 26
Tryptophan Operon	11, 12
Model Systems	13, 15, 16, 17
Eukaryotic Regulation	19, 20, 21, 22, 24, 25, 26, 27, 28, 29, 30

Vocabulary: Organization and Listing of Terms and Concepts

Structures and Substances

Lactose

  structural genes

  lac operon

    cis-acting

    trans-acting

    lac Z

      β-galactosidase

    lac Y

      permease

    lac A

      transacetylase

polycistronic mRNA

gratuitous inducers

  isopropylthiogalactoside (IPTG)

constitutive mutants

lac I⁻

lac O^c

  merozygote

repressor gene

repressor molecule (I^+)

diffusible cellular product (F15.2)

operator region

  no diffusible product (O^+)

  adjacent control (F15.2)

  lac I^s

  lac I^q

  catabolite activating protein (CAP)

  promoter region

  glucose

  CAP binding site

cyclic adenosine monophosphate (cAMP)

    adenyl cyclase

Tryptophan

    tryptophan synthetase

    trp R⁻, trp R⁺

        co-repressor

    structural genes

        trp E, D, C, B, A

    trp P-*trp* O region

    leader sequence

        attenuator

        tRNA^{trp}

        antitermination hairpin

Chromosome territory

    interchromosome compartment

    histone

    histone acetyltransferase enzyme

    promoter

    TATA box, CAAT box, GC box

    core promoter

    enhancer

    silencer

    transcription factor

    metallothionein IIA

DNA-binding domain

    helix-turn-helix

    homeobox

    homeodomain

    basic lucine zipper

    lucine zipper

    pre-initiation complex

    enhanceosome

    proteome

Processes/Methods

Genetic regulation

    adaptive

        inducible

            inducer

            lactose

    repressible

        tryptophan

            attenuation, ribosome "stall"

        negative, positive control

            catabolite repression

        constitutive

    allosteric

    superrepression

RNA splicing

    capping

Concepts

polyadenylation

t$_{1/2}$

 chromatin remodeling

histone modification

DNA methylation

mRNA stability

gene silencing

RNA interference (RNAi)

microRNA

RNA-directed DNA methylation

Genetic regulation

efficiency

Cis-acting, *trans*-acting

Positive control (F15.1)

catabolite repression

Negative control (F15.1)

lactose operon

tryptophan operon

repression

attenuation

"stalling"

Eukaryotic

pretranscriptional

posttranscriptional

alternative splicing

gene silencing

F15.1 Illustration of general processes of *negative* and *positive* control. If *negative* control is operating, the regulatory protein inhibits transcription. With *positive* control, transcription is stimulated.

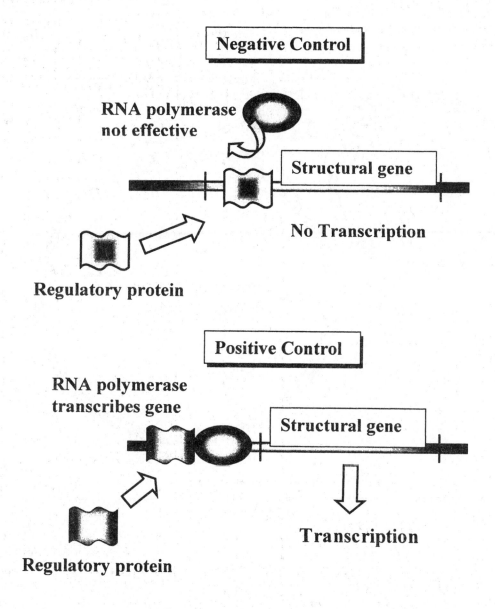

F15.2 Illustration of the nature of the product of the *I* gene. It can act "at a distance" because it is a protein that can diffuse through the cytoplasm and thus act in *trans*. There is no protein product of the operator gene, therefore, it can only act in *cis*.

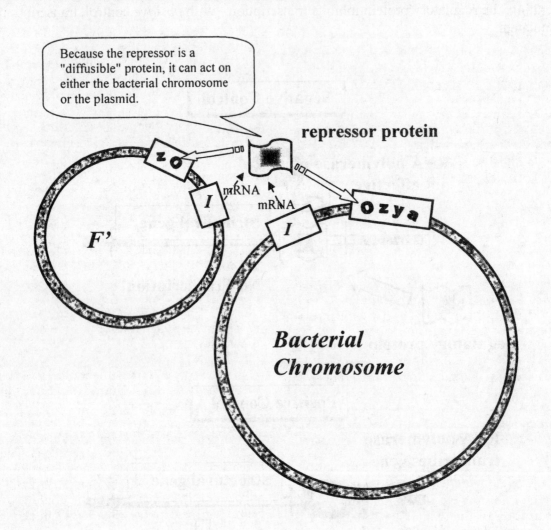

Solutions to Problems and Discussion Questions

1. The answer to this question is a key to enhancing a student's understanding of the Jacob-Monod model as related to lactose and tryptophan metabolism. The enzymes of the lactose operon are needed to break down and use lactose as an energy source. If lactose is the sole carbon source, the enzymes are synthesized to use that carbon source. With no lactose present, there is no "need" for the enzymes. The tryptophan operon contains structural genes for the *synthesis* of tryptophan. If there is little or no tryptophan in the medium, the tryptophan operon is "turned on" to manufacture tryptophan. If tryptophan is abundant in the medium, then there is no "need" for the operon to be manufacturing "tryptophan synthetases."

2. Refer to F15.1 to see that under *negative* control, the regulatory molecule interferes with transcription, while in *positive* control, the regulatory molecule stimulates transcription. Negative control is seen in the *lactose* and *tryptophan* systems. Catabolite repression is an example of positive control. Negative control requires a molecule to be removed from the DNA for transcription to occur. Positive control requires a molecule to be provided to the DNA for transcription to occur.

3. In an *inducible system*, the repressor that normally interacts with the operator to inhibit transcription is inactivated by an *inducer*, thus permitting transcription. In a *repressible system*, a normally inactive repressor is *activated* by a *co-repressor*, thus enabling it (the activated repressor) to bind to the operator to inhibit transcription. Because the interaction of the protein (repressor) has a negative influence on transcription, the systems described here are forms of *negative control* (see F15.1).

4. (a) Due to the deletion of a base early in the *lac* Z gene there will be "frameshift" of all the reading frames downstream from the deletion. It is likely that either premature chain termination of translation will occur (from the introduction of a nonsense triplet in a reading frame) or the normal chain termination will be ignored. Regardless, a mutant condition for the Z gene will be likely. If such a cell is placed on a lactose medium, it will be incapable of growth because β-galactosidase is not available. **(b)** If the deletion occurs early in the A gene, one might expect impaired function of the A gene product, but it will not influence the use of lactose as a carbon source.

5. Refer to the text and to F15.1,2 to get a good understanding of the lactose system before starting.

$I^+ O^+ Z^+$ = **Inducible** because a repressor protein can interact with the operator to turn off transcription.

$I^- O^+ Z^+$ = **Constitutive** because the repressor gene is mutant, therefore no repressor protein is available.

$I^+ O^c Z^+$ = **Constitutive** because even though a repressor protein is made, it cannot bind with the mutant operator.

$I^- O^+ Z^+ / F' I^+$ = **Inducible** because even though there is one mutant repressor gene, the other I^+ gene, on the F factor, produces a normal repressor protein that is diffusible and capable of interacting with the operon to repress transcription. (See F16.2 in this book.)

$I^+ O^c Z^+ / F' O^+$ = **Constitutive** because there is a constitutive operator (O^c) next to a normal Z gene. Remembering that this operator functions in cis and is not influenced by the repressor protein, constitutive synthesis of β-galactosidase will occur.

$I^s\,O^+\,Z^+$ = **Repressed** because the product of the I^s gene is *insensitive* to the inducer lactose and thus cannot be inactivated. The repressor will continually interact with the operator and shut off transcription regardless of the presence or absence of lactose.

$I^s\,O^+\,Z^+\,/F'\,I^+$ = **Repressed** because, as in the previous case, the product of the I^s gene is insensitive to the inducer lactose and thus cannot be inactivated. The repressor will continually interact with the operator and shut off transcription regardless of the presence or absence of lactose. The fact that there is a normal I^+ gene is of no consequence because once a repressor from I^s binds to an operator, the presence of normal repressor molecules will make no difference.

6. Refer to the text and to F15.2 to get a good understanding of the lactose system before starting.

$I^+\,O^+\,Z^+$ = Because of the function of the active repressor from the I^+ gene, and no lactose to influence its function, there will be **No Enzyme Made**.

$I^+\,O^c\,Z^+$ = There will be a **Functional Enzyme Made** because the constitutive operator is in *cis* with a Z gene. The lactose in the medium will have no influence because of the constitutive operator. The repressor cannot bind to the mutant operator.

$I^-\,O^+\,Z^-$ = There will be a **Nonfunctional Enzyme Made** because with I^- the system is constitutive, but the Z gene is mutant. The absence of lactose in the medium will have no influence because of the nonfunctional repressor. The mutant repressor cannot bind to the operator.

$I^-\,O^+\,Z^-$ = There will be a **Nonfunctional Enzyme Made** because with I^- the system is constitutive, but the Z gene is mutant. The lactose in the medium will have no influence because of the nonfunctional repressor. The mutant repressor cannot bind to the operator.

$I^-\,O^+\,Z^+\,/F'\,I^+$ = There will be **No Enzyme Made** because in the absence of lactose, the repressor product of the I^+ gene will bind to the operator and inhibit transcription.

$I^+\,O^c\,Z^+\,/F'\,O^+$ = Because there is a constitutive operator in *cis* with a normal Z gene, there will be **Functional Enzyme Made**. The lactose in the medium will have no influence because of the mutant operator.

$I^+\,O^+\,Z^-\,/F'\,I^+\,O^+\,Z^+$ = Because there is lactose in the medium, the repressor protein will not bind to the operator and transcription will occur. The presence of a normal Z gene allows a **Functional and Nonfunctional Enzyme to be Made**. The repressor protein is diffusible, working in *trans*.

$I^-\,O^+\,Z^-\,/F'\,I^+\,O^+\,Z^+$ = Because there is no lactose in the medium, the repressor protein (from I^+) will repress the operators and there will be **No Enzyme Made**.

$I^s\,O^+\,Z^+\,/\,F'\,O^+$ = With the product of I^s there is binding of the repressor to the operator and therefore **No Enzyme Made**. The lack of lactose in the medium is of no consequence because the mutant repressor is insensitive to lactose.

$I^+\,O^c\,Z^+\,/F'\,O^+\,Z^+$ = The arrangement of the constitutive operator (O^c) with the Z gene will cause a **Functional Enzyme to be Made**.

7. The mutations described are consistent with the structure of the lac repressor. The N-terminal portion of the repressor is involved in DNA binding, while the C-terminal portion is more involved in association with lactose and its analogs.

8. Catabolite repression is a mechanism whereby glucose, a catabolite of lactose, inhibits the synthesis of β-galactosidase. When glucose and lactose are both present, glucose is preferentially used as the energy source. When glucose is exhausted, β-galactosidase synthesis occurs and lactose is metabolized. Thus, catabolite repression balances the use of glucose and lactose through regulation of β-galactosidase synthesis.

9. Generally, cooperative binding occurs when the final outcome is greater than the simple sum of its parts. In the case of transcription factors, each factor has little impact on transcription; however, when all components are present, a cooperative interaction (binding) occurs and a functional complex is made.

10. In order to understand this question, it is necessary that you understand the negative regulation of the *lactose* operon by the *lac* repressor as well as the positive control exerted by the CAP protein. Remember, if lactose is present, it inactivates the *lac* repressor. If glucose is present, it inhibits adenyl cyclase, thereby reducing, through a lowering of cAMP levels, the positive action of CAP on the *lac* operon.

(a) With no lactose and no glucose, the operon is off because the *lac* repressor is bound to the operator and although CAP is bound to its binding site, it will not override the action of the repressor.

(b) With lactose added to the medium, the *lac* repressor is inactivated and the operon is transcribing the structural genes. With no glucose, the CAP is bound to its binding site, thus enhancing transcription.

(c) With no lactose present in the medium, the *lac* repressor is bound to the operator region, and since glucose inhibits adenyl cyclase, the CAP protein will not interact with its binding site. The operon is therefore "off."

(d) With lactose present, the *lac* repressor is inactivated; however, since glucose is also present, CAP will not interact with its binding site. Under this condition transcription is severely diminished and the operon can be considered to be "off."

11. (a) Because activated CAP is a component of the cooperative binding of RNA polymerase to the *lac* promoter, absence of a functional *crp* would compromise the positive control exhibited by CAP.

(b) Without a CAP binding site there would be a reduction in the inducibility of the *lac* operon.

12. Attenuation functions to reduce the synthesis of tryptophan when it is in full supply. It does so by reducing transcription of the *tryptophan* operon. The same phenomenon is observed when tryptophan activates the repressor to shut off transcription of the *tryptophan* operon.

13. It is likely that attenuation evolved as yet another means to regulate gene output. It provides a fine level of control over gene expression and attests to the complex measures that organisms have taken to effectively regulate their genomes. Attenuation can be achieved in a rather straightforward manner with amino acids, since their availability determines the availability of corresponding charged tRNAs. It is the availability, or lack of, those charged tRNAs that regulate transcription. Overall, then, attenuation provides a direct route for amino acids to control gene expression.

14. First, notice that in the first row of data, the presence of tm in the medium causes the production of active enzyme from the wild type arrangement of genes. From this one would conclude that the system is *inducible*. To determine which gene is the structural gene, look for the *IE* function and see that it is related to *C*. Therefore, *C* codes for the **structural gene**. Because when *B* is mutant, no enzyme is produced, *B* must be the **promoter**.

Notice that when genes *A* and *D* are mutant, constitutive synthesis occurs; therefore, one must be the operator and the other gene codes for the repressor protein. To distinguish these functions, one must remember that the repressor operates as a diffusible substance and can be on the host chromosome or the F factor (functioning in *trans*). However, the operator can only operate in *cis*. In addition, in *cis*, the constitutive operator is dominant to its wild type allele, while the mutant repressor is recessive to its wild type allele.

Notice that the mutant *A* gene is dominant to its wild type allele, whereas the mutant *d* allele is recessive (behaving as wild type in the first row). Therefore, the *A* locus is the **operator** and the *D* locus is the **repressor** gene.

15. Because the deletion of the regulatory gene causes a loss of synthesis of the enzymes, the regulatory gene product can be viewed as one exerting *positive control*. When tis is present, no enzymes are made; therefore, tis must inactivate the positive regulatory protein. When tis is absent, the regulatory protein is free to exert its positive influence on transcription. Mutations in the operator negate the positive action of the regulator. On the next page (F15.3) is a model that illustrates these points.

F15.3 Model of regulatory system described in problem #15. This is an example of *positive* control.

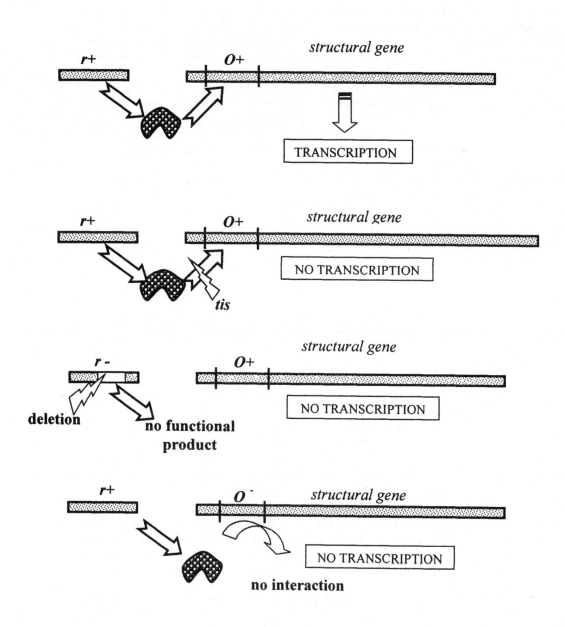

16. The first two sentences in the problem indicate an inducible system where oil stimulates the production of a protein, which turns on (positive control) genes to metabolize oil. The different results in strains #2 and #4 suggest a *cis*-acting system. Because the operon by itself (when mutant as in strain #3) gives constitutive synthesis of the structural genes, *cis*-acting system is also supported. The *cis*-acting element is most likely part of the operon.

17. (a) Call one constitutive mutation *lex*A⁻ (mutation in the repressor gene product) and the other O*uvrA*⁻ (mutation in the operator).

(b) One can make partial diploid strains using F'. O*uvrA*⁻ will (given the other genes brought in by the F' element) be dominant to O*uvrA*⁺ and *lex*A⁻ will be recessive to *lex*A⁺. O*uvrA*⁻ will act in *cis*.

18. If one could develop an assay for the other gene products under SOS control, with a *lex*A⁻ strain, the other gene products should be present at induced levels.

19. There are several reasons for anticipating a variety of different regulatory mechanisms in eukaryotes as compared with prokaryotes. Eukaryotic cells contain greater amounts of DNA and this DNA is associated with various proteins, including histones and nonhistone chromosomal proteins. *Chromatin* as such does not exist in prokaryotes. In addition, whereas there is usually only one chromosome in prokaryotes, eukaryotes have more than one chromosome all enclosed in a nuclear envelope. This nuclear envelope separates, both temporally and spatially, the processes of transcription and translation, thus providing an opportunity for post-transcriptional, pre-translational regulation.

While prokaryotes respond genetically to changes in their external environment, cells of multicellular eukaryotes interact with each other as well as the external environment. The structural and functional diversity of cells of a multicellular eukaryote, coupled with the finding that all cells of an organism contain a complete complement of genes, suggests that in some cells certain genes are active that are not active in other cells.

It is often difficult to study eukaryotic gene regulation because of the complexities mentioned above, especially tissue specificity and the various levels at which regulation can occur (as indicated in question #2 below). Obtaining a homogeneous group of cells from a multicellular organism often requires a significant alteration of the natural environment of the cell. Thus, results from studies on isolated cells must be interpreted with caution. In addition, because of the variety of intracellular components (nuclear and cytoplasmic) it is difficult to isolate, free of contamination, certain molecular species. Even if such isolation is accomplished, it is difficult to interpret the actual behavior of such molecules in an artificial environment.

20. *Chromatin remodeling*: Changes in DNA/chromosome structure can influence overall gene output. DNA methylation also influences transcription efficiency. While not specifically discussed in this chapter, ***gene amplification*** refers to cases where an increase in gene products is achieved by an increase in the number of genes producing those products. Such amplification can be achieved intrachromosomally (chorion genes) or extrachromosomally (rRNA genes in some amphibians).

Transcription: There are several factors that are known to influence transcription: *promoters*, TATA, CAAT, and GC boxes, as well as other upstream regulatory sequences: *enhancers*, which are *cis*-acting sequences that act at various locations and orientations; *transcription factors*, with various structural motifs (zinc fingers, homeodomains, and leucine zippers) which bind DNA and influence transcription; and *receptor-hormone complexes* that influence transcription. Enhancers and silencers are also often involved in regulation. Various transcription factors provide specificity and cooperative interactions with DNA targets.

Processing and transport types of regulation involve the efficiency of hnRNA maturation as related to capping, polyA tail addition, and intron removal. The stability of the mRNAs appears to be an additional regulatory control point. Certain factors, such as protein subunits, may influence a variety of steps in the translational mechanism. For instance, a protein or protein subunit may activate an RNase, which will degrade certain mRNAs or a particular regulatory element may cause a ribosome to stall, thus decreasing the speed of translation and increasing the exposure of an mRNA to the action of RNAses. Alternative splicing and various forms of RNA interference offer additional points of regulation. RNA-directed DNA methylation is also involved in some organisms.

21. *Promoters* are conserved DNA sequences that influence transcription from the "upstream" side (5') of mRNA coding genes. They are usually fixed in position and within 100 base pairs of the initiation site for mRNA synthesis. Examples of such promoter sites are the following: TATA, CAAT, and GC boxes.

Enhancers are *cis*-acting sequences of DNA that stimulate the transcription from most, if not all, promoters. They are somewhat different from promoters in that the position of the enhancer need not be fixed; it may be significantly upstream, downstream, or within the gene being regulated. The orientation may be inverted without significantly influencing its action. Enhancers can work on different genes, that is, they are not gene-specific.

22. Transcription factors are proteins that are *necessary* for the initiation of transcription. However, they are not *sufficient* for the initiation of transcription. To be activated, RNA polymerase II requires a number of transcription factors. Transcription factors contain at least two functional domains: one binds to the DNA sequences of promoters and/or enhancers, while the other interacts with RNA polymerase or other transcription factors. Some transcription factors bind to other transcription factors without themselves binding to DNA.

23. Your essay should deal with the following issues:

- differences in basic chromosome structure
- chromosome remodeling
- histone acetylation
- differences in gene structure
- cell structure (nucleus in eukaryotes)
- genomic aspects (amplification, *etc.*)
- biological context in terms of multicellular interactions *versus* single cell survival

24. The work of Cleveland and colleagues allowed selective changes to be made in the *met-arg-glu-lys* sequence. Only the engineered mRNA sequences that caused an amino acid substitution negated the autoregulation, indicating that it is the sequence of the amino acids, not the mRNA that is critical in the process of autoregulation. Notice that code degeneracy allows for changes in mRNA sequence without changes in the amino acid sequence. Therefore, the model that depicts binding of factors to the nascent polypeptide chain is supported. There are a variety of experiments that could be used to substantiate such a model. One might stabilize the proposed MREI-protein complex with "crosslinkers," treat with RNAse to digest mRNA and to break up polysomes, then isolate individual ribosomes. One may use some specific antibody or other method to determine whether tubulin subunits contaminate the ribosome population.

25. (a) There is no place for the TFIID to bind.

(b) There is more transcription in the nuclear extracts. Perhaps other factors not present in the purified system are present in the nuclear extracts.

(c) There is a region probably in the -81 to -50 area that responds to a component in the nuclear extract to bring about high efficiency transcription.

26.

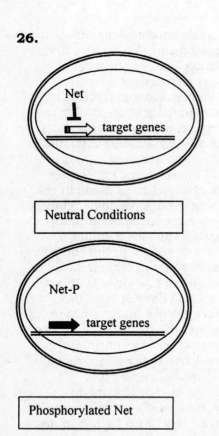

Neutral Conditions

Phosphorylated Net

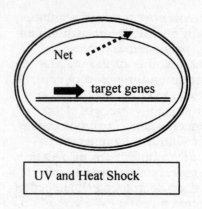

UV and Heat Shock

Sketches modified from Ducret et al. *Molecular and Cellular Biology* 1999 19:7076-7087.

27. While the mechanism of enhancer action over long distances is unknown, supercoiling may bring about the pattern below:

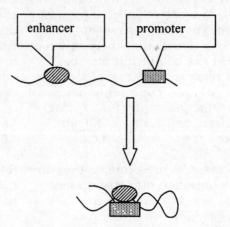

28. Methylation of CpGs causes a reduction in luciferase expression, which is somewhat proportional to the amount of methylation and patch size. Methylation within the transcription unit more drastically reduces luciferase expression compared with methylation outside the transcription unit. A high degree of methylation outside the transcription unit (593 CpGs) has as great of an impact on depressing transcription as the same degree of methylation within the transcription unit.

29. Given that DNA methylation plays a role in gene expression in mammals, any change in DNA methylation, plus or minus, can potentially have a negative impact on progeny development. In addition, since $m^5C >>>$ thymine, transitions are likely to cause mutations in coding regions of DNA, when methylation patterns change, new sites for mutation arise. Should mutations occur at a higher rate in previously unmethylated sites (genes), embryonic development is likely to be affected.

30. If the exon 45 deletion causes a reading frameshift leading to reduced dystrophin production and the removal of exon 46 reestablishes the reading frame, then one would expected enhanced production of dystrophin.

Chapter 16: Cell-Cycle Regulation and Cancer

Concept Areas	Corresponding Problems
Inherited Cancer	1, 6, 22, 29, 30
Cell Cycle Mechanisms	2, 3, 4, 5, 12, 18, 23
Cancer and the Environment	7, 16, 20, 21, 28
Apoptosis	8
Tumor Suppressors and Oncogenes	9, 10, 11, 13, 14, 27
Chromosome Structure	15, 17, 26
Viruses and Cancer	19
Cancer Biology	24, 25, 26

Vocabulary: Organization and Listing of Terms and Concepts

Structures and Substances

Tumor

  benign

  malignant

  carcinoma *in situ*

  chronic myelogenous leukemia (CML)

    BCR-ABL

  Philadelphia chromosome

    protein kinase

  hereditary nonpolyposis colorectal cancer (HNPCC)

Burkitt's lymphoma

Carcinogen

Mutator phenotype

Cell cycle components

  cyclins

  cyclin-dependent kinases (CDKs)

  cyclin/CDK complexes

  caspases

Bcl2, Bcl2-BAX

p53

  Mdm2

RB1

  pRB

  E2F

Proto-oncogene

  cyclin D1

  ras

  GTP-GDP

  Raf, Mek, Map kinase

Chapter 16 Cell-Cycle Regulation and Cancer

Transcription factors

Oncogene

Tumor suppressor gene

Cellular components

    extracellular matrix

    basal lamina

    metalloproteinases

    inhibitors of metalloproteinases (TIMPS)

Familial adenomatous polyposis (FAP)

    polyp

Viruses

    retrovirus

    acute transforming virus

    Rous sarcoma virus (RSV)

    reverse transcriptase

    provirus

    c-onc

    v-onc

    papillomavirus (HPV)

    human T-cell leukemia virus (HTLV-1)

Environmental agents

    tobacco smoke

    ras, p53

    X-rays

Processes/Methods

Cell proliferation

    metastasis

Tumorigenesis

Cell cycle

    signal transduction

    quiescent

    G1, G0, S, G2, M

    checkpoints

        G1/S, G2/M, M

    apoptosis

Cell-cell contact

Loss of heterozygosity

Concepts

Genetic basis of cancer

Loss of heterozygosity

Predisposition to some cancers

Viral involvement in cancer

Environmental agents and cancer

Solutions to Problems and Discussion Questions

1. Familial retinoblastoma is inherited as an autosomal dominant gene with 90% penetrance; that is, 90% of the individuals that inherit the gene will develop eye tumors. The gene usually expresses itself in youngsters. Because the husband's sister has RB, one of the husband's parents has the gene for RB and the husband has a 50:50 chance of inheriting that gene. However, because the husband is past the usual age of onset, it is quite likely that he was lucky and did not receive the RB gene. In that case, the chance that a child born to this couple having RB is no higher than the frequency of sporadic occurrence. However, because the gene is 90% penetrant, there is a chance that the husband has the gene but does not express it. The probability of that occurrence would be 0.50 (of inheriting the gene) X 0.10 (not expressing the gene) = 0.05. The chance of the husband then passing this non-expressed gene to his child would be again 0.5, so 0.50 X 0.05 = 0.025 for the child inheriting this gene. If the child inherits the RB gene, he/she has a 90% chance of expressing it. Therefore, the overall probability of the child having RB (using this logic) would be 0.025 X 0.9 = 0.0225 or just over 2% (or about 1 in 50).

To test the presence of the RB gene in the husband, it is possible in some forms of RB to identify (by molecular probes) a defective or missing DNA segment. Otherwise, one might attempt to assay the RB product in cells to see if it is present and functional at normal levels.

2. Review <u>Chapter 2</u> in the text and note that the following stages of the cell cycle are discussed: G1, G0, S, and G2. The G1 stage begins after mitosis and is involved in the synthesis of many cytoplasmic elements. In the S phase DNA synthesis occurs. G2 is a period of growth and preparation for mitosis. Most cell cycle time variation is caused by changes in the duration of G1. G0 is the non-dividing state.

3. The major regulatory points of the cell cycle include the following:

1. late G1 (G1/S)
2. the border between G2 and mitosis (G2/M)
3. in mitosis (M)

4. Kinases regulate other proteins by adding phosphate groups. Cyclins bind to the kinases, switching them on and off. CDK4 binds to cyclin D, moving cells from G1 to S. At the G2/mitosis border a CDK1 (cyclin-dependent kinase) combines with another cyclin (cyclin B). Phosphorylation occurs, bringing about a series of changes in the nuclear membrane *via* caldesmon, cytoskeleton, and histone H1.

5. The retinoblastoma gene (*RB1*), located on chromosome 13, encodes a protein designated pRB. Cells progress through the G1/S transition when pRB is phosphorylated and CDK4 binds to cyclin D. In the absence of phosphorylation of pRB, it binds to members of the E2F family of transcription factors, which controls the expression of genes required to move the cell from G1 to S. When E2F and other regulators are released by pRB, they are free to induce the expression of over 30 genes whose products are required for the transition from G1 into S phase. After cells traverse S, G2, and M phases, pRB reverts to a nonphosphorylated state, binds to regulatory proteins such as E2F and keeps them sequestered until required for the next cell cycle.

6. To say that a particular trait is inherited conveys the assumption that when a particular genetic circumstance is present, it will be revealed in the phenotype. For instance, albinism is inherited in such a way that individuals who are homozygous recessive, express albinism. When one discusses an inherited predisposition, one usually refers to situations where a particular phenotype is expressed in families in some consistent pattern. However, the phenotype may not always be expressed or may manifest itself in different ways. In retinoblastoma, the

186

gene is inherited as an autosomal dominant and those that inherit the mutant *RB* allele are predisposed to develop eye tumors. However, approximately 10% of the people known to inherit the gene do not actually express it and in some cases expression involves only one eye, rather than two.

7. Cancer is a complex alteration in normal cell cycle controls. Even if a major "cancer-causing" gene is transmitted, other genes, often new mutations, are usually necessary in order to drive a cell towards tumor formation. Full expression of the cancer phenotype is likely to be the result of an interplay among a variety of genes and therefore show variable penetrance and expressivity.

8. Apoptosis, or programmed cell death, is a genetically controlled process that leads to death of a cell. It is a natural process involved in morphogenesis and a protective mechanism against cancer formation. During apoptosis, nuclear DNA becomes fragmented, cellular structures are disrupted, and the cells are dissolved. Caspases are involved in the initiation and progress of apoptosis.

9. A tumor suppressor gene is a gene that normally functions to suppress cell division. Since tumors and cancers represent a significant threat to survival and therefore Darwinian fitness, strong evolutionary forces would favor a variety of co-evolved and perhaps complex conditions in which mutations in these suppressor genes would be recessive. Looking at it in another way, if a tumor suppressor gene makes a product that regulates the cell cycle favorably, cellular conditions have evolved in such a way that sufficient quantities of this gene product are made from just one allele (of the two present in each diploid individual) to provide normal function.

10. There are a number of ways in which protooncogenes are converted to oncogenes: point mutations in which a mutant gene acts as a positive "switch" in the cell cycle, translocations where a hybrid gene might be formed, and overexpression where a gene might acquire a new promoter and/or enhancer. In the case of RSV, an oncogene (*c-src*) was captured from the chicken genome.

11. Imbedded in the plasma membrane, Ras proteins act as molecular switches that transmit molecular signals from outside to inside the cell. Activated Ras proteins tranduce a signal, which activates the transcription of genes that start cell division. Mutant Ras proteins are locked into the "on" position, continually signaling cell division.

12. Various kinases can be activated by breaks in DNA. One kinase, called ATM and/or a kinase called Chk2, phosphorylates BRCA1 and p53. The activated p53 arrests replication during the S phase to facilitate DNA repair. The activated BRCA1 protein, in conjunction with BRCA2, mRAD51, and other nuclear proteins is involved in repairing the DNA.

13. Oncogenes are genes that induce or maintain uncontrolled cellular proliferation associated with cancer. They are mutant forms of protooncogenes, which normally function to regulate cell division. Oncogenes may be formed through point mutations, gene amplification, translocations, repositioning of regulatory sequences, or other mechanisms.

14. Mutations that produce oncogenes alter gene expression either directly or indirectly and act in a dominant capacity. Proto-oncogenes are those which normally function to promote or maintain cell division. In the mutant state (oncogenes), they induce or maintain uncontrolled cell division, that is, there is a gain-of-function. Generally this gain-of-function takes the form of increased or abnormally continuous gene output. On the other hand, loss-of-function is generally attributed to mutations in tumor suppressor genes, which function to halt passage through the cell cycle. When such genes are mutant, they have lost their capacity to halt the cell cycle. Such mutations are generally recessive.

15. A translocation involving exchange of genetic material between chromosomes 9 and 22 is responsible for the generation of the "Philadelphia chromosome." Genetic mapping established that certain genes were combined to form a hybrid oncogene (*BCR/ABL*) that encodes a 200kDa protein that has been implicated in the formation of chronic myelogenous leukemia.

16. Unfortunately, it is common to spend enormous amounts of money dealing with diseases after they occur rather than concentrating on disease prevention. Too often pressure from special interest groups or lack of political stimulus retards advances in education and prevention. Obviously, it is less expensive, both in terms of human suffering and money, to seek preventive measures for as many diseases as possible. However, having gained some understanding of the mechanisms of disease, in this case cancer, it must also be stated that no matter what preventive measures are taken it will be impossible to completely eliminate disease from the human population. It is extremely important, however, that we increase efforts to educate and protect the human population from as many hazardous environmental agents as possible.

17. Several approaches are used to combat CML. One includes the use of a tyrosine kinase inhibitor that binds competitively to the ATP binding site of ABL kinase, thereby inhibiting phosphorylation of BCR-ABL and preventing the activation of additional signaling pathways. In addition, real-time quantitative reverse transcription-polymerase chain reaction (Q-RT-PCR) allows one to monitor drug responses of cell populations in patients so that less toxic and more effective treatments are possible. Being able to distinguish leukemic cells from healthy cells allows one to not only target therapy to specific cell populations, but it also allows for the quantification of responses to therapy. Because such cells produce a hybrid protein, it may be possible to develop a therapy, perhaps an immunotherapy, based on the uniqueness of the BCR/ABL protein.

18. Normal cells are often capable of withstanding mutational assault because they have checkpoints and DNA repair mechanisms in place. When such mechanisms fail, cancer may be a result. Through mutation, such protective mechanisms are compromised in cancer cells and as a result they show higher than normal rates of mutation, chromosomal abnormalities, and genomic instability.

19. An acute transforming virus is a retrovirus that carries an oncogene(s), while a nonacute virus can induce the activity of cellular genes that bring about tumor formation.

20. Certain environmental agents such as chemicals and X-rays cause mutations. Since genes control the cell cycle, mutations in cell cycle control genes, or those that impact cell cycle control, can lead to cancer.

21. Radiotherapy is often administered externally or internally to damage the cell cycle machinery, thus shrinking the cancer or killing cells of the cancer. It may be completely or partially effective. Because cells have natural defenses against mutagenic insult, drugs that increase a cell's sensitivity to radiation may be administered. Radiosensitizers and radioprotectors are chemicals that alter a cell's response to radiotherapy. Radiosensitizers make cells more sensitive to therapy, whereas radioprotectors are drugs that protect normal cells from the damage caused by radiation therapy. Radiotherapy kills cells; therefore, side effects are expected.

22. No, she will still have the general population risk of about ten percent. In addition, it is possible that genetic tests will not detect all breast cancer mutations.

23. p53 is a tumor suppressor gene that protects cells from multiplying with damaged DNA. It is present in its mutant state in more than fifty percent of all tumors. Since the immediate control of a critical and universal cell cycle checkpoint is mediated by p53, mutation will influence a wide range of cell types. p53's action is not limited to specific cell types.

24. A benign tumor is a multicellular cell mass that is usually localized to a given anatomical site. Malignant tumors are those generated by cells that have migrated to one or more secondary sites. Malignant tumors are more difficult to treat and can be life-threatening.

25. Proteases in general and serine proteases, specifically, are considered tumor-promoting agents because they degrade proteins, especially those in the extracellular matrix. When such proteolysis occurs, cellular invasion and metastasis is encouraged. Consistent with this observation are numerous observations that metastatic tumor cells are associated with higher than normal amounts of protease expression. Inhibitors of serine proteases are often tested for their anticancer efficacy.

26. As with many forms of cancer, a single gene alteration is not the only requirement. The authors (Bose et al.) state "but only infrequently do the cells acquire the additional changes necessary to produce leukemia in humans." Some studies indicate that variations (often deletions) in the region of the breakpoints may influence expression of CML.

27. (a) Because one is working with somatic cells, the usual tests for heterozygosity through crosses are not available. Therefore, one must rely on chemical/physical approaches to answer the question. A genomic library could be constructed of both osteosarcoma cell DNA and noncancerous cells from the same organism. You could then screen the library using labeled probes from the clones carrying the *RB1* gene available to you as stated in the problem. At this point, some indications might emerge because if there is a significant alteration in mutant *RB1* genes, probes may not successfully hybridize to any clones in the cancerous cell DNA library. Assuming that control hybridization occurs in the noncancerous cells, lack of hybridization in the library derived from the osteosarcoma cell line might indicate deletions. However, assuming that hybridization does allow one to identify clones containing putative *RB1* alleles, subcloning into appropriate vectors would allow sequencing to reveal sequence changes in the *RB1* alleles when compared with nonmutant genes. A second approach combines an immunoassay described in part (b) of this problem. Assuming that one can successfully make antibodies to the normal RB1 gene product (pRB), lack of cross-reactivity of the pRB antibodies to proteins from the cancerous cell line would indicate that both *RB1* alleles are mutant.

(b) As indicated in the last portion of part (a) above, one can make antibodies to pRB from the noncancerous cells and test these antibodies for reactivity against proteins from the cancerous cell lines. A pRB-antibody reaction would indicate that the pRB protein is made.

(c) To determine whether addition of a normal *RB1* gene will change the cancer-causing potential of osteosarcoma cells, one could transfer the cloned normal *RB1* gene into the cells by transformation or transfection (often by electroporation or ultrasound). Transformed cells would then be introduced into the cancer-prone mice to determine whether their cancer-causing potential had been altered.

28. Any agent that causes damage to DNA is a potential carcinogen since cell cycle control is achieved by gene (DNA) products, proteins. Since cigarette smoke is known to contain an agent that changes DNA, in this case transversions, numerous modified gene products (including cell cycle controlling proteins) are likely to be produced. The fact that many cancer patients have such transversions in *p53* strongly suggests that cancer is caused by agents in cigarette smoke.

29. (a) The mRNA triplet for Gln is CAG(A). The mRNA triplet that specifies a stop is one of three: UAA, UAG, or UGA. The strand of DNA that codes for the CAG(A) would be the following: 3'-GTC(T)-5'. Therefore, if the G mutated to an A (transition), then the DNA strand would be 3'-ATC(T)-5', which would cause a UAG(A) triplet to be produced and this would cause the stop.

(b) It is likely to be a tumor suppressor gene because loss-of-function causes predisposition to cancer.

(c) Some women may carry genes (perhaps mutant) that "spare" for the *BRCA1* gene product. Some women may have immune systems that recognize and destroy precancerous cells or they may have mutations in breast signal transduction genes so that cell division suppression occurs in the absence of *BRCA1*.

30. (a, b) Even though there are changes in the *BRCA1* gene, they do not always have physiological consequences. Such neutral polymorphisms make screening difficult in that one cannot always be certain that a mutation will cause problems for the patient.

(c) The polymorphism in *PM2* is probably a silent mutation because the third base of the codon is involved.

(d) The polymorphism in *PM3* is probably a neutral missense mutation because the first base is involved. However, because there is some first codon position degeneracy, it is possible for the mutation to be silent.

Chapter 17: Recombinant DNA Technology

Concept Areas	Corresponding Problems
Overview	1, 5, 9, 10
Making DNA Clones	1, 3, 8, 9, 12, 28
Restriction Endonucleases	4, 6, 7, 9, 10, 11, 20, 24, 26
Constructing DNA Libraries	2, 8, 13, 15, 16, 17, 18, 21, 25
Identifying Specific Cloned Sequences	12, 13, 18, 19, 20, 23
Methods of Analysis of Cloned Sequences	12, 14, 19, 20, 23, 24, 25
DNA Sequencing	19, 30, 31
Polymerase Chain Reaction	27, 28, 29
Applications	22, 24, 25

Vocabulary: Organization and Listing of Terms and Concepts

Structures and Substances

Recombinant DNA, clone

   E. coli

Restriction endonucleases

   recognition sequence, 4^n

   restriction fragment

   "sticky" ends

   EcoR1

Vector

   cloning vehicle, plasmids

      pUC18

         polylinker site

         lacZ, X-gal

bacteriophage, λ

expression vector

Yeast artificial chromosome (YAC)

Probe

Reverse transcriptase

Oligonucleotide

   primers

      gene specific, random

   Taq polymerase

Restriction map

Dideoxynucleotide (ddNTP)

Chapter 17 Recombinant DNA Technology

Processes/Methods

Recombinant DNA technology

gene splicing

genetic engineering

selection (antibiotic resistance)

DNA sequencing

cloning

amplification

antibiotic resistance

hosts, *E. coli* transformation

polymerase chain reaction (PCR)

library construction

genomic libraries

N = ln(1-P)/ln(1-f)

cDNA libraries

reverse transcriptase

oligo-dT

DNA polymerase I

selection of recombinant clones

probing

Analytical methods

restricting mapping

restriction fragment length
polymorphism (RFLP)

gel electrophoresis

nucleic acid blotting

Southern blot

northern blot

western blot

PCR analysis

denaturation

annealing of primers

extension of primers

heat stable polymerase

Taq polymerse

DNA sequencing

gene mapping

Genome projects

Celera, Human genome project

Concepts

Cloning

selection strategies

Polymerase chain reaction

sensitivity, limitations

Probes, blotting

Chromosome walking, jumping

Restriction mapping

Gene mapping

DNA sequencing

Gene engineering

Solutions to Problems and Discussion Questions

1. Recombinant DNA technology, also called genetic engineering or gene splicing, involves the creation of associations of DNA that are not typically found in nature. Particular enzymes, called *restriction endonucleases*, cut DNA at specific sites and often yield "sticky" ends for additional interaction with DNA molecules cut with the same class of enzyme.

Isolated from bacteria, restriction enzymes fall into several classes, each having peculiarities as to structure and interaction with DNA. A vector may be a plasmid, bacteriophage, or cosmid which receives, through ligation, a piece or pieces of foreign DNA. The recombinant vector can transform (or transfect) a host cell (bacterium, yeast cell, etc.) and be amplified in number.

2. *Reverse transcriptase* is often used to promote the formation of cDNA (complementary DNA) from a mRNA molecule. Eukaryotic mRNAs typically have a 3' polyA tail as indicated in the diagram below. The poly-dT segment provides a double-stranded section which serves to prime the production of the complementary strand.

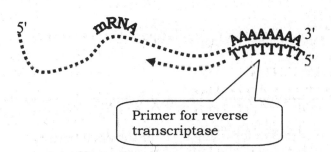

Primer for reverse transcriptase

3. Even though the human gene coding for insulin contains a number of introns, a cDNA generated from insulin mRNA is free of introns. Plasmids containing insulin genes (from cDNA) are free of introns so no processing issue surfaces.

4. The question of protein/DNA recognition and interaction is a difficult one to answer. Much research has been done to attempt to understand the nature of the specificity of such interactions. It is believed that the protein interacts with the major groove of the DNA helix. This information comes from the structure of the proteins which have been sufficiently well studied to suggest that the DNA major groove and "fingers" or extensions of the protein form the basis of interaction.

5. There are several reasons, some stemming from the original use of bacteria as the "workhorse" of molecular biologist as well as the ease with which bacteria and yeast can be manipulated. In addition, there is intense interest in understanding the biology of mammalian cells for obvious reasons and such cells have been manipulated in culture for many years. Perhaps one of the most important reasons is the fact that higher plants lack a suitable variety of vectors which are common to the other cell types mentioned above.

6. This segment contains the palindromic sequence of GGATCC which is recognized by the restriction enzyme *Bam*HI. The double-stranded sequence is the following

CCTAGG
GGATCC

7. The simple answer to this question is to assume that one is asking about the advantage to the scientist of having restriction enzyme sites recognize palindromic sites. In this case the answer would be that single-stranded overhanging ends are often generated which allow DNA from different sources cut with the same restriction enzyme to generate complementary overhangs which can anneal to form recombinant molecules.

If one considers the question from a bacterial standpoint, the answer is much more involved. In fact, bacterial chromosomes actually have fewer palindromic sites than expected based on chance. This adaptation stems from the fact that restriction sites cleave at palindromic sequences and one way to keep them from cleaving the host DNA is to evolve away from such sequences. So why do restriction enzymes often cleave at palindromic sites in the first place? First, the classical Type II restriction enzymes are dimers of identical units that recognize identical sequences. To protect such sequences in the bacterial chromosome from attack, a modification enzyme, a methyltransferase must fully methylate certain bases on both strands of the DNA at the site of a particular restriction endonuclease attack.

Methyltransferases are typically monomers consistent with the process of methylating newly replicated DNA strands. In order for both strands to be protected by methylation, the sequence must be read the same in both directions on the double helix. So, returning to the original question, the advantage to the bacterium of having palindromic sites for restriction enzymes is more related to the protection of such sites from cleavage.

8. Plasmids were the first to be used as cloning vectors and they are still routinely used to clone relatively small fragments of DNA. Because of their small size, they are relatively easy to separate from the host bacterial chromosome and they have relatively few restriction sites. They can be engineered fairly easily (*i.e.*, polylinkers and reporter genes added). For cloning larger pieces of DNA such as entire eukaryotic genes, cosmids are often used. For instance, when modifications are made in the bacterial virus lambda (λ) relatively large inserts of about 20kb can cloned. This is an important advantage when one needs to clone a large gene or generate a genomic library from a eukaryote. In addition, some cosmids will only accept inserts of a limited size, which means that small, less meaningful perhaps, fragments will be cloned unnecessarily. Both plasmids and cosmids suffer from the limitation that they can only use bacteria as hosts.

YACs (yeast artificial chromosomes) contain telomeres, an origin of replication, and a centromere and are extensively used to clone DNA in yeast. With selectable markers (TRP1 and URA3) and a cluster of restriction sites, DNA inserts ranging from 100kb to 1000kb can be cloned and inserted into yeast. Since yeast, being eukaryotes, undergo many of the typical RNA and protein processing steps of other, more complex eukaryotes, the advantages are numerous when working with eukaryotic genes.

9. Assuming a random distribution of all four bases and an equal percentage of A-T and G-C base pairs, the four-base sequence would occur (on average) every 256 base pairs (4^4), the six-base sequence every 4096 base pairs (4^6).

10. This problem can be solved by the following expressions:

*Not*I 4^8
*Hin*fI $4 \times 4 \times 1 \times 4 \times 4$
*Xho*II $2 \times 4 \times 4 \times 4 \times 4 \times 2$

The reason for using a "1" in the *Hin*fI portion is that any of the four bases can be inserted for the "N" whereas only two bases can be used for "Pu" and "Py" in the *Xho*II portion.

11. One might use an eight-base restriction enzyme to produce a relatively few large fragments. If one wanted to construct a eukaryotic genomic library, such large fragments would have to be cloned into special vectors, such as yeast artificial chromosomes.

12. (a) Because the *Drosophila* DNA has been cloned into the *Pst*I site in the ampicillin resistance gene of the plasmid, the gene will be mutated and any bacterium with the recombinant plasmid will be ampicillin sensitive. The tetracycline resistance gene remains active, however. Bacteria which have been transformed with the recombinant plasmid will be resistant to tetracycline and therefore tetracycline should be added to the medium.

(b) Colonies which grow on a tetracycline medium should be tested for growth on an ampicillin medium either by replica plating or some similar controlled transfer method. Those bacteria which do not grow on the ampicillin medium probably contain the *Drosophila* DNA insert.

(c) Resistance to both antibiotics by a transformed bacterium could be explained in several ways. First, if cleavage with the *Pst*I was incomplete, then no change in biological properties of the uncut plasmids would be expected. Also, it is possible that the cut ends of the plasmid were ligated together in the original form with no insert.

13. Since pBR322 has a size of 4361 base pairs, the average size of the inserts must be about 700 base pairs. Apply the formula:

$$N = \ln(1-P)/\ln(1-f)$$

$$= \ln(1- 0.99)/\ln[1- (700/1.5 \times 10^8)]$$

$$= \ln(.01)/\ln(.99999534)$$

$$= -4.605/-0.00000466$$

$$= 9.88 \times 10^5$$

14. Given that there is only one site for the action of *Hind*III, then the following will occur. Cuts will be made such that a four base single-stranded set of sticky ends will be produced. For the antibiotic resistance to be present, the ligation will reform the plasmid into its original form. However, two of the plasmids can join to form a dimer as indicated in the diagram below.

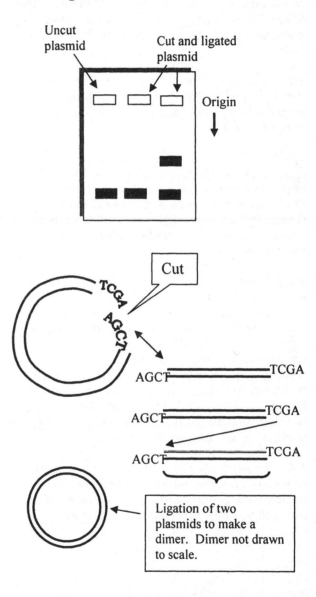

15. Using the human nucleotide sequence, one can produce a probe to screen the library of the African okapi. Second, one can use the amino acid sequence and the genetic code to generate a complementary DNA probe for screening of the library.   The probe is used, through hybridization, to identify the DNA which is complementary to the probe and allow one to identify the library clone containing the DNA of interest. Cells with the desired clone are then picked from the original plate and the plasmid is isolated from the cells.

16. Because of complementary base pairing, the 3' end of the DNA strand often loops back onto itself, thereby providing a primer for DNA polymerase I.

17. All other factors being equal (appropriate cloning sites and selectable markers), it is important to consider the size of the foreign DNA which can be cloned into the vector. Generally, for large genomes it is best to use a vector which will accept relatively large fragments.

18. A typical procedure is outlined in the text. A filter is used to bind the DNA from the colonies containing recombinant plasmids. A labeled probe is constructed for the protein sequence of EF1a. Since it is highly conserved, it should show considerable complementation to the human EF-1a cDNA. It is used to detect, through hybridization, the DNA of interest. Cells with the desired clone are then picked from the original plate and the plasmid is isolated from the cells.

19. The genomic clone most likely contains numerous introns which are spliced out during RNA processing. Such sections of DNA (introns) are not represented in cDNAs.

20. The problem can be best solved by drawing out the strands, then placing the restriction sites in the appropriate positions as follows:

enzyme I   __350_|____950_____

enzyme II 200|_____1100_____

To determine the orientation of the restriction sites to each other, examine the results of the double digested DNA and note that there is a 150bp fragment meaning that enzyme II cuts within the 350bp fragment of enzyme I. Therefore the final map is as follows:

      II I
200 _|__|_____950_____
     150

21. There may be several factors contributing to the lack of representation of the 5' end of the mRNA. One has to deal with the possibility that the reverse transcriptase may not completely synthesize the DNA from the RNA template. The other reason may be that the 3' end of the copied DNA tends to fold back on itself thus providing a primer for the DNA polymerase. Additional preparation of the cDNA requires some digestion at the folded region. Since this folded region corresponds to the 5' end of the mRNA, some of the message is often lost.

22. Option (b) fits the expectation because the thick band in the offspring probably represents the bands at approximately the same position in both parents. The likelihood of such a match is expected to be low in the general population.

23. (a) Starting with zero at the top, the various patterns tell us that there is an E site at 1000bp because a new E site was brought in by the *Drosophila* fragment. By comparing the lanes of the double digests, one can see that there is an A site at 500bp, and a B site at 2500bp. For the 2000bp band of the E + B double digest, there are actually two fragments.

(b) Notice that the probe hybridizes consistently to the 2000bp fragment between the A and B restriction sites so the *rosy* gene is somewhere in that region.

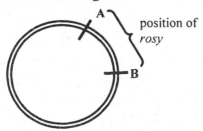

24. (a) The overall size of the fragment is 12kb. From the A + N digest, sites A and N must be 1kb apart. N must be 2kb from an E site. Pattern #5 is the likely choice. Notice that digest A + N breaks up the 6kb E fragment.

(b) By drawing lines though sections that hybridize to the probe, one can see that the only place of consistent overlap to the probe is the 1kb fragment between A and N.

25. Assuming that one has knowledge of the amino acid sequence of the protein, using the genetic code a DNA strand can be made which can be prepared for cloning into an appropriate vector or amplified by PCR. A variety of labeling techniques can then be used to identify complementary base sequences contained in the genomic library. One must know at least a portion of the amino acid sequence of the protein in order for the procedure to be applied.

Some problems can occur through degeneracy in the genetic code (not allowing construction of an appropriate probe), pseudogenes in the library (hybridizations with inappropriate fragments in the library), and variability of DNA sequences in the library due to introns (causing poor or background hybridization).

To overcome some of these problems, one can construct a variety of relatively small probes of different types that take into account the degeneracy in the code. By varying the conditions of hybridization (salt and temperature) one can reduce undesired hybridizations.

26. Taking the number of bases recognized by *Bam*HI as 6, there would be approximately 4096 base pairs between sites. Given that lambda DNA contains approximately 48,500 base pairs, there would be about 11.8 sites (48,500/4096).

27. Heating to 90-95^0 C denatures the double-stranded DNA so that it dissociates into single strands. It usually takes about five minutes, depending on the length and GC content of the DNA. Lowering the temperature to 50-70^0 C allows the primers to bind to the denatured DNA. Bringing the temperature to 70-75^0 C allows the heat stable DNA polymerase an opportunity to extend the primers by adding nucleotides to the 3' ends of each growing strand. Each PCR is designed with specific temperatures (not ranges) based on the characteristics of the DNAs (template and primers).

28. $T_m(^oC) = 81.5 + 0.41(\%GC) - (675/N) = 81.5 + 0.41(33.3) - (675/21) =$ about 63^{0}C. Subtracting 5^{0}C gives us a good starting point of about 58^{0}C for PCR with this primer. Notice that as the %GC and length increase, the $T_m(^oC)$ increases. GC pairs contain three hydrogen bonds rather than two as between AT pairs.

29. *Taq* polymerase is from a bacterium called *Thermus aquaticus* which typically lives in hot springs. It is heat stable like some other enzymes used in PCR which are isolated from thermal vents in the ocean floor.

30. ddNTPs are analogs of the "normal" deoxyribonucleotide triphosphates (dNTPs) but they lack a 3'-hydroxyl group. As DNA synthesis occurs, the DNA polymerase occasionally inserts a ddNTP into a growing DNA strand. Since there is no 3'-hydroxyl group, chain elongation cannot take place and resulting fragments are formed which can be separated by electrophoresis. Where the ddNTP was incorporated, the length of each strand and therefore the position of the particular ddNTP is established and used to eventually provide the base sequence of the DNA.

31. It is likely that the DNA which served as the template in the sequencing reaction was not pure so that at the same position (length) more than one type of ddNTP could be incorporated. This could be due to natural polymorphisms, often called single nucleotide polymorphisms (or SNPs) or impure sample.

Chapter 18: Genomics and Proteomics

Concept Areas	Corresponding Problems
Genome Annotation	1, 2, 3, 4, 5, 6, 7, 8, 17, 26, 28
Genomic Organization	6, 10, 11, 13, 15, 18, 24, 26
Genomics	9, 13, 14, 24
Essential Genes	12, 19, 20
Gene Duplication	16
Multigene Families	21, 22, 23, 27
Proteomics	17, 25

Vocabulary: Organization and Listing of Terms and Concepts

Structures and Substances

Genome

Proteome

Bacterial chromosomes

   DNA

   double-stranded

   circular, linear

   plasmids

   high density

      approximately one gene/kb

   operons

   Pseudomonas aeruginosa

   E. coli, Mycoplasma genitalium

Aquifex aeolicus

Borrelia burgdorferi, Vibrio cholerae

Bacillus sp., Haemophilus influenzae

Eukaryote

   variable gene density

   introns

   repetitive sequences

   intergenic spacer DNA

   Drosophila melanogaster

   Caenorhabditis elegans

   higher plants

      Arabidopsis thaliana

      rice and others

   humans

      3 billion nucleotides

protein-coding about 5%

transposable elements (LINE, *Alu*)

gene desert

about 25,000 genes

paralog

multigene families

alpha-globin, zeta

pseudogene

beta-globin

paralogous

intergenic regions

epsilon, gamma (Gγ, Aγ)

Immunoglobulin genes

antigen, antibody

B-cell, lymphocyte

IgM, IgD, IgG, IgA, IgE

heavy chain (H)

variable region

constant region (C)

light chain (L)

kappa, lambda

antibody-combining site

leader variable region (L-V)

joining region (J)

constant region (C)

Inteins

Indels

Orthologous genes

Bacterial proteome

Processes/Methods

Genomics

Proteomics

Human Genome Project (HGP)

map-based sequence

shotgun method

ELSI (ethical, legal, and social aspects)

TIGR (The Institute for Genome Research)

annotation

open reading frame (ORF)

ATG

TAA, TAG, TGA

Sequence verification

multiple coverage compiling

Genome evolution

Genome duplication

Gene duplication

Imprecise joining

Break-nibble-add

Sequence conservation

Proteomics

    2DGE two-dimensional gel electrophoresis

    MALDI

    high-throughput technology

Bacterial proteome changes

Concepts

Bioinformatics

Genomics

Proteomics

Annotation

Homology search

Genome organization comparisons

Unfinished tasks

Genome evolution

Minimum genome size (265-300 genes)

Comparative genomics (model organisms):

    Archaea

    Eubacteria

    Eukaryotes

        multigene families

        globin genes

        immunoglobin genes

Gene number *vs* protein number

Sequence conservation

Solutions to Problems and Discussion Questions

1. 0.8^5 = 33%

2. Knowing the sequence of DNA in an organism is only the beginning. Annotating the DNA is a significant challenge. Even at that, knowing how gene products interact in time and space (proteomics) will take additional rounds of technological advances as yet unconsidered. The work of Haas et al. identified variation in intron/exon splice sites, micro-exons, and alternative transcription start sites. Correlating various transcriptional and translational schemes with the phenotype will be an interesting adventure.

3. Aneuploidy in humans occurs for the sex chromosomes (X and Y) and three of the autosomes (13, 18, and 21). Other aneuploids are apparently not compatible with survival. Extra or missing X chromosomes are apparently tolerated because of dosage compensation, while Y chromosome aneuploids are most likely compatible with survival because of general paucity of Y-linked genes. Notice that the number of genes on chromosomes 13, 18, and 21 are the lowest for the autosomes. It is probably not coincidental that chromosomes with the fewest number of genes expressed in embryos and no known mechanism for dosage compensation are the only ones which survive as human aneuploids.

4. (a) Assuming an average gene size of 5,000 base pairs there would be about 6.7×10^7 base pairs comprising genes. Subtracting this value from 116.8 Mb gives 49.8 Mb between genes. Dividing 49.8 Mb by 13,379 genes gives about 3700 bases between genes.

(b) 54,934/13,379 = 4.11 exons per gene

(c) 48,257/13,379 = 3.61 introns per gene

(d) There is a marked increase in the number of genes that produce alternative transcripts.

5. Accurate annotation of genomes will not be a simple, straightforward process. Limitations on interpretation of sequence data will mean that new, uncharted levels of genomic, transcriptomic, and proteomic complications will be discovered. Since computer programs can only identify what is already predicted, manual verification and examination will be needed to bridge the gap between what we think we know and what has actually evolved over a few billion years. All the information will be highly significant in terms of understanding how organisms go about daily living and how we manage our relationships among them. For instance, one clinical application of genome sequence information is based on the development of antisense DNA to nullify the function of harmful RNAs and proteins within a cell. Opposite strand RNA transcription overlap generates the possibility of natural antisense interactions for gene regulation *in vivo* and may provide insight to the development of antisense therapies presently being developed.

6. First, calculate the number of base pairs in heterochromatic regions of the human genome: 0.15 X 3000Mb = 450 X 10⁶ bp

Since there is one gene for 69,697 bp in the *Drosophila* there could be:

450,000,000/69,697 = 6,456.5

genes in the heterochromatic region of humans. In all likelihood this number is an overestimate because overall gene density in *Drosophila* is approximately 10X higher than in humans. Applying this information to the above calculation, perhaps as many as 650 genes are located in human heterochromatin. If these simple calculations are correct, then a considerable number of genes are yet to be identified. In addition, because these genes are located in heterochromatin, they may possess unique properties.

7. Generally one can examine conserved sequences in other organisms to indicate that an ORF is likely a coding region. One can also match a sequence to previously described sequences which are known to code for proteins. The problem is not easily solved; that is, deciding which ORF is actually a gene. The shorter the ORF scan the more likely the overestimate of genes because ORFs longer than 200 are less likely to occur by chance.

8. Open reading frames are identified by computer programs based on identification of start (ATG) and stop (TAA, TGA, TAG) codons. Notice that the percentage of GC pairs compared to AT pairs is quite low in such punctuation triplets. Therefore, when scanning DNA sequences for ORFs with high AT content, many short sequences are obtained which are clearly not likely to be involved in protein production. However, when DNA is GC-rich, the likelihood of long ORFs similar to protein-coding size is increased. Therefore, the likelihood of falsely considering a sequence "protein-coding" increases with increasing GC content as indicated in the figure.

9. Functional genomicists seek to understand functional similarities of genomes across phylogenetic and evolutionary distances. Comparative genomicists analyze the arrangement and organization of families of genes within and among genomes.

10. Genomes of both types of organisms are composed of double stranded DNA (larger in eukaryotes) associated with proteins (more transient in prokaryotes). Both contain open reading frames, but those of prokaryotes are more densely packed. Both have some genes in clusters, but much more pronounced in prokaryotes (operons). There are a few repetitive sequences in prokaryotes, but this trend is much more common in eukaryotes. Both contain informational sequences but those of eukaryotes are often interrupted (introns).

11. Operons are genomic entities in which clusters of often functionally related genes are under coordinate control. In *A. aeolicus*, one operon contains six genes with widely varying functions. This finding and others like it merits reconsidering the classical definition of an operon.

12. The question as to how to define an organism's genome is complicated by a variety of symbiotic relationships which are known to exist in virtually all organisms. Plasmids are capable of carrying both essential and non-essential genes of the host. To complicate the matter, it is likely that all cells contain non-essential genes. In all likelihood, an organism's genome will probably come to encompass all genetic elements which can be shown to be stable cellular inhabitants.

13. General similarities and differences:

Yeast	Bacteria (E.coli)
DNA	DNA
double-stranded	double-stranded
chromosomes	circular (*E. coli*)
12.1 Mb	naked nucleic acid
6200 genes	4.6 Mb
	4397 genes

14. While greater DNA content per cell is associated with eukaryotes, one cannot universally equate genomic size with an increase in organismic complexity. There are numerous examples where DNA content per cell varies considerably among closely related species. Because of the diverse cell types of multicellular eukaryotes, a variety of gene products is required, which may be related to the increase in DNA content per cell. In addition, the advantage of diploidy automatically increases DNA content per cell. However, seeing the question in another way, it is likely that a much higher *percentage* of the genome of a prokaryote is actually involved in phenotype production than in a eukaryote. Eukaryotes have evolved the capacity to obtain and maintain what appears to be large amounts of "extra," perhaps "junk," DNA.

In contrast, prokaryotes, with their relatively short life cycles, are extremely efficient in their accumulation and use of their genomes. Given the larger amount of DNA per cell in eukaryotes and the requirement that the DNA be partitioned in an orderly fashion to daughter cells during cell division, certain mechanisms and structures (mitosis, nucleosomes, centromeres, etc.) have evolved for *packaging* the DNA. In addition, the genome is divided into separate entities (chromosomes) to perhaps facilitate the partitioning process in mitosis and meiosis.

15. Bacterial genes are densely packed in the chromosome. The protein-coding genes are mostly organized in polycistronic transcription units without introns. Eukaryotic genes are less densely packed in chromosomes and protein-coding genes are mostly organized as single transcription units with introns.

16. The relatively small compact genome of *Arabidopsis* resembles those of *Drosophila* and *C. elegans*. Both coding and noncoding DNA loss can account for the compact genome of *Arabidopsis*. Compared with rice, maize, and barley, there are fewer "gene-empty" repetitive DNA regions in intergenic areas and many copies of transposable elements (intergenic also) have been lost.

17. Increased protein production from approximately 25,000 genes is probably related to alternative splicing and various posttranslational processing schemes. In addition, a particular DNA segment may be read in a variety of ways and in two directions.

18. The human genome is composed of over 3 billion nucleotides in which about 5% code for genes. At least 50% of the genome is derived of transposable elements. Genes are unevenly distributed over chromosomes with clusters of gene-rich separated by gene-poor ones (deserts). Human genes tend to be larger and contain more and larger introns than do genes in invertebrates such as

Drosophila. Hundreds of genes have been transferred from bacteria into vertebrates. Duplicated regions which may facilitate chromosomal rearrangement are common. The human genome appears to contain approximately 20,000 to 25,000 protein-coding genes.

19. The issue here is whether the organism under consideration is independent and self-reproducing. It appears that the minimum number of genes for a free-living organism is in the range of 265-300. Symbionts can have much smaller genomes and exist with fewer genes because of materials supplied by the host cell. As long as one defines the life style (free-living or symbiont) of the organism in question, it is informative to consider how many genes are needed to accomplish the task of "living."

20. Assuming that the APS strain is the ancestral strain, the remaining strains appear to have smaller genome sizes indicating genome reduction. The smallest *Buchnera* genome is approximately 448kb compared to a genome size of *M. genitalium* of about 600 kb with about 480 protein-coding genes. The APS genome codes for about 564 genes in its 641kb genome. A gene is coded every 1136 bp (641,000/564) for the APS strain and every 1250 bp (600,000/480) for *M. genitalium*. Given these data, the CCE species should code for approximately (448,000/1193) = 375.5 genes. (Note: 1193 was obtained as the average gene spacing of the two bacterial species mentioned above.) Using these calculations, the CCE strain would contain fewer genes than *M. genitalium*. There are other possible approaches to determine minimum genome size to sustain life. Among them would include computational studies whereby one might estimate the number of essential chemical reactions that are needed for life. Another would be to take an organism with a small number of genes, then systematically mutate genes to see if elimination of genes caused reduced survival. By eliminating individual and groups of genes by mutation, the minimum number might be obtainable.

21. V_L = variable region of the light chain, C_H = constant region of the heavy chain, IgG = an immunoglobin class which represents approximately 80% of the antibodies in the blood. J = genes that specify a portion of the V region which includes a portion of the hypervariable region. D = a region between V and J in the heavy immunoglobin chain.

22. The number of combinations is determined by a simple multiplication of the number of genes in each class: V X D X J X C. Thus, in this case the answer would be 10 V X 30 D X 50 J X 3 C = 45,000.

23. Again, notice in the *Insights and Solutions* section in this chapter, the total number of combinations is determined by simple multiplication. In this case, for the heavy chain 5 V X 10 D X 20 J = 1000, and for the light chain 10 V X 100 J = 1000. The final total would be 1000 X 1000 = 10^6.

24. Selection for gene order might occur as a result of any one or combination of the following: functional and/or structural interaction of proteins coded in a gene cluster, similar localization of gene transcripts in a cell, and operon structure or common regulation. In addition, horizontal gene transfer resulting from transformation and/or transduction disseminates gene combinations in forms different from those generated by typical vertical transfer (parent to offspring).

25. In general, one would expect certain factors (such as heat or salt) to favor evolution to increase protein stability: distribution of ionic interactions on the surface, density of hydrophobic residues and interactions, number of hydrogen and disulfide bonds. By examining the codon table, a high GC ratio would favor amino acids Ala, Gly, Pro, Arg, and Trp and minimize the use of Ile, Phe, Lys, Asn, and Tyr. How codon bias influences actual protein stability is not yet understood.

Most genomic sequences change by relatively gradual responses to mild selection over long periods of time. They strongly resemble their patterns of common descent. While the same can be said for organisms adapted to extreme environments, extraordinary physiological demands may dictate unexpected sequence bias.

26. Pseudogenes are nonfunctional versions of genes that resemble gene sequences but contain significant nucleotide changes which prevent their expression. They are formed by gene duplication and subsequent mutation.

27. While the β-globin gene family is a relatively large (60kb) sequence and restriction analyses show that it is composed of six genes, one is a pseudogene and therefore does not produce a product. The five functional genes each contain two similarly-sized introns which, when included with non-coding flanking regions (5' and 3') and spacer DNA between genes, account for the 95% mentioned in the question.

28. Since structural and chemical factors determine the function of a protein, it is likely to have several proteins share a considerable amino acid sequence identity but not be functionally identical. Since the *in vivo* function of such a protein is determined by secondary and tertiary structures as well as local surface chemistries in active or functional sites, the nonidentical sequences may have considerable influence on function. Note that the query matches to different positions within the target proteins. A number of other factors suggesting different functions include: associations with other molecules (cytoplasmic, membrane, or extracellular), chemical nature and position of binding domains, post-translational modification, or signal sequences.

Chapter 19: Applications and Ethics of Genetic Engineering

Concept Areas	Corresponding Problems
Use of Genetically Engineered Products	1, 2, 3, 4, 18
Genetic Engineering	5, 6, 7, 21
Diagnosing and Screening Genetic Disorders	12, 13, 14, 15, 16, 19, 20, 24, 25
Gene Therapy	6, 7, 8, 9, 10, 11, 17, 22
Genome Analysis	12
Ethical Issues	23

Vocabulary: Organization and Listing of Terms and Concepts

Structures and Substances

Recombinant DNA molecules

Transgenic organisms

Plants

    herbicide resistance

    glyphosate

    EPSP synthase

    Agrobacterium tumifaciens

        Ti plasmid

        corn, soybeans, cotton

        rice, canola

        β-carotene

Animals

    livestock, salmon

Pharmaceutical products

    insulin

fusion polypeptide

Pombe disease

edible vaccines

    inactivated vaccines

    attenuated vaccines

    subunit vaccine

    hepatitis B

Allele-specific oligonucleotides

    cystic fibrosis

    transmembrane conductance regulator (CFTR)

DNA chip

p53

Processes/Methods

Genetic engineering

Transgenesis

Organismic enhancement

Chapter 19 Applications and Ethics of Genetic Engineering

Vaccine production

Medical diagnosis

Genetic screening

   amniocentesis

   chorionic villus sampling

      RFLP

Microarrays

   high-throughput methods

   genotyping microarray

   single-nucleotide polymorphism (SNP)

   PCR

   gene expression microarray

   cDNA

      DLBCL

Targeted medical therapy

   CML, BCR

Pharmacogenomics

   rational drug design

Gene therapy

   retroviral vectors (and others)

   severe combined immunodeficiency (SCID)

      adenosine deaminase (ADA)

      somatic gene therapy

      germ-line gene therapy

      enhancement gene therapy

Gene testing

   RFLP

DNA profiling

   DNA fingerprints

   minisatellites

   variable number tandem repeats (VNTR)

   applications

      forensic

        cold cases

   short tandem repeats (STR)

   (CODIS)

   capillary gel electrophoresis

Concepts

Genetically modified organisms

Environmental concerns

Diagnostics

Therapy

   somatic gene therapy

   germline gene therapy

   enhancement gene therapy

   associated problems

   guidelines

Ethical (ELSI) Transgenic systems

Vaccine administration

Solutions to Problems and Discussion Questions

1. The nature of the digestion process is the breakdown of foodstuffs for eventual absorption by the small intestine. Antigens are usually quite large molecules, and in the process of digestion, they are sometimes broken down into smaller molecules, thus becoming ineffective in stimulating the immune system. Some individuals are allergic to the food they eat, testifying to the fact that all antigens are not completely degraded or modified by digestion. In some cases ingested antigens do indeed stimulate the immune system (oral polio vaccine) and provide a route for immunization. Localized (intestinal) immunity can sometimes be stimulated by oral introduction of antigens and in some cases this can offer immunity to ingested pathogens.

2. Kleter and Peijnenburg used the BLAST tool from the

http://www.ncbi.nlm.nih.gov/BLAST

website to conduct a series of alignment comparisons of transgenic sequences with sequences of known allergenic proteins. Of 33 transgenic proteins screened for identities of at least six contiguous amino acids found in allergenic proteins, 22 gave positive results.

3. From a purely scientific viewpoint, there will be no added danger to consuming cow's milk from cloned animals. However, some individuals may have an aversion to organismic cloning and supporting such activities through consumption of products of cloned organisms may be viewed negatively on moral grounds. It is likely that public sentiment will pressure for labeling of "cloned products" on the grounds that consumers should be able to make an informed choice as to the origin of such products.

4. (a) Both the saline and column extracts of Lkt50 appear to be capable of inducing at least 50% neutralization of toxicity when injected into rabbits. (b) In order for a successful edible vaccine to be developed, numerous hurdles must be overcome. First, the immunogen must be stably incorporated into the host plant hereditary material and the host must express only that immunogen. During feeding, the immunogen must be transported across the intestinal wall unaltered, or altered in such a way as to stimulate the desired immune response. There must be guarantees that potentially harmful byproducts of transgenesis have not been produced. In other words, broad ecological and environmental issues must be addressed to prevent a transgenic plant from becoming an unintended vector for harm to the environment or any organisms feeding on the plant (directly or indirectly).

5. Glyphosate (a herbicide) inhibits EPSP, a chloroplast enzyme involved in the synthesis of the amino acids phenylalanine, tyrosine, and tryptophan. To generate glyphosate resistance in crop plants, a fusion gene was created which introduced a viral promoter to control the EPSP synthetase gene. The fusion product was placed into the Ti vector and transferred to *A. tumifaciens* which was used to infect crop cells. Calluses were selected on the basis of their resistance to glyphosate. Resistant calluses were later developed into transgenic plants.   There is a remote possibility that such an "accident" can occur as suggested in the question. However, in retracing the steps to generate the resistant plant in the first place, it seems more likely that the trait will not "escape" from the plant; rather that the engineered *A. tumifaciens* may escape, infect and transfer glyphosate resistance to pest species.

6. Enhancement therapy using gene products benefits from the application of modern biotechnology without being burdened by alteration of the genome. Enhancement gene therapy, however, opens the door to a variety of ethical issues. What limits can/should be imposed on individuals or institutions seeking to improve human qualities? What qualities should be open for enhancement? Gene therapy is not without medical and ethical risks.

7. As with all therapies, the cure must be less hazardous than the disease. In the case of viral-mediated gene therapy, the antigenicity of the virus must not interfere with the delivery system; such antigenicity can cause inflammation or more severe immunologic responses. Combating the host immune response may involve the use of immunosuppressive drugs or modification of the vector. The duration of desired gene expression at the diseased site is an issue. Short-period expression may require repeated exposure to the vehicle which may present undesired responses. For some diseases, local gene therapy through inhalation or injection may produce fewer side effects than systemic exposure. Adenoviruses appear to be particularly useful for gene therapy because they can infect non-dividing cells and they can accept relatively large amounts of additional DNA (30kb or more).

8. Somatic gene therapy involves attempts to alter the genetic material in non-germ line cells. Clinical trials are currently underway. Germ line therapy, while certainly being more efficient (although perhaps more difficult technically) alters the germ line and is transmitted to offspring. There are considerable ethical problems associated with germ plasm therapy. It recalls previous attempts of the eugenics movements of past decades which involved the use of selective breeding to purify the human stock. Some present-day biologists have said publicly that germ line gene therapy will *not* be conducted.

Enhancement gene therapy raises a considerable ethical dilemma. Should genetic techniques be used to enhance human potential? It is generally felt that enhancement gene therapy, like germ line therapy is unacceptable.

9. A major problem with engineering the capsid to specifically engage target cells is that the capsid itself is now altered. A reconfigured capsid, either by size or shape, may no longer serve its packaging and infecting role properly. One may end up with a very specific viral-target interaction, but the virus may be incapable of replicating efficiently. A nongenetic approach is to use bispecific molecules to conjugate vectors with target cells. Such approaches often employ desired electrostatic bridges or monoclonal antibody conjugates. While such approaches often work in the test tube, their application *in vivo* is often limited due to instability.

10. p53 and pRB are tumor suppressor proteins and are required by the cell to effectively monitor the cell cycle. Reduction in their activity would diminish normal cell cycle controls and most likely lead to cancer. It would be especially important if such viral vectors are intended to treat cancer where cell cycle control is likely already compromised.

11. (a,b) One of the main problems with gene therapy is delivery of the desired virus to the target tissue in an effective manner. Several of the problems involving the use of retroviral vectors are the following. (1) Integration into the host must be cell specific so as not to damage non-target cells. (2) Retroviral integration into host cell genomes only occurs if the host cell is replicating. (3) Insertion of the viral genome might influence non-target but essential genes. (4) Retroviral genomes have a low cloning capacity and cannot carry large inserted sequences as are many human genes. (5) There is a possibility that recombination with host viruses will produce an infectious virus that may be harmful.

(c) The question posed here plays on the practical versus the ethical. It would certainly be more efficient (although perhaps more difficult technically) to engineer germ tissue, for once it is done in a family, the disease would be eliminated. However, there are considerable ethical problems associated with germ plasm therapy. It recalls previous attempts of the eugenics movements of past decades which involved the use of selective breeding to purify the human stock. Some present-day biologists have said publically that germ line gene therapy will *not* be conducted.

12. (a) A microarray is a solid support containing an orderly arrangement of DNA samples. A typical array contains thousands of DNA spots that may contain small oligonucleotides, cDNAs or short genomic sequences. Labeled sequences hybridize to the immobilized DNAs by standard base pairing. Such technology allows a method for monitoring RNA expression levels of thousands of genes in virtually any cell population. **(b)** Using microarray technology, researchers can observe the overall behavior of the genome in cancer and normal cells and by comparison, determine which genes are active or inactive under various circumstances. It is possible to identify the set of genes whose expression or lack thereof defines the properties of each tumor type. This application can therefore lead to precise diagnosis and refine possible therapies. In addition, microarray profiling can be used to determine the efficacy of particular therapies. For instance, one can monitor responses to radiation and/or chemotherapy to determine the degree to which cells are responding.

13. Short tandem repeats are very similar to VNTRs except that the repeat motif is much shorter (2 to 9 base pairs). STRs have been used to generate a marker panel for DNA profiling. STR typing is less expensive, less labor intensive, and quicker to perform than traditional DNA typing.

14. *Drosophila* is a unique experimental organism in that there is a vast knowledge of its genetics, it is easily cultured and genetically manipulated, and it contains unique chromosomes, polytene chromosomes, which allow visual landmarks. Coupled with probe-labeling (sequence tagged sites), that provide visible landmarks (chromomeres) and ease of manipulation, one can actually see where important genes are located in chromosomes. The *Drosophila* genome also contains P elements which allow sequence markers to be inserted into the genome. Microdissection of chromosomes is also useful in developing specific clones for sequencing. In addition, techniques (*in situ* hybridization) have been developed to allow scientists to actually determine the distributions of gene activities in all tissues of the organism.

15. Even though you have developed a method for screening seven of the mutations described, it is possible that negative results can occur when the person carries the gene for CF. In other words, the specific probes (or allele-specific oligonucleotides) that have been developed will not necessarily be useful for screening all mutant genes. In addition, the cost-effectiveness of such a screening proposal would need to be considered.

16. Since both mutations occur in the CF gene, children that possess both alleles will suffer from CF. With both parents heterozygous, each child born will have a 25% chance of developing CF.

17. In the case of haplo-insufficient mutations, gene therapy holds promise; however for "gain-of-function" mutations it is likely that the mutant gene's activity or product must be compromised. Addition of a normal gene probably will not help.

18. In general, bacteria do not process eukaryotic proteins in the same manner as eukaryotes. Transgenic eukaryotes are more likely to correctly process and express eukaryotic proteins, thus increasing the likelihood of their normal biological activity.

19. It will hybridize by base complementation to the normal DNA sequence.

20. The answer provided here is based on the condition that individual I-2 is a carrier and the son, II-4, has the disorder. The 3kb fragment occurs in the normal I-1 father and the normal son II-1. The affected son, II-4, has the 4kb fragment. One daughter, II-2, is a carrier while the other daughter, II-3, is not a carrier.

21. One method is to use the amino acid sequence of the protein to produce the gene synthetically. Alternatively, since the introns are spliced out of the hnRNA in the production of mRNA, if mRNA can be obtained, it can be used to make DNA (cDNA) through the use of reverse transcriptase.

22. The two major problems described here are common concerns related to genetic engineering. The first is the localization of the introduced DNA into the target tissue and target location in the genome. Inappropriate targeting may have serious consequences. In addition, it is often difficult to control the output of introduced DNA. Genetic regulation is complicated and subject to a number of factors including upstream and downstream signals as well as various post-transcriptional processing schemes. Artificial control of these factors will prove difficult.

23. At this point there is considerable reluctance to allow the open sharing of genetic information among institutions. In general, the establishment of governmental databases containing our most intimate information is viewed with skepticism. It is likely considerable time and discussion will elapse before such databases are established.

24. Using restriction enzyme analysis to detect point mutations in humans is a tedious trial-and-error process. Given the size of the human genome and the relatively low number of unique restriction enzymes, the likelihood of matching a specific point mutation, separate from other normal sequence variations, to a desired gene is low.

25. The child in question is a carrier of the deletion in the beta-globin gene, just as the parents are carriers. Its genotype is therefore $\beta^A\beta^o$.

Chapter 20: Developmental Genetics

Concept Areas	Corresponding Problems
Developmental Concepts	1, 3, 14
Methods	2, 8, 9, 10, 16, 17, 21
Differential Transcription in Development	9, 10
Maternal-Effect Genes and Body Plans	4, 5,
Zygotic and Homeotic genes	6, 7, 11, 12, 13, 18, 19, 20
Genetics of Arabidopsis	22, 23
Cell-Cell Interactions in C. elegans	24, 25, 26

Vocabulary: Organization and Listing of Terms and Concepts

Structures and Substances

Zygote

Drosophila

  master regulator

  maternal-effect genes

    positional information

  zygotic genes

  segmentation genes

    gap genes

    pair-rule genes

    segment polarity genes

homeotic genes

  selector

  homeobox

  homeodomain

Arabidopsis

  MADS box proteins

Caenorhabditis elegans

  male, hermaphrodite

  lin, let, etc.

  vulva

Maternal cytoplasm

Blastoderm

Processes/Methods

Development

  specification

  determination

  differentiation

  cascades of gene action

  cytoplasmic localization

  cell-cell interaction

    intercellular communication

Chapter 20 Developmental Genetics

Analyses

    Drosophila

        oogenesis

        syncytial cellular blastoderm

        posterior pole

        germ cells

        Hox genes

        segmentation

            homeotic mutants

            positional cues

        signaling pathways

    Arabidopsis thaliana

    C. elegans

        vulval formation

Concepts

    Development (F20.1)

        transcriptional events

            different cells

            different times

        cell and tissue interactions

        cytoplasmic localization

    Maternal influences

        anterior-posterior gradient

        positional information

    Zygotic gene influences s

    Homeotic genes

    Homology among organism

    Evolutionary relationships

––––––––––––––

F20.1 Illustration of the relationship between determination and differentiation. Determination sets the program which will later be revealed by differentiation. The variable gene activity hypothesis suggests that different sets of genes are transcriptionally active in differentiated cells.

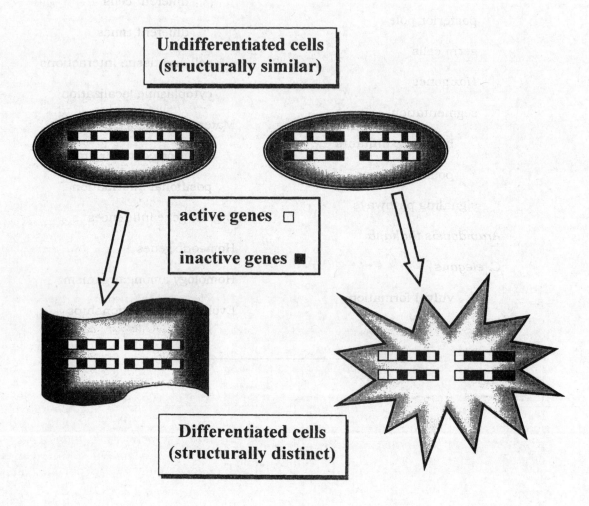

Solutions to Problems and Discussion Questions

1. *Determination* refers to early developmental and regulatory events which set eventual patterns of gene activity. Determination is not the end result of the regulatory activity, rather, it is the process by which the developmental fate of a particular cell type is fixed. *Differentiation* on the other hand follows determination and is the manifestation, in terms of genetic, physiological, and morphological changes, of the determined state.

2. The fact that nuclei from almost any source remain transcriptionally and translationally active substantiates the fact that the genetic code and the ancillary processes of transcription and translation are compatible throughout the animal and plant kingdoms. Because the egg represents an isolated, "closed" system which can be mechanically, environmentally, and to some extent biochemically manipulated, various conditions may be developed which allow one to study facets of gene regulation. For instance, the influence of transcriptional enhancers and suppressors may be studied along with factors which impact on translational and post-translational processes. Combinations of injected nuclei may reveal nuclear-nuclear interactions which could not normally be studied by other methods.

3. The syncytial blastoderm is formed as nuclei migrate to the egg's outer margin or cortex, where additional divisions take place. Plasma membranes organize around nuclei, thus creating the cellular blastoderm.

4. Genes that control early development are often dependent on the deposition of their products (mRNA, transcription factors, various structural proteins, etc.) in the egg by the mother. Such maternal effect genes control early events such as defining anterior-posterior polarity. Such products are placed in eggs during oogenesis and are activated immediately after fertilization.

5. It is possible that your screen was more inclusive, that is, it identified more subtle alterations than the screen of Wieschaus and Schüpbach. In addition, your screen may have included some zygotic effect mutations which were dependent on the action of maternal effect genes.

6. Zygotic genes are activated or repressed depending on their response to maternal-effect gene products. Three subsets of zygotic genes divide the embryo into segments. These segmentation genes are normally transcribed in the developing embryo and their mutations have embryonic lethal phenotypes. The maternal genotype contains zygotic genes and these are passed to the embryo as with any other gene.

7. The three main classes of zygotic genes are (a) *gap* genes which specify adjacent segments, (2) *pair-rule* genes which specify every other segment and a part of each segment, and (3) *segment polarity* genes which specify homologous parts of each segment.

8. Because the polar cytoplasm contains information to form germ cells, one would expect such a transplantation procedure to generate germ cells in the anterior region. Work done by Illmensee and Mahowald in 1974 verified this expectation.

9. There are several somewhat indirect methods for determining transcriptional activity of a given gene in different cell types. First, if protein products of a given gene are present in different cell types, it can be assumed that the responsible gene is being transcribed. Second, if one is able to actually observe, microscopically, gene activity, as is the case in some specialized chromosomes (such as polytene chromosomes), gene activity can be inferred by the presence of localized chromosomal puffs.   A more direct and common practice to assess transcription of particular genes is to use labeled probes. If a labeled probe can be obtained which contains base sequences that are complementary to the transcribed RNA, then such probes will hybridize to that RNA if present in different tissues. This technique is called *in situ* hybridization and is a powerful tool in the study of gene activity during development.

10. There are a variety of approaches to determine the level of control of a particular gene. First, one may determine whether levels of hnRNA are consistent among various cell types of interest. This is often accomplished by either direct isolation of the RNA and assessment by northern blotting or by use of *in situ* hybridization. If the hnRNA pools for a given gene are consistent in various cell types, then transcriptional control can be eliminated as a possibility. Support for translational control can be achieved directly by determining, in different cell types, the presence of a variety of mRNA species with common sequences. This can be accomplished only in cases where sufficient knowledge exists for specific mRNA trapping or labeling. Clues as to translational control *via* alternative splicing can sometimes be achieved by examining the amino acid sequence of proteins. Similarities in certain structural/functional motifs may indicate alternative RNA processing.

11. *Hox* genes are clustered and have particular properties which include the encoding of a DNA-binding domain and a homeodomain. Such genes are organized into clusters. All *homeobox* genes are not *Hox* genes because they do not occur in clusters.

12. The "gain-of-function" *Antp* mutation causes the wild type *Antennapedia* gene to be expressed in the head and mutant flies have legs on the head in place of antenna. In general, such gain-of-function mutations cause new or enhanced activity on a gene product.

13. Many of the appendages of the head, including the mouth parts and the antennae, are evolutionary derivatives of ancestral leg structures. In *spineless aristapedia,* the distal portion of the antenna is replaced by its ancestral counterpart, the distal portion of the leg (tarsal segments). Because the replacement of the arista (end of the antenna) can occur by a mutation in a single gene, one would consider that one "selector" gene distinguishes aristal from tarsal structures. Notice that a "one-step" change is involved in the interchange of leg and antennal structures.

14. Because of the regulatory nature of *homeotic* genes in fundamental cellular activities of determination and differentiation, it would be difficult to ignore their possible impact on oncogenesis. Homeotic genes encode DNA binding domains which influence gene expression and any factor which influences gene expression may, under some circumstances, influence cell cycle control. However attractive this model, there have been no homeotic transformations noted in mammary glands, so the typical expression of mutant homeotic genes in insects is not revealed in mammary tissue according to Lewis (2000). A substantial number of experiments will be needed to establish a functional link between homeotic gene mutation and cancer induction. Mutagenesis and transgenesis experiments are likely to be most productive in establishing a cause-effect relationship.

15. Because in *ftz/ftz* embryos, the engrailed product is absent and in *en/en* embryos *ftz* expression is normal, one can conclude that the *ftz* gene product regulates, either directly or indirectly, *en*. Because the *ftz* gene is expressed normally in *en/en* embryos, the product of the *engrailed* gene does not regulate expression of *ftz*.

16. Two coupled approaches might be used. First, one could make transgenic flies which contain a series of deletions spanning all segments of the *bicoid* mRNA; the coding region, 5' and 3' untranslated regions. Comparison of stabilities of individual, deleted mRNAs with controls would indicate whether a particular segment of the mRNA contains a degradation signal sequence. If a degradation-sensitive region or signal sequence is located by deletion, that same intact region, when ligated to a non-involved, non-degraded mRNA (like a ribosomal protein or tubulin mRNA) should foster degradation in a manner similar to the *bicoid* mRNA.

17. First, it would be interesting to know whether inhibitors of mitochondrial-ribosomal translation would interfere with germ cell formation. Second, I would like to know what types of mRNAs are being translated with these ribosomes.

18.

Pre- cell cycle remodeling:

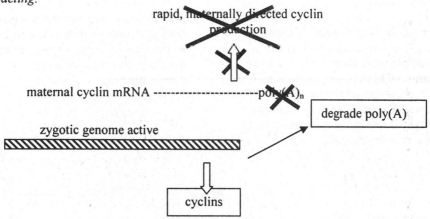

Post- cell cycle remodeling:

217

19. The typical developmental sequence for axis and segment formation in *Drosophila* proceeds from the gap genes to the pair-rule genes to the segment polarity genes. The fact that *fushi-tarazu* (*ftz*) is affected by early (anterior-posterior determining genes) and gap genes indicates that *ftz* functions after those genes. That segment polarity genes are influenced by *ftz* indicates that *ftz* functions earlier, thus placing *ftz* in the pair-rule group of genes.

20. Given the information in the problem, it is likely that this gene normally controls the expression of BX-C genes in all body segments. The wild type product of *esc* stored in the egg may be required to interpret the information correctly stored in the egg cortex.

21. (a) The term "rescued" is often used when the introduction of genes from an outside source (within or among species) restores the wild type phenotype from a mutant organism.

(b) Results such as these, and there are many like them, indicate the extreme conservation of protein structure and function across phylogenetically distant organisms. Such results attest to the conservation from a distant common ancestor of fundamental molecular species during development. Failure to adhere to a common developmental theme is rewarded by death.

22. Three classes of flower *homeotic* genes are known that are activated in an overlapping pattern to specify various floral organs. Class *A* genes give rise to sepals. Expression of *A* and *B* class genes specify petals, *B* and *C* genes control stamen formation and expression of *C* genes gives rise to carpels.

23. The *Polycomb* gene family induces changes in chromatin that influence *Hox* gene expression. A gene in *Arabidopsis* has significant homology to the *Polycomb* gene family and works by altering chromatin structure. Such parallel functions indicate that mechanisms of regulation are conserved over vast evolutionary distances.

24. Because signal-receptor interactions depend on membrane-bound structures, the pathway can only work with adjacent cells. The advantage of such a system is that only cells in a certain location will be influenced --- those in contact. A disadvantage would occur if large groups of cells are to be induced into a particular developmental pathway or if cells not in contact need to be induced.

25. Since *her-1*⁻ mutations cause males to develop into hermaphrodites, and *tra-1*⁻ causes hermaphrodites to develop into males, one may hypothesize that the *her-1*⁺ gene produces a product which suppresses hermaphrodite development, while the *tra-1*⁺ gene product is needed for hermaphrodite development. Information provided in Problem 26 supports this hypothesis.

26. (a) If the *her-1*⁺ product acts as a negative regulator, then when the gene is mutant, suppression over *tra-1*⁺ is lost and hermaphroditism would be the result. This hypothesis fits the information provided.

(b) The double mutant should be male because even though there is no suppression from *her-1*⁻, there is no *tra-1*⁺ product to support hermaphrodite development.

Chapter 21: Quantitative Genetics

Concept Areas	Corresponding Problems
Phenotypic Expression	1, 2, 10, 21, 22, 24, 26, 30
Continuous Variation and Polygenes	1, 2, 3, 4, 5, 6, 7, 23, 24, 25, 27, 28, 29
Heritability	2, 8, 9, 12, 13, 14, 16, 17, 18, 19, 20
Statistics	11, 15
Twin Studies	2, 8, 9

Vocabulary: Organization and Listing of Terms and Concepts

Structures and Substances

Threshold traits

Meristic traits

QTLS

RFLP

Dizygotic twin (fraternal)

Monozygotic twin (identical)

Processes/Methods

Transmission genetics

Quantitative, polygenic inheritance

Discontinuous traits

Continuous traits

   multiple-factor hypothesis

   additive (cumulative, quantitative)

alleles

   nonadditive alleles

   polygenic

$1/4^n$

Statistical analysis

   descriptive summary

   statistical inference

   statistics

   parameters

      mean

         central tendency

      frequency distribution

      variance

      standard deviation

      standard error of the mean

      covariance

Heritability

   broad-sense heritability

      phenotypic variation

      environmental variance

219

genetic variance

interaction (genotype by environment)

narrow-sense heritability

additive variance

dominance variance

interactive variance

artificial selection

response

selection differential

realized heritability

twin studies

monozygotic (identical) twins

dizygotic (fraternal) twins

concordant, discordant

Concepts

Transmission genetics

Quantitative inheritance

Heredity and environment

Mapping quantitative traits

restriction fragment length polymorphism

quantitative trait loci

Heritability

inbred lines

heritability index (H^2)

broad-sense heritability

narrow-sense heritability

Twin studies

Chapter 21 Quantitative Genetics

Solutions to Problems and Discussion Questions

1. In *discontinuous* variation the influences of each gene pair are not additive and more typical Mendelian ratios such as 9:3:3:1 and 3:1 result. In *continuous* variation, different gene pairs interact (usually additively) to produce a phenotype that is less "stepwise" in distribution. Inheritance involving polygenic systems follows a more continuous distribution.

2. (a) *Polygenes* are sets of genes that are involved in determining continuously varying or multiple factor traits.

(b) *Additive alleles* are those alleles which account for the hereditary influence on the phenotype in an additive way.

(c) *Correlation* is a statistic that varies from -1 to +1 and describes the extent to which variation in one trait is associated with variation in another. It does not imply that a cause-and-effect relationship exists between two traits.

(d) *Monozygotic twins* are derived from a single fertilized egg and are thus genetically identical to each other. They provide a method for determining the relative influences of genetics and environment on certain traits. *Dizygotic twins* arise from two eggs fertilized by two sperm cells. They have the same genetic relationship as siblings.
The role of genetics and the role of the environment can be studied by comparing the expression of traits in monozygotic and dizygotic twins. The higher concordance value for monozygotic twins as compared with the value for dizygotic twins indicates a significant genetic component for a given trait.

(e) *Heritability* is a measure of the degree to which the phenotypic variation of a given trait is due to genetic factors. A high heritability indicates that genetic factors are major contributors to phenotypic variation, while environmental factors have little impact.

(f) QTL stands for Quantitative Trait Loci, which are multiple genes that have a major contribution to a quantitative trait.

3. (a) Since 1/256 of the F_2 plants are 20 cm and 1/256 are 40 cm, there must be 4 gene pairs involved in determining flower size.

(b) Since there are nine size classes, one can conduct the following backcross:

$$AaBbCcDd \quad X \quad AABBCCDD$$

The frequency distribution in the backcross would be:

1/16	=	40 cm
4/16	=	37.5 cm
6/16	=	35 cm
4/16	=	32.5 cm
1/16	=	30 cm

(c) The mean is the sum of the individual values divided by the number of values:

$$mean = 35.0 \text{ cm}$$

The variance is the sum of the squared differences between the individual values and the mean, divided by n-1:

$$variance = 6.67 \text{ cm}$$

The standard deviation is the square root of the variance:

$$standard \ deviation = 2.58 \text{ cm}$$

4. If you add the numbers given for the ratio, you obtain the value of sixteen, which is indicative of a dihybrid cross. The distribution is that of a dihybrid cross with additive effects.

(a) Because a dihybrid result has been identified, two loci are involved in the production of color. There are two alleles at each locus for a total of four alleles.

(b, c) Because the description of red, medium red, *etc.*, gives us no indication of a *quantity* of color in any form of units, we would not be able to actually quantify a unit amount for each change in color. We can say that each additive allele provides an equal unit amount to the phenotype and the colors differ from each other in multiples of that unit amount. The number of additive alleles needed to produce each phenotype is given below:

1/16	= dark red	=	AABB
4/16	= medium-dark red	=	2AABb
			2AaBB
6/16	= medium red	=	AAbb
			4AaBb
			aaBB
4/16	= light red	=	2aaBb
			2Aabb
1/16	= white	=	aabb

(d)

F$_1$ = all light red
F$_2$ = 1/4 medium red
    2/4 light red
    1/4 white

5. (a) It is *possible* that two parents of moderate height can produce offspring that are much taller or shorter than either parent because segregation can produce a variety of gametes as illustrated below:

rrSsTtuu   X   RrSsTtUu
(moderate)   (moderate)

Offspring from this cross can range from very tall *RrSSTTUu* (14 "tall" units) to very short *rrssttuu* (8 "small" units).

(b) If the individual with a minimum height, *rrssttuu*, is married to an individual of intermediate height *RrSsTtUu*, the offspring can be no taller than the height of the tallest parent. Notice that there is no way of having more than four uppercase alleles in the offspring.

6. As you read this question, notice that the strains are inbred, therefore homozygous, and that approximately 1/250 represent the shortest and tallest groups in the F$_2$ generation. See 1/4^n formula in the text.

(a, b) Referring to the text, see that where four gene pairs act additively, the proportion of one of the extreme phenotypes to the total number of offspring is 1/256. The same may be said for the other extreme type. The extreme types in this problem are the 12cm and 36cm plants. From this observation one would conclude that there are four gene pairs involved.

(c) If there are four gene pairs, there are nine (2n+1) phenotypic categories and eight increments between these categories. Since there is a difference of 24cm between the extremes, 24cm/8 = 3cm for each increment (each of the additive alleles).

(d) A typical F$_1$ cross that produces a "typical" F$_2$ distribution would be where all gene pairs are heterozygous (*AaBbCcDd*), independently assorting, and additive. There are many possible sets of parents that would give an F$_1$ of this genotype.

The limitation is that each parent has genotypes that give a height of 24cm as stated in the problem. Because the parents are inbred, it is expected that they are fully homozygous. An example:

AABBccdd   X   aabbCCDD

(e) Since the *aabbccdd* genotype gives a height of 12cm and each uppercase allele adds 3cm to the height, there are many possibilities for an 18cm plant:

AAbbccdd,

AaBbccdd,

aaBbCcdd, etc.

Any plant with seven uppercase letters will be 33cm tall:

AABBCCDd,

AABBCcDD,

AABbCCDD, for example.

7. (a) There is a fairly continuous range of "quantitative" phenotypes in the F$_2$ and an F$_1$ that is between the phenotypes of the two parents; therefore, one can conclude that some phenotypic blending is occurring that is probably the result of several gene pairs acting in an additive fashion. Because the extreme phenotypes (6cm and 30cm) each represent 1/64 of the total, it is likely that there are three gene pairs in this cross. Remember, trihybrid crosses that show independent assortment of genes have a denominator (4^3) of 64 in ratios. Also, the fact that there are seven categories of phenotypes, which, because of the relationship 2n+1 = 7, would give the number of gene pairs (n) of 3. The genotypes of the parents would be combinations of alleles that would produce a 6cm (*aabbcc*) tail and a 30cm (*AABBCC*) tail, while the 18cm offspring would have a genotype of *AaBbCc*.

(b) A mating of an *AaBbCc* (for example) pig with the 6cm *aabbcc* pig would result in the following offspring:

Gametes (18cm tail)	Gamete (6cm tail)	Offspring
ABC	abc	AaBbCc (18cm)
ABc	abc	AaBbcc (14cm)
AbC	abc	AabbCc (14cm)
Abc	abc	Aabbcc (10cm)
aBC	abc	aaBbCc (14cm)
aBc	abc	aaBbcc (10cm)
abC	abc	aabbCc (10cm)
abc	abc	aabbcc (6cm)

In this example, a 1:3:3:1 ratio is the result. However, had a different 18cm tailed-pig been selected, a different ratio would occur:

AABbcc X *aabbcc*

Gametes (18cm tail)	Gamete (6cm tail)	Offspring
ABc	abc	AaBbcc (14cm)
Abc	abc	Aabbcc (10cm)

8. For height, notice that average differences between MZ twins reared together (1.7 cm) and those MZ twins reared apart (1.8 cm) are similar (meaning little environmental influence) and considerably less than differences of DZ twins (4.4 cm) or sibs (4.5) reared together. These data indicate that genetics plays a major role in determining height.

However, for weight, notice that MZ twins reared together have a much smaller (1.9 kg) difference than MZ twins reared apart, indicating that the environment has a considerable impact on weight. By comparing the weight differences of MZ twins reared apart with DZ twins and sibs reared together one can conclude that the environment has almost as much an influence on weight as genetics.

For ridge count, the differences between MZ twins reared together and those reared apart are small. For the data in the table, it would appear that ridge count and height have the highest heritability values.

9. Comparison of phenotypic variances between monozygotic and dizygotic traits provides an estimate of broad-sense heritability (H^2).

10. Many traits, especially those we view as quantitative are likely to be determined by a polygenic mode with possible environmental influences. The following are some common examples: height, general body structure, skin color, and perhaps most common behavioral traits including intelligence.

11. At first glance, this problem looks as if it will be an arithmetic headache, however, the problem can be simplified.

(a) The mean is computed by adding the measurements of all of the individuals, then dividing by the number of individuals. In this case there are 760 corn plants. To keep from having to add 760 numbers, merely multiply each height group by the number of individuals in each group. Add all the products then divide by n (760). This gives a value for the mean of 140cm.

(b) For the variance, use the formula given below (as in the text):

$$s^2 = V = n\Sigma f(x^2) - (\Sigma fx)^2 / n(n - 1)$$

To simplify the calculations, determine the square of each height group (100cm, for example), then multiply the value by the number in each group.

For the first group (100cm) we would have:

$$100 \quad X \quad 100 \quad X \quad 20 = 200000$$

The rest of the groups are as follows:

$$
\begin{array}{ll}
110 \text{ X } 110 \text{ X } 60 & = 726000 \\
120 \text{ X } 120 \text{ X } 90 & = 1296000 \\
130 \text{ X } 130 \text{ X } 130 & = 2197000 \\
140 \text{ X } 140 \text{ X } 180 & = 3528000 \\
150 \text{ X } 150 \text{ X } 120 & = 2700000 \\
160 \text{ X } 160 \text{ X } 70 & = 1792000 \\
170 \text{ X } 170 \text{ X } 50 & = 1445000 \\
180 \text{ X } 180 \text{ X } 40 & = 1296000 \\
 & = 15180000
\end{array}
$$

Now, the mean squared, multiplied by n is as follows:

$$140 \text{ X } 140 \text{ X } 760 = 14896000$$

Completing the calculations gives the following: (15180000 - 14896000)/759
= 284000/759
$s^2 = V = 374.18$

(c) The *standard deviation* is the square root of the variance or 19.34.

(d) The *standard error* of the mean is the standard deviation divided by the square root of n, or about 0.70. The plot approximates a normal distribution. Variation is continuous.

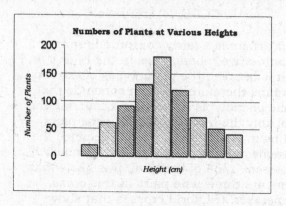

12. (a) Using the following equations, H^2 and h^2 can be calculated as follows.

For back fat:

Broad-sense heritability = H^2 = 12.2/30.6 = .398

Narrow-sense heritability = h^2 = 8.44/30.6 = .276

For body length:

Broad-sense heritability = H^2 = 26.4/52.4 = .504

Narrow-sense heritability = h^2 = 11.7/52.4 = .223

(b) For a trait that is quantitatively measured, the relative importance of genetic *versus* environmental factors may be formally assessed by examining the heritability index (H^2 or broad-sense heritability). In animal and plant breeding, a measure of potential response to selection based on additive variance and dominance variance is termed narrow-sense heritability (h^2). A relatively high narrow-sense heritability is a prediction of the impact selection may have in altering an initial randomly breeding population. Therefore, of the two traits, selection for back fat would produce more response.

Chapter 21 Quantitative Genetics

13. The formula for estimating broad-sense heritability is

$$H^2 = V_G/V_P$$

where V_G and V_P are the genetic and phenotypic components of variation, respectively. The main issue in this question is obtaining some estimate of two components of phenotypic variation: genetic and environmental. V_P is the combination of genetic and environmental variance. Because the two parental strains are inbred, they are assumed to be homozygous and the variances of 4.2 and 3.8 are considered to be the result of environmental influences. The average of these two values is 4.0. The F_1 is also genetically homogeneous and gives us an additional estimation of the environmental factors.

By averaging with the parents

$$[(4.0 + 5.6)/2 = 4.8]$$

we obtain a relatively good idea of environmental impact on the phenotype. The phenotypic variance in the F_2 is the sum of the genetic (V_G) and environmental (V_E) components. We have estimated the environmental input as 4.8, so 10.3 (V_P) minus 4.8, gives us an estimate of (V_G), which is 5.5. Heritability then becomes 5.5/10.3 or 0.53. This value, when viewed in percentage form indicates that about 53% of the variation in plant height is due to genetic influences.

14. (a) For Vitamin A:

$$h_A^2 = V_A/V_P = V_A/(V_E + V_A + V_D) = 0.097$$

For Cholesterol: $h_A^2 = 0.223$

(b) Cholesterol content should be influenced to a greater extent by selection.

15. (a) Taking the sum of the values and dividing by the number in the sample gives the following means:

mean sheep fiber length = 7.7 cm
mean fleece weight = 6.4 kg

The variance for each is:

variance sheep fiber length = 6.097
variance fleece weight = 3.12

The standard deviation is the square root of the variance:

sheep fiber length = 2.469
fleece weight = 1.766

(b,c) The covariance for the two traits is 30.36/7, or 4.34, while the correlation coefficient is + 0.998.

(d) There is a very high correlation between fleece weight and fiber length and it is likely that this correlation is not by chance. Even though correlation does not mean cause-and-effect, it would seem logical that as you increased fiber length, you would also increase fleece weight. It is probably safe to say that the increase in fleece weight is directly related to an increase in fiber length.

16. Given that both narrow-sense heritability values are relatively high, it is likely that a farmer would be able to alter both milk protein content and butterfat by selection. The value of 0.91 for the correlation coefficient between protein content and butterfat suggests that if one selects for butterfat, protein content will increase. However, correlation coefficients describe the extent to which variation in one quantitative trait is associated with variation in another and does not reveal the underlying causes of such variation. Assuming that these dairy cows had been selected for high butterfat in the past and increased protein content followed that selection (for butterfat) it is likely that selection for butterfat would continue to correlate with increased protein content. However, there may well be a point where physiological circumstances change and selection for high butterfat may be at the expense of protein content.

17. $h^2 = (7.5 - 8.5/6.0 - 8.5) = 0.4$

(realized heritability)

18. Given the realized heritability value of 0.4 it is unlikely that selection experiments would cause a rapid and/or significant response to selection. A minor response might result from intense selection.

19. $h^2 = 0.3 = (M_2 - 60/80 - 60)$

$M_2 = 66$ grams

20. Since the rice plants are genetically identical, V_G is zero and $H^2 = V_G/V_P$ = zero. Broad-sense heritability is a measure to which the phenotypic variance is due to genetic factors. In this case, with genetically identical plants, H^2 is zero, and the variance observed in grain yield is due to the environment. Selection would not be effective in this strain of rice.

21. Chromosome 2 seems to confer considerable resistance to the insecticide, somewhat in the heterozygous state and more in the homozygous state. Thus, some partial dominance is occurring.

22. (a) The most direct explanation would involve two gene pairs, with each additive gene contributing about 1.2mm to the phenotype. **(b)** The fit to this backcross supports the original hypothesis. **(c)** These data do not support the simple hypothesis provided in part (a). **(d,e)** With these data, one can see no distinct phenotypic classes suggesting that the environment may play a role in eye development or that there are more genes involved.

23. The best way to approach this problem is to first determine the number of gene pairs involved. Notice that all the F_1 plants are uniform and are in the middle of the extremes of 3" and 15", therefore the parents must each be homozygous and at the extremes. Notice also that there are thirteen classes in the F_2 so, there must be six gene pairs. See the text for an explanation of the $2n+1$ formula. **(a)** There are two ways to answer this section, a hard way and an easy way. The hard way would be to take a big sheet of paper, make the cross ($AaBbCcDdEeFf$ X $AaBbCcDdEeFf$), collect the genotypes, and calculate the ratios.

This method would be very laborious and error-prone. The easy way would be to reread the material on the binomial expansion and note the pattern preceding each expression. Notice that all numbers other than the 1's are equal to the sum of the two numbers directly above them. By enlarging the numbers to include six gene pairs, you can arrive at the thirteen classes and their frequencies:

3" =	1	4" =	12	5" =	66
6" =	220	7" =	495	8" =	792
9" =	924	10" =	792	11" =	495
12" =	220	13" =	66	14" =	12
15" =	1				

To check your calculations, be certain that your frequencies total 4096. You will also notice an additional shortcut in that since the distribution is symmetrical, you need only calculate to the center and the remainder will be in the reverse order.

(b) To determine the outcome of a cross of the F_1 plants in the test cross, apply the formula that allows you to calculate any set of components: $n!/(s!t!)$ where n = total number of events (6), s = number of events of outcome a and t = number of events of outcome b. For example, to determine how many 6" plants would be recovered from the cross $AaBbCcDdEeFf$ X $aabbccddeeff$, we are really asking how many will have three additive alleles (uppercase) and three non-additive alleles (lowercase).

$6!/(3!3!) = 20$

Applying this formula throughout gives the following frequencies:

3" = 1   4" = 6   5" = 15
6" = 20   7" = 15   8" = 6
9" = 1

And the total is 64. You can check your logic by considering that there should be only 1/64 with no additive alleles (3") and 1/64 with all additive alleles (9").

24. *Monozygotic twins* are derived from a single fertilized egg and are thus genetically identical to each other. They provide a method for determining the influence of genetics and environment on certain traits. *Dizygotic twins* arise from two eggs fertilized by two sperm cells. They have the same genetic relationship as siblings. The role of genetics and the role of the environment can be studied by comparing the expression of traits in monozygotic and dizygotic twins. The higher concordance value for monozygotic twins as compared with the value for dizygotic twins indicates a significant genetic component for a given trait. Notice that for traits including blood type, eye color, and mental retardation, there is a fairly significant difference between MZ and DZ groups. However, for measles, the difference is not as significant, indicating a greater role of the environment. Hair color has a significant genetic component as do idiopathic epilepsy, schizophrenia, diabetes, allergies, cleft lip, and club foot. The genetic component to mammary cancer is present but minimal according to these data.

25. The solution to these types of problems rests on determining the ratio of individuals expressing the extreme phenotype to the total number of individuals. In this case, 8:2028 is equal to 1:253, which is close to 1:256. If there are three gene pairs the ratio is 1:64, four gene pairs 1:256, or five gene pairs 1:1024. Therefore, these data indicate that there are four gene pairs that influence size in these guinea pigs.

26. As with many traits that are caused by numerous loci acting additively, some genes have more influence on expression than others. Environmental factors may also play a role in the expression of some polygenic traits. With brachydactyly, there are numerous modifier genes in the genome that can influence brachydactyly expression. Examination of OMIM through http://www.ncbi.nlm.nih.gov/ will illustrate this point.

27. (a,b) Because there are nine phenotypic classes in the F_2, there must be four gene pairs involved. The genotypes of the parents could be symbolized as *AABBCCDD* X *aabbccdd*, and the F_1 as *AaBbCcDd*.

28. It is likely that the flies maintained in the *Drosophila* repository are more highly inbred and less heterozygous than those recently obtained from the wild. Response to selection is dependent on genetic variation. The greater the genetic variation in a species, the more likely and dramatic the response to selection. Therefore, one would expect a greater response to selection in the wild population.

29. $6 \times 5 \times 4 \times 3 \times 2 \times 1/(2 \times 1)(4 \times 3 \times 2 \times 1) = 15$ of 64.

30. Breeders attempt to "select" out this disorder by first maintaining complete and detailed breeding records of afflicted strains. Second, they avoid breeding dogs whose close relatives are afflicted. The molecular-developmental mechanism that causes the "month of birth" effect in canine hip dysplasia is unknown. However, with many, perhaps all quantitative traits, it is clear that there is a significant environmental influence on both the penetrance and/or expression of the phenotype. With many genes acting in various ways to influence a phenotype, there are opportunities for varied molecular and developmental intraorganismic microenvironments. Stated another way, the longer and more complex the molecular distance from the genome to the phenotype, the greater the likelihood for environmental factors to be involved in expression.

Chapter 22: Population Genetics

Concept Areas	Corresponding Problems
Populations and Gene Pools	4
Calculating Allele Frequencies	1, 2, 3, 5, 6, 7, 8, 17, 19
The Hardy-Weinberg Law	4, 17, 18
Extensions of the Hardy-Weinberg Law	8, 9, 10, 21, 23, 24
Using the Hardy-Weinberg Law	11, 12, 14, 15, 16, 20, 22
Factors that Alter Allele Frequencies	8, 9, 10, 11, 12, 13, 22, 24, 25, 26

Vocabulary: Organization and Listing of Terms and Concepts

Historical

Charles Darwin

> *The Origin of Species* (1859)

> Alfred Russell Wallace

> Hardy and Weinberg

Structures and Substances

Population

Species

Gene pool

> HIV-1

> *CCR5*

> *CCR5-Δ32*

> *1/Δ32*

> major histocompatibility complex

> (MHC)

> *I* locus (ABO blood groups)

acetylcholinesterase (ACE), *Ace^R*

aspartate amino transferase 1

cystic fibrosis (*CFTR*)

FY-NULL

founder

bottleneck

> prairie chickens

Processes/Methods

Natural selection

> fitness

Gene frequencies

> mutation

> migration

> selection

> random genetic drift

ABO blood group genetics

Symbolism

p, q

$p + q = 1$

$p^2 + 2pq + q^2 = 1$

Multiple alleles

$p + q + r = 1$

$p^2 + 2pq + 2pr + q^2 + 2qr + r^2 = 1$

Heterozygote frequency

$\sqrt{q^2}$

$p = 1 - q$

$2pq$

Demonstrating equilibrium

expected frequencies

observed frequencies

selection coefficient (s)

directional selection

stabilizing selection

disruptive selection

Drosophila

Changes in gene frequencies

mutation (generates variability)

recessive

dominant

achondroplasia

migration

genetic drift

small populations

population size

founder effect

genetic bottleneck

Drosophila

forked bristles

isolated subpopulations

inbreeding and heterosis

assortative

positive

negative

inbreeding

self-fertilization

consanguineous marriages

coefficient of inbreeding

inbreeding depression

hybrid vigor

dominance hypothesis

overdominance

Chapter 22 Population Genetics

Concepts

Population genetics

   genetic structure

Gene pool

   gene (allelic) frequencies (F22.1)

Population

Hardy-Weinberg Law

   multiple alleles

   allelic frequencies

   genotypic frequencies

Hardy-Weinberg assumptions

   infinitely large

   no drift

   random mating

   no selection

   no mutation

   no migration

Natural selection

Genetic equilibrium

   genetic variability

Inbreeding and hybrid vigor (F22.2)

Fitness

F22.1 Simple illustration of the relationships among populations, individuals, alleles, and allelic frequencies (*p* and *q*).

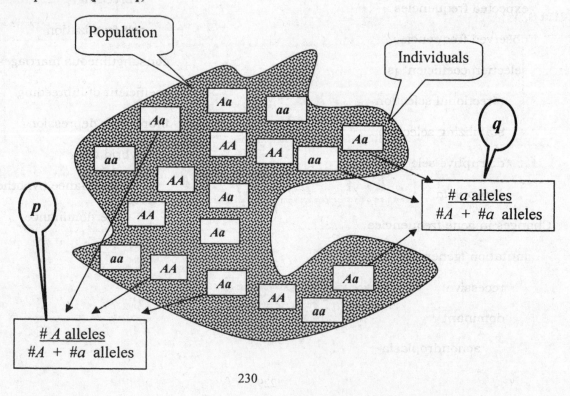

230

F22.2 Diagram of the relationships among inbreeding, heterosis, and homozygosity. Note that as inbreeding occurs, heterosis decreases and homozygosity increases.

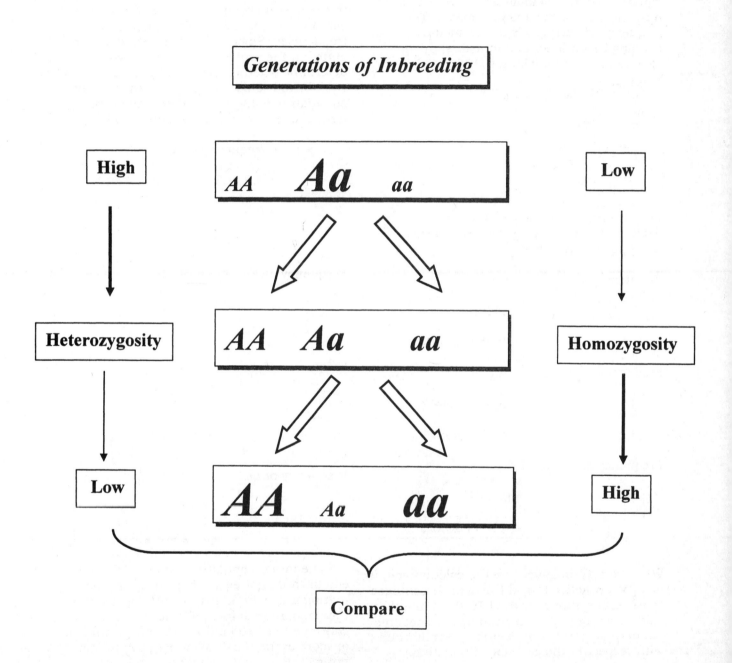

Solutions to Problems and Discussion Questions

1. Because the alleles follow a dominant/recessive mode, one can use the equation $\sqrt{q^2}$ to calculate q from which all other aspects of the answer depend. The frequency of aa types is determined by dividing 37 (number of nontasters) by the total number of individuals (125).

q^2 = 37/125 = .296

q = .544

p = 1 - q

p = .456

The frequencies of the genotypes are determined by applying the formula $p^2 + 2pq + q^2$ as follows:

Frequency of AA = p^2

= (.456)^2

= .208 or 20.8%

Frequency of Aa = $2pq$

= 2(.456)(.544)

= .496 or 49.6%

Frequency of aa = q^2

= (.544)^2

= .296 or 29.6%

When completing such a set of calculations, it is a good practice to add the final percentages to be certain that they total 100%. (Note that calculation requires the assumption that this population is in Hardy-Weinberg equilibrium with respect to the gene for PTC tasting.)

2. Understanding the Hardy-Weinberg equilibrium allows us to state that if a population is in equilibrium, the genotypic frequencies will not shift from one generation to the next unless there are factors such as selection or migration which alter gene frequencies. Since none of these factors are stated in the problem, we need only to determine whether the initial population is in equilibrium. Calculate p and q, then apply the equation $p^2 + 2pq + q^2$ to determine genotypic frequencies in the next generation.

p = frequency of A

= 0.2 + .3

= 0.5

q = 1 - p = 0.5

Frequency of AA = p^2

= (. 5)^2

= .25 or 25%

Frequency of Aa = $2pq$

= 2(.5)(.5)

=.5 or 50%

Frequency of aa = q^2

= (.5)^2

= .25 or 25%

The initial population was not in equilibrium, however, after one generation of mating under the Hardy-Weinberg conditions the population is in equilibrium and will continue to be so (and not change) until one or more of the Hardy-Weinberg conditions is not met. Note that *equilibrium* does not necessarily mean p and q equal 0.5.

3. For each of these values, one merely takes the square root to determine q, then one computes p, then one "plugs" the values into the $2pq$ expression.

(a) $q = .08;$ $2pq$ $= 2(.92)(.08)$

$= .1472$ or 14.72%

(b) $q = .009;$ $2pq$ $= 2(.991)(.009)$

$= .01784$ or 1.78%

(c) $q = .3;$ $2pq$ $= 2(.7)(.3)$

$= .42$ or 42%

(d) $q = .1;$ $2pq$ $= 2(.9)(.1)$

$= .18$ or 18%

(e) $q = .316;$ $2pq$ $= 2(.684)(.316)$

$= .4323$ or 43.23%

(Depending how one rounds off the decimals, slightly different answers will occur.)

4. In order for the Hardy-Weinberg equations to apply, the population must be in Hardy-Weinberg equilibrium.

5. Assuming that the population is in Hardy-Weinberg equilibrium, if one has the frequency of individuals with the dominant phenotype, the remainder have the recessive phenotype (q^2). With q^2 one can calculate q and from this value one can arrive at p. Applying the expression $p^2 + 2pq + q^2$ will allow a solution to the question.

6. (a) For the CCR5 analysis, first determine p and q. Since one has the frequencies of all the genotypes, one can add

.6 and .351/2 to provide p (= .7755)

q will be

.049 and .351/2 = .2245

The equilibrium values will be as follows:

Frequency of $l/l = p^2$ $= (.7755)^2$

$= .6014$ or 60.14%

Frequency of $l/\Delta32$ $= 2pq$

$= 2(.7755)(.2245)$

$= .3482$ or 34.82%

Frequency of $\Delta32 /\Delta32 = q^2 = (.2245)^2$

$= .0504$ or 5.04%

Comparing these equilibrium values with the observed values strongly suggests that the observed values are drawn from a population in Assuming that the population is in Hardy-Weinberg equilibrium, equilibrium.

(b) For the AS (sickle-cell) analysis, first determine p and q. Since one has the frequencies of all the genotypes, one can add

.756 and .242/2 to provide p (= .877)

q will be

1 - .877 or .123

The equilibrium values will be as follows:
Frequency of AA $= p^2$ $= (.877)^2$

$= .7691$ or 76.91%

Frequency of AS $= 2pq$ $= 2(.877)(.123)$

$= .2157$ or 21.57%

Frequency of SS $= q^2$ $= (.123)^2$

$= .0151$ or 1.51%

Comparing these equilibrium values with the observed values suggests that the observed values may be drawn from a population that is not in equilibrium. Notice that there are more heterozygotes than predicted, and fewer SS types.

To test for a Hardy-Weinberg equilibrium, apply the chi-square test as follows.

$$\chi^2 = \frac{\Sigma(o-e)^2}{e}$$

$(75.6-76.9)^2 / 76.9 +$

$(24.2 - 21.6)^2 / 21.6 +$

$(0.2 - 1.51)^2 / 1.5 = 1.47$

In calculating degrees of freedom in a test of gene frequencies, the "free variables" are reduced by an additional degree of freedom because one estimated a parameter (p or q) used in determining the expected values. Therefore, there is one degree of freedom even though there are three classes. Checking the χ^2 table with 1 degree of freedom gives a value of 3.84 at the 0.05 probability level.

Since the χ^2 value calculated here is smaller, the null hypothesis (the observed values fluctuate from the equilibrium values by chance and chance alone) should not be rejected. Thus, the frequencies of *AA, AS,* and *SS* sampled a population that is probably in Hardy-Weinberg equilibrium.

7. Given that $q^2 = .04$, then $q = .2$, $2pq = .32$, and $p^2 = .64$. Of those not expressing the trait, only a mating between heterozygotes can produce an offspring that expresses the trait, and then only at a frequency of 1/4. The different types of matings possible (those without the trait) in the population, with their frequencies, are given below:

$AA \times AA$ = $.64 \times .64$ = $.4096$

$AA \times Aa$ = $.64 \times .32$ = $.2048$

$Aa \times AA$ = $.64 \times .32$ = $.2048$

$Aa \times Aa$ = $.32 \times .32$ = $.1024$

$Aa \times Aa$ = $.32 \times .32$ = $.1024$

Notice that of the matings of the individuals who do not express the trait, only the last two (about 20%) are capable of producing offspring with the trait. Therefore, one would arrive at a final likelihood of 1/4 X 20% or 5% of the offspring with the trait.

8. The following formula calculates the frequency of an allele in the next generation for any selection scenario, given the frequencies of *a* and *A* in this generation and the fitness of all three genotypes.

$$q_{g+1} = [w_{Aa}p_g q_g + w_{aa}q_g^2]/[w_{AA}p_g^2 + w_{Aa}2p_g q_g + w_{aa}q_g^2]$$

where q_{g+1} is the frequency of the *a* allele in the next generation, q_g is the frequency of the *a* allele in this generation, p_g is the frequency of the *A* allele in this generation, and each "w" represents the fitness of its respective genotype.

(a)

$$q_{g+1} = [.9(.7)(.3)+.8(.3)^2/[1(.7)^2 +.9(2)(.7)(.3)+.8(.3)^2]$$

$q_{g+1} = .278$ $p_{g+1} = .722$

(b) $q_{g+1} = .289$ $p_{g+1} = .711$

(c) $q_{g+1} = .298$ $p_{g+1} = .702$

(d) $q_{g+1} = .319$ $p_{g+1} = .681$

9. The general equation for responding to this question is

$$q_n = q_0 /(1 + nq_0)$$

where n = the number of generations, q_0 = the initial gene frequency, and q_n = the new gene frequency.

(a) n = 1

$q_n = q_0 / (1 + n q_0)$

$q_n = 0.5 / [1 + (1 \times 0.5)]$

$q_n = .33 \qquad p_n = .67$

(b) n = 5

$q_n = q_0 / (1 + n q_0)$

$q_n = 0.5 / [1 + (5 \times 0.5)]$

$q_n = .143 \qquad p_n = .857$

(c) n = 10

$q_n = q_0 / (1 + n q_0)$

$q_n = 0.5 / [1 + (10 \times 0.5)]$

$q_n = .083 \qquad p_n = .917$

(d) n = 25

$q_n = q_0 / (1 + n q_0)$

$q_n = 0.5 / [1 + (25 \times 0.5)]$

$q_n = .037 \qquad p_n = .963$

(e) n = 100

$q_n = q_0 / (1 + n q_0)$

$q_n = 0.5 / [1 + (100 \times 0.5)]$

$q_n = .0098 \qquad p_n = .9902$

(f) n = 1000

$q_n = q_0 / (1 + n q_0)$

$q_n = 0.5 / [1 + (1000 \times 0.5)]$

$q_n = .00099 \qquad p_n = .99901$

10. Since a dominant lethal gene is highly selected against, it is unlikely that it will exist at too high a frequency, if at all. However, if the gene shows incomplete penetrance or late age of onset (after reproductive age) it may remain in a population.

11. For this question, apply the equations

$$\Delta p = m(p_m - p)$$

and $p_1 = p + \Delta p$

Substituting, gives: $p_1 = p + m(p_m - p)$.

    (a) $p_1 = 0.6 + 0.2(0.1 - 0.6) = 0.5$

    (b) $p_1 = 0.2 + 0.3(0.7 - 0.2) = 0.35$

    (c) $p_1 = 0.1 + 0.1(0.2 - 0.1) = 0.11$

12. What one must do is predict the probability of one of the grandparents being heterozygous in this problem. Given the frequency of the disorder in the population as 1 in 10,000 individuals (0.0001), then $q^2 = 0.0001$, and $q = 0.01$. The frequency of heterozygosity is $2pq$ or approximately .02 as also stated in the problem. The probability for one of the grandparents to be heterozygous would therefore be 0.02 + 0.02 or 0.04 or 1/25. (Note: if one considers the probability of both parents being carriers, 0.02 X 0.02 --- the answer differs slightly). If one of the grandparents is a carrier, then the probability of the offspring from a first-cousin mating being homozygous for the recessive gene is 1/16. Multiplying the two probabilities together gives 1/16 X 1/25 = 1/400.

Following the same analysis for the second-cousin mating gives 1/64 X 1/25 = 1/1600. Notice that the population at large has a frequency of homozygotes of 1/10,000; therefore, one can easily see how inbreeding increases the likelihood of homozygosity.

13. *Inbreeding depression* refers to the reduction in fitness observed in populations that are inbred. With inbreeding comes an increase in the number of homozygous individuals (see F25.2 in this book) and a decrease in genetic variability. Genetic variability is necessary for a genetic response to environmental change. As deleterious alleles become homozygous, more individuals are less fit in the population.

14. Because heterozygosity tends to mask expression of recessive genes that may be desirable in a domesticated animal or plant, inbreeding schemes are often used to render strains homozygous so that such recessive genes can be expressed. In addition, assume that a particularly desirable trait occurs in a domesticated plant or animal. The best way to increase the frequency of individuals with that trait is by self-fertilization (not often possible) or by matings to blood relatives (inbreeding). In theory, one increases the likelihood of a gene "meeting itself" by various inbreeding schemes. There are disadvantages to increasing the degree of homozygosity by inbreeding. *Inbreeding depression* is a reduction in fitness often associated with an increase in homozygosity.

15. While inbreeding increases the frequency of homozygous individuals in a population, it does not change the *allele* frequencies. There will be fewer heterozygotes in the population to compensate for the additional homozygotes. There will be no change in the frequency of recessive alleles. See F22.2 in this book.

16. The quickest way to generate a homozygous line of an organism is to *self-fertilize* that organism. Because this is not always possible, brother-sister matings are often used.

17. Given that the recessive allele *a* is present in the homozygous state (q^2) at a frequency of 0.0001, the value of q is 0.01 and $p = 0.99$.

(a) q is 0.01

(b) $p = 1 - q$ or .99

(c) $2pq = 2(.01)(.99)$
$\quad\quad = 0.0198$ (or about 1/50)

(d) $2pq \times 2pq$

$\quad\quad = 0.0198 \times 0.0198$
$\quad\quad = 0.000392$ or about 1/255

18. The frequency of an allele is determined by a number of factors including the fitness it confers, mutation rate, and input from migration. There is no tendency for a gene to reach any artificial frequency such as 0.5. In fact, you have seen that rare alleles tend to remain rare even when they are dominant -- unless there is very strong selection for the allele. The distribution of a gene among individuals is determined by mating (population size, inbreeding, etc.) and environmental factors (selection, etc.). A population is in Hardy-Weinberg equilibrium when the distribution of genotypes occurs at or around the $p^2 + 2pq + q^2 = 1$ expression. Equilibrium does not mean 25% *AA*, 50% *Aa*, and 25% *aa*. This confusion often stems from the 1:2:1(or 3:1) ratio seen in Mendelian crosses.

19. Because three of the affected infants had affected parents, only two "new" alleles, from mutation, enter into the problem. The allele is dominant, therefore each new case of achondroplasia arose from a single new mutation. There are 50,000 births, therefore 100,000 gametes (genes) are involved. The frequency of mutation is therefore given as follows: 2/100,000 or 2×10^5.

20. The probability that the woman (with no family history of CF) is heterozygous is $2pq$ or $2(1/50)(49/50)$. The probability that the man is heterozygous is 2/3. The probability that a child with CF will be produced by two heterozygotes is 1/4. Therefore the overall probability of the couple producing a CF child is $98/2500 \times 2/3 \times 1/4 = .00653$ or about 1/153.

21. Since $r1 = 0.81$ and $r2 = 0.19$ the expected frequency of heterozygotes would be $2pq \times 125$ or $2(0.81 \times 0.19) \times 125 = 38.475$. Given the following equation and substituting the values:

$$F = (H_e - H_o)/H_e$$
$$F = (38.475 - 20)/38.475 = 0.48$$

22. Given that only 10% of the sensitive (bb) corn borer larvae feeding on Bt corn plants survive, the selection coefficient against them would be 0.9. The B allele for resistance exists at an initial frequency of 0.02 (represent at p), therefore, $q = 0.98$. The frequency of the b allele after one generation of corn borers fed on Bt corn would be computed as follows:

$$q' = q(1-sq)/1-sq^2$$
$$q' = .98[1-(0.9)(.98)]/1-[(0.9)(.98)(.98)]$$
$$q' = 0.852 \text{ and } p' = 0.148$$

23. The following distribution of genotypes occurs among the fifty desert bighorn sheep in which the normal dominant C allele produces straight coats.

$CC = 29$ = straight coats
$Cc = 17$ = straight coats
$cc = 4$ = curled coats

Computing,

$p = .75$ and $q = .25$ and $2pq = 0.375$ for the expected frequency of heterozygotes. Since 17/50 or (0.34) are observed as heterozygotes, the following equation applies:

$$F = (H_e - H_o)/H_e$$
$$F = (.375 - .34)/.375 = 0.093$$

This problem could also be solved using the actual numbers of sheep in each category where there would be 18.75 heterozygotes expected $(2pq)(50)$:

$$F = (18.75 - 17)/18.75 = 0.093$$

24. The equation for determining the impact of immigration on the gene pool of an existing population is estimated by the following equation:

$$p_i' = (1- m)p_i + mp_m$$

Substituting in the appropriate values one obtains the following expression. Note that the value of 0.2 comes from that fact that 10 sheep out of 50 or 20% are being introduced and there are no cc alleles in the introduced population, so $p_m = 1.0$.

$$p_i' = (1-0.2)(0.75) + (0.2)(1.0)$$
$$p_i' = 0.8$$

25. (a) The gene is most likely recessive because all affected individuals have unaffected parents and the condition clearly runs in families. For the population, since $q^2 = .002$, then $q = .045$, $p = .955$, and $2(pq) = 0.086$. For the community, since $q^2 = .005$, then $q = .07$, $p = .93$, and $2(pq) = 0.13$.

(b) The "founder effect" is probably operating here. Relatively small, local populations that are relatively isolated in a reproductive sense tend to show differences in gene frequencies when compared with larger populations. In such small populations, homozygosity is increased as a gene has a higher probability of "meeting itself" due to inbreeding.

26. Given small populations and very similar environmental conditions, it is more likely that "sampling error" or genetic drift is operating. Under such conditions (small population sizes) large fluctuations in gene frequency are likely, regardless of selection pressures. Since the same gene is behaving differently under similar environmental conditions, selection is an unlikely explanation.

Chapter 23: Evolutionary Genetics

Concept Areas	Corresponding Problems
Evolution and Speciation	1, 2, 3, 4, 13, 14
Chromosomal Polymorphism	7, 8
Models of Speciation	4, 5, 9, 16
Measuring Genetic Variation	6, 10, 12, 21, 22, 23, 24, 25, 27
Formation of Species	2, 5, 17, 18, 19
Molecular Techniques	10, 11, 15, 21, 22, 23, 24, 25, 26
Human Evolution	20, 21, 22, 23, 28

Vocabulary: Organization and Listing of Terms and Concepts

Structures and Substances

Origin of Species (1859)

Allozyme

   alcohol dehydrogenase

   CFTR

Cytochrome c

Polytene chromosome

Drosophila pseudoobscura

Fundulus heteroclitus (mummichog)

   lactate dehydrogenase

   ectotherm

Arabidopsis thaliana

Mitochondrial DNA

HIV

Neanderthals

SSU (small-subunit rRNA)

Rickettsia

Processes/Methods

Species definition

Speciation

Artificial selection

Reproduction and speciation

   birds, plants

Evolutionary divergence (F23.1)

Genetic divergence

Genetic diversity

   heterozygosity

    protein polymorphism

    allozymes (F23.1)

     molecular phylogenetic trees

    amino acid sequence homology

     cytochrome c

    chromosomal polymorphism

     inversions

DNA sequence polymorphism

mitochondrial DNA

Ecological diversity

niche

Drosophila heteroneura, etc.

Hawaii

Minulus cardinalis

Cichlids

SINES

Speciation

stasis

phyletic evolution (anagenesis)

cladogenesis

neutralist theory

reproductive barriers

physiological

behavioral

mechanical

isolating mechanisms

reproductive

prezygotic

postzygotic

Gel electrophoresis

protein polymorphism

nucleic acid sequence variation

UPGMA

Concepts

Species definition and concept

Evolutionary divergence

molecular clock

minimal mutational distance

minimal genetic divergence

rates of speciation

polyploidy

divergence dendrograms

evolutionary trees

Artificial selection

Species formation (speciation)

isolating mechanisms

Phylogenetic reconstruction

Sequence homology

amino acid, nucleic acid

Sequence conservation

Parsimony

Maximum likelihood

Mutation and speciation

Origin of mitochondria

F23.1 The diagram below is meant to illustrate the meaning of the term allozyme. Notice that alleles A^1 and A^2 produce protein products that differ electrophoretically, but that accomplish the same function.

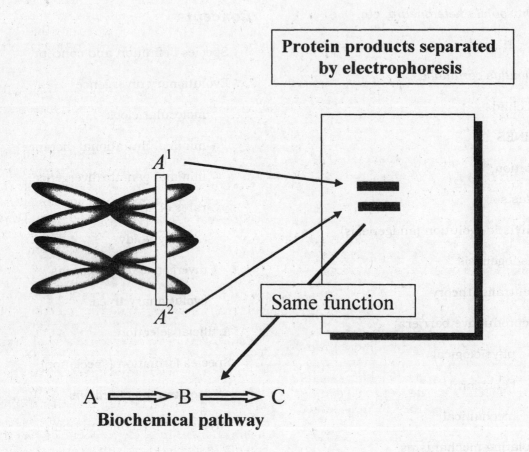

Solutions to Problems and Discussion Questions

1. Neo-Darwinism is defined as the explanation of natural selection in terms of changes in allelic frequencies or the combining of Darwin's theory of evolution with that of Mendelian genetics.

2. A species is a group of interbreeding or potentially interbreeding populations that is reproductively isolated from all other such groups. Speciation is the process that leads to the formation of species. Evolution is the change in a population over time. Speciation is one of many results of evolution.

3. Darwin and Wallace could not explain the origin of species variation nor the manner in which such variations were passed from parent to offspring.

4. Organisms may appear to be similar but be reproductively isolated for a sufficient period to justify their species identity. If significant genetic differences occur, they may be considered separate species.

5. Natural selection is usually viewed as a gradual process that leads to genetic differences over time. However, more dramatic forms of speciation may involve more rapid genomic changes in the form of transposable elements or polyploidy. New species can be formed by hybridization and chromosome doubling.

6. The subterranean niche is less broad and less dynamic than above ground niche. The underground microhabitat consists of a narrower range of climatic changes, thus genetic polymorphism is not selected. This conclusion has been supported by additional studies indicating that genetic diversity is positively correlated with niche-width.

7. Assume that a chromosome in the "standard arrangement" undergoes an inversion (*pericentric* or *paracentric*). The following are possible consequences of such an inversion:

(a) change in gene order with possible introduction of position effects,

(b) breakage within a structural gene or other functional element, and

(c) reduction in the recovery of crossover gametes in heterokaryotypes (those which carry an inversion as well as a standard homologue). While (c) may reduce the production of variation, the first two (a and b) may introduce variation.

At the population level, different populations with different inversion polymorphisms are genetically distinct.

8. Results from laboratory studies indicated that there was a selective advantage in having the two inversions present, rather than either one. Specifically, different inversions were favored at different times of the year. Thus, natural selection favored the maintenance of both inversions over the loss of either.

9. During speciation, individuals or groups of potentially interbreeding organisms become genetically distinct from other members of the species. Members of different populations with substantial genetic divergence are, at first, not reproductively isolated from each other, although gene flow may be restricted. The distinction between such groups is not absolute in that one group may blend with other groups of the species. Any process that favors changes in allele frequencies has the potential of generating substantial genetic differences among different populations.

Factors such as selection, migration, genetic drift, or even mutation may be important in generating significant genetic change. One would certainly include geographic isolation as a major barrier to gene flow and thus an important process in such formation.

Natural selection occurs when there is nonrandom elimination of individuals from a population. Since such selection is a strong force in changing allele frequencies, it should also be considered as a significant factor in subspecies formation.

10. (a) Missense mutations cause amino acid changes.

(b) Horizontal transfer refers to the process of passing genetic information from one organism to another without producing offspring. In bacteria, plasmid transfer is an example of horizontal transfer.

(c) The fact that none of the isolates shared identical nucleotide changes indicates that there is little genetic exchange among different strains. Each alteration is unique, most likely originating in an ancestral strain and maintained in descendents of that strain only.

11. Because of degeneracy in the code, there are some nucleotide substitutions, especially in the third base, that do not change amino acids. In addition, if there is no change in the overall charge of the protein, it is likely that electrophoresis will not separate the variants. If a positively charged amino acid is replaced by an amino acid of like charge, then the overall charge on the protein is unchanged. The same may be said for other negatively charged and neutral amino acid substitutions.

12. The approximate similarity of mutation rates among genes and lineages should provide more credible estimates of divergence times of species and allow for broader interpretations of sequence comparisons. It also provides for increased understanding of the mutational processes that govern evolution among mammalian genomes. For instance, if the rate of mutation is fairly constant among lineages or cells that have a more rapid turnover, it indicates that replication-related errors do not make a significant contribution to mutation rates.

13. The text lists several cornerstones of the *neutral mutation theory:*

(a) there is a relatively uniform rate of amino acid substitution in different organisms (under different types of selection);

(b) there is no particular pattern to the substitutions indicating that selection is not eliminating some variations;

(c) the rate of mutation is relatively high and has remained relatively constant for millions of years even though environments have fluctuated greatly over that period of time;

(d) certain regions of molecules and certain functions of those molecules should logically be less likely to have amino acid substitutions influence the phenotype;

(e) the rate of amino acid substitution in some proteins is much too high to have been produced by selection. The *selectionists* suggest that even though amino acid substitutions *appear* to be neutral, it is more likely that their influence has just not been determined. In addition, they point out that many polymorphisms are clearly maintained in the population *by* selection. Thus, the issues listed above do not really challenge present views of genetic variation.

Like many other debates that surround the nature of evolution, it is important to see that debate is a natural component of scientific understanding. It is likely that some genes (like histone genes) will not tolerate nucleotide substitutions to a significant degree and the neutral mutation theory will not hold. However, there are other genes that produce quite variable products and provide support for the neutral mutation theory. Usually controversy is resolved as one dives deeper into the problem and seeks to define the variables and complexities of the process. It is controversy that stimulates a desire to seek answers.

14. In general, speciation involves the gradual accumulation of genetic changes to a point where reproductive isolation occurs. Depending on environmental or geographic conditions, genetic changes may occur slowly or rapidly. They can involve point mutations or chromosomal changes.

15. The *Ldh-B^b* allele is more efficient in cold waters, while the *Ldh-B^a* allele is more efficient in warm waters. There is a correlation between allele frequency and water temperature. Both catalytic efficiency and transcription of the *Ldh-B^b* allele are higher in cold water; transcriptional rate of *Ldh-B^b* is also higher than the *Ldh-B^a* allele.

16. Reproductive isolating mechanisms are grouped into prezygotic and postzygotic and include the following:

- geographic or ecological
- seasonal or temporal
- behavoral
- mechanical
- physiological
- hybrid inviability or weakness
- developmental hybrid sterility
- segregational hybrid sterility
- F_2 breakdown

17. Reproductive isolating mechanisms are grouped into prezygotic and postzygotic. Prezygotic mechanisms are most efficient because they occur before resources are expended in the processes of mating.

18. Polyploid plants that result from the hybridization of two species would be expected to be more heterozygous than the diploid parental species because two distinct genomes are combined. Generally, genetic variation is an advantage unless a significant degree of that variation is outside acceptable physiological tolerance.

19. With some exceptions, plants tolerate departures from diploidy more successfully than animals. Some vertebrate exceptions include amphibians. It is possible that such genomic restrictions in animals are the result of narrow physiological limits on development of a complex nervous system and the resulting characteristics of that system.

20. Somatic gene therapy, like any therapy, allows some individuals to live more normal lives than those not receiving therapy. As such, the ability of such individuals to contribute to the gene pool increases the likelihood that less fit alleles will enter and be maintained in the gene pool. This is a normal consequence of therapy, genetic or not, and in the face of disease control and prevention, societies have generally accepted this consequence. Germline therapy could, if successful, lead to limited, isolated, and infrequent removal of an allele from a gene lineage. However, given the present state of the science, its impact on the course of human evolution will be diluted and negated by a host of other factors that afflict mankind.

21. All of the amino acid substitutions

(Ala - Gly, Val - Leu, Asp - Asn, Met - Leu)

require only one nucleotide change. The last change from

Pro (CC-) - Lys (AAA,G)

requires two changes (the minimal mutational distance).

22. Approach this problem by writing the possible codons for all the amino acids (except Arg and Asp, which show no change) in the human cytochrome c chain. Then determine the minimum number of nucleotide substitutions required for each changed amino acid in the various organisms. Once listed, count up the numbers for each organism: horse, 3; pig, 2; dog, 3; chicken, 3; bullfrog, 2; fungus, 6.

23. Construct a chart similar to the one below, which indicates the number of base changes between each pair:

	H	C	G	O
H	-	-	-	-
C	1	-	-	-
G	3	2	-	-
O	7	6	4	-
B	12	11	9	10

Following the instructions given in the text, develop the relationships in the following manner:

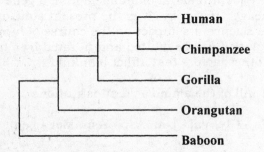

- Human
- Chimpanzee
- Gorilla
- Orangutan
- Baboon

24. The classification of organisms into different species is based on evidence (morphological, genetic, ecological, etc.) that they are reproductively isolated. That is, there must be evidence that gene flow does not occur among the groups being called different species. Classifications above the species level (genus, family, etc.) are not based on such empirical data. Indeed, classification above the species level is somewhat arbitrary and based on traditions that extend far beyond DNA sequence information. In addition, recall that DNA sequence divergence is not always directly proportional to morphological, behavioral, or ecological divergence. While the genus classifications provided in this problem seem to be invalid, other factors, well beyond simple DNA sequence comparison, must be considered in classification practices. As more information is gained on the meaning of DNA sequence differences in comparison to morphological factors, many phylogenetic relationships will be reconsidered and it is possible that adjustments will be needed in some classification schemes.

25. There are many sections of DNA in a eukaryotic genome that are not reflected in a protein product. Indeed, there are many sections of DNA that are not even transcribed and/or have no apparent physiological role. Such regions are more likely to tolerate nucleotide changes compared with those regions with a necessary physiological impact. Introns, for example, show sequence variation, which is not reflected in a protein product. Exons, on the other hand, code for products that are usually involved in production of a phenotype and, as such, are subject to selection.

26. (a) Since noncoding genomic regions are probably silent genetically, it is likely that they contribute little, if anything, to the phenotype. Selection acts on the phenotype, therefore, such noncoding regions are probably selectively neutral.

(b) These polymorphism data indicate that all the Lake Victoria area (lake and contributing rivers) cichlids are related by recent ancestry, whereas those from neighboring lakes are more distantly related. In addition, since Lake Victoria dried out about 14,000 years ago, it is likely that it was repopulated by a relatively small sample of cichlids.

27. A number of studies using SINES, repetitive DNA, and neutral polymorphisms (see above problem) indicate that most, if not all, cichlid species in Lake Victoria evolved from a single ancestral species. If that is the case, then this finding would represent the most rapid evolutionary radiation ever documented for vertebrates.

28. The pattern of genetic distances through time indicates that from the present to about 25,000 years ago, modern humans and Cro-Magnons show an approximately constant number of differences. Conversely, there is an abrupt increase in genetic distance seen in comparing modern humans and Cro-Magnons with Neanderthals. The results indicate a clear discontinuity between modern humans, Cro-Magnons, and Neanderthals with respect to genetic variation in the mitochondrial DNAs sampled. Assuming that the sampling and analytical techniques used to generate the data are valid, it appears that Neanderthals made little, if any, genetic contributions to the Cro-Magnon or modern European gene pool.

It could be argued that the absence of Neanderthal mtDNA lineages in living humans is a consequence of random drift or lineage extinction since the disappearance of Neanderthals. However, the examination of mtDNA in ancient Cro-Magnon mtDNA shows no evidence of a historical relationship and suggests that Neanderthals were not genetically related to the ancestors of modern humans.

Chapter 24: Conservation Genetics

Concept Areas	Corresponding Problems
Population Dynamics	1, 3, 11
Genetic Assessment of Threatened Species	1, 12, 14, 15, 17, 20, 21, 22, 23
Management of Threatened Species	2, 5, 6, 7, 9, 10, 15, 16, 18, 19, 24
Inbreeding and Drift in Small Populations	3, 4, 6, 8, 13

Vocabulary: Organization and Listing of Terms and Concepts

Structures and Substances

Grey wolf (*Canis lupus*)

California condors

   (*Gymnogyps californianus*)

Antarctic fur seal (*Arctocephalus sp.*)

Cheetah (*Acinonyx jubatus*)

Red-cockaded woodpecker (*Picoides borealis*)

North American brown bear (*Ursus arctos*)

Fruit fly (*Drosophila melanogaster*)

Black-footed ferret (*Mustela nigripes*)

Native rock grape (*Vitis rupestris*)

Domesticated species

Allozyme

DNA profile

   nuclear

   mitochondrial

   chloroplast

Gene bank

Core collection

Metapopulation

Processes/Methods

Human population growth

Biodiversity

   human impact

Conservation genetics

Intraspecific diversity

   interpopulation

   intrapopulation

Chapter 24 Conservation Genetics

Interspecific diversity

Loss of genetic diversity

    reduced population size

    habitat loss

    population fragmentation

Detection of genetic diversity

    allozyme analysis

    RFLP

    PCR

Absolute population size (N)

    effective populaton size (N_e)

    $N_e = 4(N_m N_f)/(N_m + N_f)$

    $N_e = 1/(1/t)(1/N_1 + 1/N_2 + 1/N_3 \ldots)$

Population bottleneck

Founder effect

Genetic drift

Inbreeding

Concepts

Vulnerable and endangered species

Genetic diversity

Loss of genetic diversity

Population dynamics

    bottleneck

    founder effect

    genetic drift

    inbreeding

    gene flow

    genetic erosion

Conservation strategies

Probability of fixation $p(A)$

Inbreeding coefficient

    $F = (2pq - H)/2pq$

    $H_t = (1-1/2N_e)^t H_o$

    inbreeding depression

Genetic load

    purging genetic load

Gene flow relates to migration

Genetic erosion (loss of diversity)

Ex situ and *in situ* conservation

    captive species

    gene banks

Population augmentation

    outbreeding depression

Chapter 24 Conservation Genetics

Solutions to Problems and Discussion Questions

1. (a) Apply the formula which computes the effective population size as the harmonic mean of the numbers in each generation:

$$N_e = 1/(1/t)(1/N_1 + 1/N_2 + 1/N_3 ...)$$

Substituting the values:

$$N_e = 1/(1/4)(1/47 + 1/17 + 1/20 + 1/35)$$

$$N_e = 25.21$$

(b) Apply the formula which computes the frequency of heterozygotes after t generations as a function of effective population size:

$$H_t = (1-1/2N_e)^t H_o$$

Substituting the values:

$$H_t = (1-1/2(25.21))^4(.55)$$

$$H_t = .5073$$

(c) Apply the formula which relates the inbreeding coefficient to the frequency of heterozygotes in a population:

$$F = (2pq - H)/2pq$$
$$F = (.55 - .5073)/.55$$
$$F = 0.0776$$

2. The frequency (rough estimate because of small sample size) of the lethal allele in the captive population ($q^2 = 5/169$ and $q = .172$) is approximately double that in the gene pool as a whole ($q = 0.09$). Applying the formula

$$q_n = q_o/(1 + nq_o)$$

one can estimate that it would take 10 generations to reduce the lethal gene's frequency to .063 in the captive population with no intervention (random mating assumed). Since condors produce very few eggs per year, a more proactive approach seems justified.

First, if detailed records are kept of the breeding partners of the captive birds, then knowledge of heterozygotes should be available. Breeding programs could be established to restrict matings between those carrying the lethal gene. Such "kinship management" is often used in captive populations. If kinship records are not available, it is often possible to establish kinship using genetic markers such as DNA microsatellite polymorphisms. Using such markers, one can often identify mating partners and link them to their offspring.

By coupling knowledge of mating partners with the likelihood of producing a lethal genetic combination, selective matings can often be used to minimize the influence of a deleterious allele. In addition, such markers can be used to establish matings which optimize genetic mixing, thus reducing inbreeding depression.

3. Notice (in the text) that the probability of fixation through drift is the same as a gene's initial frequency. In this problem, the probability of A being fixed (and therefore a lost) is 0.75. The probability of B being fixed (and b being lost) is 0.8 and the probability of C being fixed (and c being lost) is 0.95. Therefore the probability that all the recessive alleles will be lost through genetic drift is

$$0.75 \times 0.80 \times 0.95 = 0.57$$

4. Both genetic drift and inbreeding tend to drive populations toward homozygosity. Genetic drift is more common when the effective breeding size of the population is low. When this condition prevails, inbreeding is also much more likely. They are different in that inbreeding can occur when certain population structures or behaviors favor matings between relatives, regardless of the effective size of the population. Inbreeding tends to increase the frequency of both homozygous classes at the expense of the heterozygotes. Genetic drift can lead to fixation of one allele or the other, thus producing a single homozygous class.

5. There are a number of dangers inherent in the management of such a small herd of endangered rhinos. Because of the small breeding pool, inbreeding depression is likely to lead to less fit individuals over time. To combat this problem, genetic markers (such as microsatellites) can be used to assess the general degree of relatedness and heterozygosity of each of the 16 rhinos. From such information, appropriate matings can be facilitated which would reduce inbreeding depression. However, additional efforts may be needed in this extreme case. It is possible to develop exchange programs whereby animals from other herds provide semen (either naturally or artificially) thereby reducing inbreeding. This practice can be successful if females are receptive and if no deleterious alleles are brought into the population (outbreeding depression).

Population augmentation, where individuals are transplanted into a declining population, can be used to increase numbers and genetic diversity. However, as stated above, outbreeding depression may accompany this practice. Sometimes drastic measures must be taken in extreme cases such as the black rhino. Dehorning is often practiced to remove the incentive for poaching and reduce lethal wounding due to fighting. This practice is only useful in areas devoid of dangerous predators.

6. Inbreeding depression, over time, reduces the level of heterozygosity, usually a selectively advantageous quality of a species. When homozygosity increases (through loss of heterozygosity) deleterious alleles are likely to become more of a load on a population. Outbreeding depression occurs when there is a reduction in fitness of progeny from genetically diverse individuals. It is usually attributed to offspring being less well-adapted to the local environmental conditions of the parents.

Even though forced outbreeding may be necessary to save a threatened species, where population numbers are low, it significantly and permanently changes the genetic make-up of the species.

7. Cloning of some highly threatened species may be the only way to save that species from extinction. However, the long-term disadvantages of cloning for this purpose are often considered self-defeating. With cloning one "short-circuits" normal processes (meiosis, gametic union, etc.) necessary to maintain genetic variation. With a loss of genetic variation come difficulties with adaptation as environments change. It may be possible to identify certain conditions in which cloning would be useful to "save" a species, however, interbreeding provides benefits that allow a species to evolve. In addition, as members of a species become more uniform (through cloning) they are more likely to suffer more severe and widespread responses to disease and environmental stress.

8. Often, molecular assays of overall heterozygosity can indicate the degree of inbreeding and/or genetic drift. Refer to Figure 22.2 in this book and notice that as inbreeding (and genetic drift for that matter) occurs, the degree of heterozygosity decreases. An allele that has its frequency dictated by inbreeding will not be uniquely influenced. That is, other alleles would be characterized by decreased heterozygosity as well. So, if the genome in general has a relatively high degree of heterozygosity, the gene is probably influenced by selection rather than inbreeding and/or genetic drift.

9. *Ex situ* conservation involves the removal of an organism from an original habitat to an artificially maintained habitat. *In situ* conservation is an attempt to preserve a species in its original habitat. Each confronts problems because while it may be possible to maintain an organism in an artificial habitat, it is no longer subject to the same selective pressures as experienced in the wild. Thus, the population will change. Attempts to maintain original habitats for *in situ* conservation are often met with failure as factors beyond a conservationist's control may dominate (air pollution, encroachment, and other aspects of habitat deterioration).

10. Generally, threatened species are captured and bred in an artificial environment until sufficient population numbers are achieved to ensure species survival. Next, genetic management strategies are applied to breed individuals in such a way as to increase genetic heterozygosity as much as possible. If plants are involved, seed banks are often used to maintain and facilitate long-term survival.

11. Genetic diversity generally increases the likelihood of long-term survival of a species by providing multiple opportunities for adaptation to environmental change. The ability of an organism to exploit varied environments and withstand environmental modification is directly related to genetic diversity.

12. Allozymes are variants of a particular protein often detected by electrophoresis. Such variation may or may not impact on the fitness of an individual. The greater the allozyme variation, the more genetically heterogeneous the individual. It is generally agreed that such genetic diversity is essential for long-term survival. All other factors being equal, allozyme variation is more likely to reflect physiological variation than RFLP variation because RFLPs region are not necessarily found in protein-coding regions of the genome. RFLP analysis allows one to detect very small amounts of genetic diversity in a population and is unlikely to encounter an organism that is not in some way variable in terms RFLP with respect to other organisms (within and among species).

13. Apply the formula:

$$N_e = 4(N_m N_f)/N_m + N_f \quad = 6.9$$

14. **(a)** The probability of being a heterozygote is $2pq = 2(.99)(.01) = 0.0198$. Multiplying this value by 20 gives the probability of being heterozygous:

$$0.0198 \times 20 = 0.396$$

(b) To determine N_e use the expression:

$$N_e/N = .42$$

$$N_e = .42 \times 50 = 21$$

$$H_t = (1-1/2N_e)^t H_o$$

$$= (1-1/42)^5 \times 0.0198$$

$$= 0.01755$$

$$H_t/H_o = .01755/.0198 = 0.886$$

Therefore there is a loss of approximately 11.4% heterozygosity after five generations.

15. The maximum genetic diversity of the population will be enhanced by using the largest possible number in the founding population and minimizing the number of generations in captivity. By keeping complete pedigree records, one can increase genetic variation by reducing inbreeding and exchanging breeding individuals among captive populations.

16. First, it will be necessary to determine whether the native habitat in the Asian steppes of the 1920s is suitable to any introduction. If the original range is supportive of reintroduction, care must be taken to introduce horses with maximum genetic diversity possible. To do so, you might monitor RFLP patterns. Since the founder breeding group included a domestic mare, it may be desirable to select those for reintroduction which are least like the domestic mare genetically. It might be desirable to release reasonably-sized breeding groups in separate locations within the range to enhance eventual genetic diversity.

17. DNA profiles indicate the degree of heterogeneity in DNA sequences and therefore the degree of genetic variation. While non-coding DNA sequences represent the bulk of sequence diversity, such information can be helpful in determining gene flow, ancestry, and overall inter- and intra-population diversity. Since diversity *per se* appears to be essential for long-term species survival in natural environments, one would expect that the assessment of diversity by any tool will be a useful predictor.

18. From a physiological standpoint, cryogenic preservation in liquid nitrogen can allow 100 years or more of seed storage for some species, however, such elaborate storage can only be offered to a small fraction of the world's seeds. Thus, seeds of most species undergo storage loss which decreases genetic diversity. Seeds of tropical plants are somewhat intolerant to cold storage and must be regenerated frequently, a practice which is prone to a loss of genetic diversity arising from genetic drift. Only a finite number of seeds can be used in each regeneration procedure and the restriction of sample size (often fewer than 100 plants) reduces genetic diversity. To somewhat counteract this problem, plants are grown under optimum conditions to reduce selection. Another problem associated with preserved seeds is the accumulation of deleterious mutations both as a result of seed storage and regeneration. Some studies indicate increased frequencies of chromosomal and mtDNA lesions, chlorophyll deficiency mutations, and decreased DNA polymerase activity associated with long term seed storage.

19. A census of population size and range would be needed to establish levels of habitat exploitation and probable number of effective breeding pairs. From this information, an estimation of long term habitat support can be provided along with the probability of genetic drift eroding genetic variability. Effective breeder estimates will also provide a method for estimating inbreeding depression. It would be helpful to conduct surveys on a season-to-season and year-to-year basis to decrease the possibility of sampling in an atypical season or year. In would be important to determine the age and stage-specific structure of the endangered population. Few young or juveniles might indicate that reproductive capacities are in decline. It would be important to determine the general level biodiversity and carrying capacity of the habitat as well as the genetic diversity of the species in question. Nuclear, mitochondrial, and chloroplast DNA profiles can be used to assess intrapopulation and interpopulation variation as well as to aid in determining migration and breeding patterns.

20. The longest bottleneck-to-present interval occurred with cheetahs and one would expect cheetahs to show the highest degree of microsatellite polymorphism. The shortest bottleneck-to-present interval occurred with the Gir Forest lions so it would be expected to have the least polymorphism. Data from Driscoll et al. (2002 *Genome Research* 12:414-423) include the following estimates of microsatellite polymorphism in the three feline groups mentioned above: cheetahs (84.1%), pumas (42.9%), and Gir Forest lions (19.3%).

21. The following graph would incorporate the expected relationship between bottlenecks and microsatellite variation.

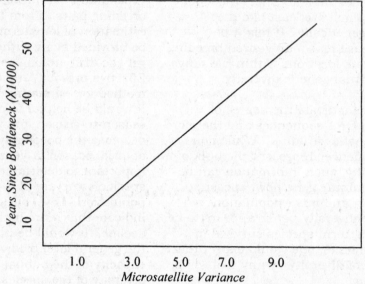

22. **(a)** The species with the greatest genetic variability, as estimated by these markers, is the domesticated cat. Domesticated cats share an immense and variable gene pool. Their staggering numbers and outbreeding behaviors allow them to maintain a high degree of genetic variability. **(b)** The lion has the least genetic variability. **(c)** Since allozymes are proteins and proteins often provide a significant function in an organism, selection is stronger and mutations are less tolerated. Selection would be expected to be more harsh on DNA segments which are related to function. In addition, by their very nature, microsatellites and minisatellites are more mutable.

23. Since there is less genetic variation in lions (according to these data), it is likely that they are the species which underwent the population crisis mentioned above. That "bottleneck" apparently reduced allelic variation considerably.

24. While flagship species (often large mammals) may make it possible to gather considerable public support and funding, they may reduce support for species which may have a greater impact on a community of species. Primary producers (plants) are a necessary component of a diverse and supportive habitat. If one focuses on a flagship species within an area, it is possible that other areas will suffer more dramatically because foundational species are lost. Using umbrella species to protect a large geographic area in hopes of protecting other species in that area is a reasonable approach. However, the size of an area is not necessarily a primary factor in determining species success. Diversity and productivity of a habitat are major contributors to species success. Since land is at a premium, it may be wiser in the long run to select umbrella species in diverse and productive habitats rather than on the basis of land size. By selecting sets of species which show considerable biodiversity, one increases the likelihood of protecting a sufficiently rich habitat to support many species. Such habitats are often of considerable economic value thereby making their availability limited.

Sample Test Questions
(detailed explanations of answers follow in next section)

How to use this section:

The purpose of these *Sample Test Questions* is to present a slightly different style of question. Set aside several hours of study time, perhaps a week before each examination. Select two questions from each chapter covered on your upcoming test. Attempt to work selected questions, five or so per hour, under test conditions. **Write down your answers**, then, *after* you have finished the entire "test," check your answers.

If you are having difficulty, then you are weak in the concept areas listed for each question. If you have made mistakes, take comfort, there are many places to make mistakes on these problems. Some of the students who made the same mistakes are now practicing geneticists!

For the questions below from Chapter 1, there are few major concepts. This chapter serves as an introduction and gives you a general overview of the content of the text and its significance. Test questions are primarily oriented toward reading retention and study effort.

Ch. 1 Ques.1 In 1859, Charles Darwin published *The Origin of Species* in which he presented ideas on the causes of organismic change through time. A primary conceptual gap existed, which left his theory open to criticism. What was that conceptual gap?

Ch. 1 Ques.2 Name the individual who, working with the garden pea in the mid 1850s, demonstrated quantitative patterns of heredity and developed a theory involving the behavior of hereditary factors.

Ch. 1 Ques.3 What does the term "genetics" mean?

Ch. 1 Ques.4 Name the substance that serves as the hereditary material in eukaryotes and prokaryotes. Is your answer the same for viruses?

Sample Test Questions

Ch. 1 Ques.5 When examining chromosomes from a single nucleus of an individual cell it is often possible to match up chromosomes on the basis of overall size, centromere position, and sometimes other physical characteristics. Chromosomes that can be matched up or paired are called _____.

Ch. 1 Ques.6 What is the difference between deoxyribonucleic acid and ribonucleic acid?

Ch. 1 Ques.7 List three components of the genetic material, DNA.

Concepts: chromosome mechanics (mitosis, meiosis), symbolism, DNA content (cell cycles)

Ch. 2, 3 Ques.8 The mosquito, *Culex pipiens*, has a diploid chromosome number of six. Assume that one chromosome pair is metacentric, and the other two pairs are acrocentric.

(a) Draw chromosomal configurations that one would expect to see at the following stages: primary oocyte (metaphase I) and secondary spermatocyte.

(b) Assuming that a G1 nucleus in *Culex* contains about 20 picograms (pg) of DNA, how much DNA would you expect in the following nuclei: primary spermatocyte, first polar body, secondary oocyte, and ootid in G1 phase.

(c) Assume that a female mosquito is heterozygous for the recessive gene *wavy bristles* (symbolized as *wb*) and this gene locus is on an acrocentric chromosome. Draw an expected mitotic metaphase with the appropriate genetic labeling pattern.

254

> **Concepts: chromosome mechanics (mitosis, meiosis), symbolism, DNA content (cell cycles)**

Chs. 2, 3 Ques.9 In humans, chromosome #1 is large and metacentric, the X chromosome is medium in size and submetacentric (submedian), and the Y chromosome is small and acrocentric. Assume that you were microscopically examining human chromosomes at the stages given below.

(a) Illustrate (draw) the above-mentioned (#1, X and/or Y) chromosomes and/or pairs at the stages given (several different configurations may be applicable in some cases):

Metaphase I (Primary Oocyte):

First Polar Body:

Secondary Spermatocyte:

Secondary Oocyte:

(b) The Rh blood group locus is on Chromosome #1. Individuals are *DD* or *Dd* if Rh⁺ and *dd* if Rh⁻. The locus for glucose-6-phosphate-dehydrogenase deficiency (*G6PD*) is located on the X chromosome. There are two alternatives at this locus, + and -. For each of the above cells, place genes (using the symbolism given) on chromosomes if the female is heterozygous at both the *Rh* and *G6PD* loci. Do the same for the secondary spermatocyte (above) assuming that the male is Rh⁻ and + for the *G6PD* locus.

(c) Assume that the average DNA content per G1 nucleus in humans is 6.5 picograms. For the nuclei (including the entire chromosome complement for each nucleus) presented, give the expected DNA content:

Metaphase I (Primary Oocyte):_____   Secondary Spermatocyte:_____

First Polar Body:_____   Secondary Oocyte:_____

Sample Test Questions

Concepts: chromosome morphology (telocentric, etc.), anaphase configurations chromosome mechanics, meiosis, mitosis, DNA content in cell cycles

Ch. 2 Ques.10 Assume that you are examining a cell under a microscope and you observe the following as the total chromosomal constituents of a nucleus. You know that $2n = 2$ in this organism, that all chromosomes are telocentric, and that each G1 cell nucleus contains 8 picograms of DNA.

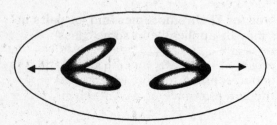

(a) Circle the correct stage for this cell:

anaphase of mitosis
anaphase of meiosis I
anaphase of meiosis II
telophase of mitosis

(b) How many picograms of chromosomal DNA would you expect in the cell shown above?_____

Concepts: chromosome mechanics (meiosis), symbolism, meiotic nondisjunction, sex-linkage

Chs. 2, 3, 4 Ques.11 The genes for *singed bristles (sn)* and *miniature wings (m)* are recessive and located on the X chromosome in *Drosophila melanogaster*. In a cross between a singed-bristled, miniature-winged female and a wild type male, all of the male offspring were singed-miniature.

> **(a)** Draw meiotic metaphase I chromosomal configurations that represent the X and/or Y chromosomes of the parental (singed-miniature female and wild type male) flies. Place gene symbols (*sn, m*) and their wild type alleles (*sn⁺, m⁺*) on appropriate chromosomes.

(b) Draw a mitotic metaphase chromosomal configuration that represents the X and/or Y chromosomes of the F_1 male. Place gene symbols (*sn, m*) on appropriate chromosomes.

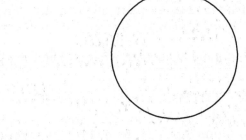

(c) Most of the female offspring from the above-mentioned cross were phenotypically wild type; however one exceptional female was recovered that had singed bristles and miniature wings. Given that meiotic nondisjunction accounted for this exceptional female, would you expect it to have occurred in the parental male or parental female?

(d) Draw a meiotic, labeled (with gene symbols) circumstance and division product(s) that could account for the exceptional female described above in part (c). (Confine your drawing to X chromosomes only.)

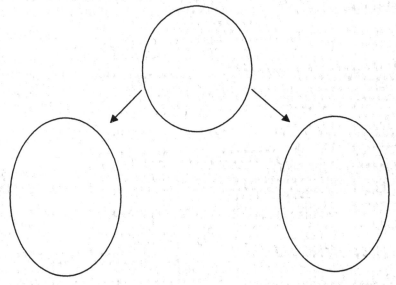

Sample Test Questions

Concepts: meiosis and chromosome numbers, DNA content

Ch. 2 Ques.12 The red fox (*Vulpes vulpes*) has 17 pairs of somewhat long chromosomes. The Arctic fox (*Alopex lagopus*) has 26 pairs of somewhat shorter chromosomes.

(a) If a female red fox is crossed with a male Arctic fox, what will be the chromosome number in the somatic tissues of the hybrid?

(b) Assume that a somatic G1 nucleus of the Arctic fox contains 12 picograms of DNA, while a somatic G1 nucleus of the red fox contains 8 picograms of DNA. How much nuclear DNA could you expect in a G2 somatic nucleus of the hybrid?

Concepts: sex-linked inheritance (X-linked), pedigree construction, probability (product rule)

Chs. 3, 4, 5 Ques.13 Red-green color blindness is inherited in man as an X-linked, recessive gene. Using the symbols below, draw a pedigree that is consistent with the following statements:

A phenotypically normal woman is married to a phenotypically normal man. The woman's parents are phenotypically normal, but her maternal grandfather is color-blind. The woman's paternal grandparents, as well as her maternal grandmother, are phenotypically normal.

male = □
female = ○
Rg = **normal color sight**
rg = **color-blind**

What is the probability that the first son born to the woman will be phenotypically normal (not be color-blind)?

Concepts: **sex-linked inheritance (X-linked), chromosome mechanics, meiosis, conventional symbolism**

Chs. 3, 4, 5 Ques.14 In a *Drosophila* experiment, a cross is made between a homozygous wild type female and a tan-bodied (mutant) male. All the resulting F_1 flies were phenotypically wild type. Adult flies of the F_2 generation (from a mating of the F_1's) had the following characteristics:

Sex	Phenotype	Number
Male	wild	346
Male	tan	329
Female	wild	702

(a) Using conventional symbolism, illustrate the genotype, *on an appropriate chromosomal configuration*, of a secondary oocyte nucleus of one of the F_1 females. Be certain to distinguish the X chromosomes from the autosomes. Note: *Drosophila melanogaster* has a diploid chromosome number of eight.

(b) Using the same conventional symbolism, give the genotype, *on an appropriate chromosomal configuration*, of a primary spermatocyte of the tan-bodied F_2 males.

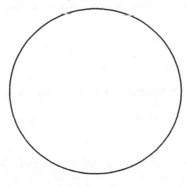

Sample Test Questions

> **Concepts: Mendelian genetics, monohybrid cross, dominance/recessiveness, 3:1 and 1:1 ratios**

Ch. 3 Ques.15 *Gray* seed color in peas is dominant to *white*. Assume that Mendel conducted a series of experiments where plants were crossed and offspring classified according to the table below. What are the most probable genotypes of each parent?

Parents			Progeny	
			gray	white
(a) gray	X	white	81	79
(b) gray	X	gray	120	42
(c) white	X	white	0	50
(d) gray	X	white	74	0

(a) gray _____ X white_____
(b) gray _____ X gray _____
(c) white _____ X white _____
(d) gray _____ X white _____

> **Concepts: sex-linkage (X-linked), autosomal inheritance, dihybrid situation incomplete dominance, complete dominance**

Chs. 3, 4, 5 Ques.16 Hemophilia (type A) is recessive and X-linked in humans, whereas the ABO blood groups locus is autosomal. Assume that the following matings were examined for the transmission of these genes. Give the expected phenotypes and numbers assuming 800 offspring are produced.

Group A: Females heterozygous for hemophilia with blood type AB mated to normal males with blood group O.

Group B: Females heterozygous for hemophilia with blood type AB mated to males with hemophilia and blood group AB.

> **Concepts: Mendelian patterns, 1:1:1:1 ratio, null hypothesis, expected values**
> **χ² analysis, interpretation of χ²**

Ch. 3 Ques.17 For the cross *PpRr* X *pprr* where complete dominance and independent assortment hold, assume that you received the following results and that you wished to determine whether they differ significantly (in a statistical sense) from expectation.

PR phenotypes	= 40
Pr phenotypes	= 10
pR phenotypes	= 20
pr phenotypes	= 30

(a) State the null hypothesis associated with this test of significance.

(b) How many degrees of freedom would be associated with this test of significance?

(c) Assuming that a Chi-Square value of 20.00 is arrived at in this test of significance, do you accept or reject the null hypothesis?

Degrees of Freedom	*p* = 0.05
1	3.84
2	5.99
3	7.82
4	9.49
5	11.07

> **Concepts: sex-linked inheritance (X-linked), gynandromorph production,**
> **sex determination in *Drosophila*, insect development mitosis,**
> **mitotic nondisjunction**

Chs. 2, 5 Ques.18 Explain the processes --- genotypic, chromosomal, and developmental --- that would lead to a bilateral gynandromorph in *Drosophila melanogaster* in which the male half of the fly has white eyes and singed bristles, while the female half is phenotypically wild type.

Sample Test Questions

> **Concepts:** **interaction of gene products, relationship between genotype and phenotype, multi-factor inheritance**

Chs. 2, 3, 21 Ques.19 Describe and exemplify similarities and differences between *discontinuous* and *continuous* traits at the *molecular* and *transmission* levels.

> **Concepts:** **crossing over mechanisms, meiosis, gene mapping, chromosome mechanics**

Chs. 2, 7 Ques.20 Assume that there are 18 map units between two loci in the mouse and that you are able to microscopically observe meiotic chromosomes in this organism. If you examined 150 primary oocytes, in how many would you expect to see a chiasma between the two loci mentioned above?

> **Concepts:** **extranuclear inheritance, maternal effects**

Ch. 4 Ques.21 Direction of shell coiling in the land snail, *Limnaea peregra*, is determined by alleles at a single locus: *dextral* (right) = *DD* or *Dd*; *sinistral* (left) = *dd*. However, a maternal effect is present such that the genotype of the mother determines the direction of coiling (phenotype) of the immediate offspring. Given the following crosses, write the genotypes and phenotypes in the spaces provided. Be certain to indicate which genotypes go with which phenotypes.

	Source of sperm	Source of egg
Cross #1	*DD*	*dd*

Offspring genotype(s): [   ]   Offspring phenotype(s): [   ]

	Source of sperm	Source of egg
Cross #2	*dd*	*Dd* (sinistral)

Offspring genotype(s): [   ]   Offspring phenotype(s): [   ]

	Source of sperm	Source of egg
Cross #3	*Dd*	*Dd*

Offspring genotype(s): [   ]   Offspring phenotype(s): [   ]

Sample Test Questions

> **Concepts: linkage and crossing over, computation of map units, complete linkage independent assortment, lack of crossing over in males**

Ch. 7 Ques.22 Given below are four dihybrid crosses between various strains of *Drosophila*. To the right of each are map distances known to exist between the genes involved. For each cross, give the phenotypes of the offspring and the percentages expected for each.

	Matings	
Female	*Male*	*Map distance*
(a) *AB/ab*	*ab/ab*	20
(b) *Pq/pQ*	*pq/pq*	50
(c) *DB/db*	*db/db*	0
(d) *ab/ab*	*AB*/ab	20

(a) *AB/ab* X *ab/ab* _____

(b) *Pq/pQ* X *pq/pq* _____

(c) *DB/db* X *db/db* _____

(d) *ab/ab* X *AB*/ab _____

> **Concepts: recombination in bacteria, transduction, transformation, lysogeny**

Ch. 8 Ques.23 Below are phrases that refer to various forms of recombination in bacteria. For each, clearly state whether you **agree** or **disagree**. If you disagree, briefly explain your reason(s).

(a) Transduction is the process in which exogenous DNA is drawn into bacteria as a single-stranded structure, then integrated into the bacterial chromosome. [____]

(b) Temperate phages are capable of entering a lysogenic cycle such that their genomes are incorporated into the bacterial chromosome. [____]

(c) During the lysogenic cycle, phages are capable of producing bacteria when exposed to U.V. light. [____]

Sample Test Questions

Chs. 9, 11, 12, 13, 14 Ques.24 The foundations of molecular genetics rest upon the assumption that a genetic material exists with the following properties:

     a. autocatalytic (can replicate itself)

     b. heterocatalytic (can direct form and function)

     c. mutable

     d. can exist in an infinite number of forms

(a) Provide a simple sketch that demonstrates the replication scheme of DNA.

(b) Briefly describe how DNA provides form and function.

(c) At the level of nucleotides, what characterizes mutant DNA?

(d) Why may we say that DNA can exist in an infinite number of forms?

Chs. 9, 11 Ques.25 On the graph below draw C$_{o}$t curves for DNA from two genomes, one lacking repetitive DNA and the other containing repetitive DNA. Indicate the point on each curve at which the renaturation is half-complete. Label the horizontal and vertical axes accordingly. Explain the molecular basis for the different curves.

Sample Test Questions

Concepts: **DNA and RNA structure, complementarity 5', 3' orientations, degradation products**

Chs. 9, 10 Ques.26 Given below is a single-stranded nucleotide sequence. Answer questions that refer to this sequence.

(a) In the circle at the bottom of this sequence, place a 5' or 3', whichever corresponds.

(b) Is the above structure an RNA or a DNA? State which_____.

(c) Assume that a complementary strand is produced in which all the innermost phosphates of the adenine triphosphonucleoside precursors are labeled with ^{32}P. What bases would be labeled if the complementary strand were completely degraded with spleen diesterase (cleaves between the phosphate and the 5'carbon)?_____.

(d) What bases would be labeled if the complementary strand were completely degraded with snake venom diesterase (cleaves between the phosphate and the 3' carbon)?_____.

Sample Test Questions

> **Concepts: semiconservative replication, labeling, centrifugation, denaturation**

Ch. 10 Ques.27 Assume that you were able to culture a strain of *E. coli* in medium containing either "normal" nitrogen or a heavy isotope of nitrogen (^{15}N). You grow the bacteria for a time in ^{15}N-containing medium, which permits one complete replication of the bacterial chromosome. You extract the DNA, calling this extraction A. You continue to grow the bacterial culture in the ^{15}N DNA for a time, which permits one more complete round of chromosome replication. You again extract the DNA, calling this extraction B. Assuming that nonlabeled DNA has a density of 1.6 and that fully labeled DNA (that is with *all* the ^{14}N replaced with ^{15}N) has a density of 1.9, construct sedimentation profiles that reflect the expected densities of DNA from extractions A and B.

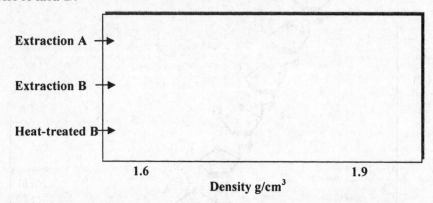

Knowing that heating DNA to 100° C causes separation of complementary strands, use a broken line (- - -) to indicate the sedimentation profile of heat denaturation of extraction B DNA.

> **Concepts: semiconservative replication, chromosome morphology, DNA structure, labeling, enzymatic digestion, 5', 3' orientations**

Ch. 10 Ques.28 Assume that you are microscopically examining mitotic metaphase cells of an organism with a $2n$ chromosome number of two (both telocentric). Assume also that the cell passed through one S phase labeling (innermost phosphate of dCTP radioactive) just prior to the period of observation.

(a) Draw this cell's chromosomes, and the autoradiographic pattern you would expect to see.

(b) Assuming that the A+T/G+C ratio of the DNA in this cell is 1.67 and that this DNA is digested with snake venom diesterase (cleaves at the 3' position), what percentages of the total radioactivity would the following products have?

Adenine_____ Guanine_____
Thymine_____ Cytosine_____

266

Concepts: overall DNA replication, 5', 3' polarity restrictions, enzymology, priming

Ch. 10 Ques.29 Drawn below is a diagram (not to scale) of DNA in the process of replication. Numbered arrows point to specific structures that you are to identify in the corresponding spaces below:

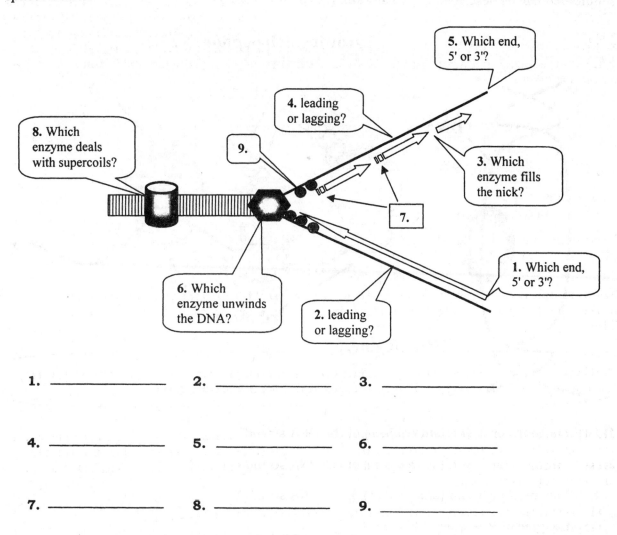

1. _____ 2. _____ 3. _____

4. _____ 5. _____ 6. _____

7. _____ 8. _____ 9. _____

Concepts: transcription 5', 3' orientations, translation tRNA orientation, general process, rRNA in ribosomes

Chs. 12, 13 Ques.30 Below is a schematic of transcription and translation occurring simultaneously as described by Miller *et al.* (1970) in *E. coli.*

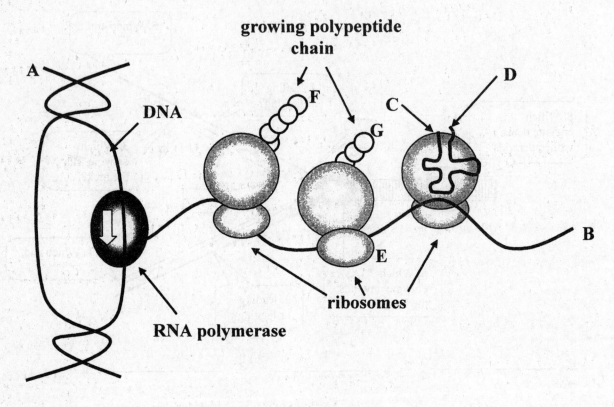

1. Is "A" at the 5' or 3' end (*state which*) of the DNA strand? _____

2. Is "B" at the 5' or 3' end (*state which*) of the RNA strand? _____

3. Is "C" at the 5' or 3' end (*state which*) of the RNA strand? _____

4. To what type of RNA does "D" point? _____

5. Would base sequences near letters "C" or "D" (*state which*) be expected to hold the amino acid? _____

6. What is the S value of the rRNA in the small subunit of the ribosome closest to letter "E"? _____

7. Is the amino acid nearest letter "F" the same type as the one nearest letter "G" (*yes or no*)? _____

> **Concepts: translation, coding, mutation**

Chs. 12, 13, 14 Ques.31 Assume that the following sequence of amino acids occurs in a protein starting from the "N" terminus (with asp) of a large polypeptide chain:

> asp-glu-ile-leu-ser-thr-met-arg-tyr-try-phe-gly

Assume that gene *X* is responsible for synthesis of this gene. Answer the questions below.

(a) Which amino acid(s) would you expect to change if gene *X* is altered by the mutagen, 2-amino purine, such that a transition mutation occurred that caused a change in the 9th base of the mRNA (counting from the 5' end of the coding region)?

(b) Which amino acid(s) would you expect to change if gene *X* is altered by mutagen, such as acridine orange, such that a frameshift mutation occurred that caused an insertion of a base between bases 3 and 4 of the mRNA (counting from the 5' end of the coding region)?

(c) Which amino acid(s) would you expect to change if gene *X* is altered by the mutagen, nitrous acid, such that a mutation occurred That caused a change in the 11th base of the mRNA (counting from the 5' end of the coding region)?

> **Concepts: pathway analysis, Beadle and Tatum "set-up",
> biochemical (nutritional) phenotype**

Ch. 13 Ques.32 Below is a set of experimental results relating the growth (+) of *Neurospora* on several media. Based on the information provided, present the biochemical pathway and the locations of the metabolic blocks.

Strain	*Medium*		
	MM	MM+A	MM+B
t409	-	+	+
t410	+	+	+
r3	-	-	+

Concepts: importance of primary structure, varieties of bonds "higher level" folding structure/function relationships

Ch. 13 Ques.33 Drawn below is a hypothetical protein that contains areas where various types of bonds might be expected to occur. For each area, a box is drawn and in that box is a number. In the corresponding spaces below, state which bond type (or interaction) is most likely illustrated **and** state how that particular type of bond (or interaction) is formed. *You may use a given bond type only once.*

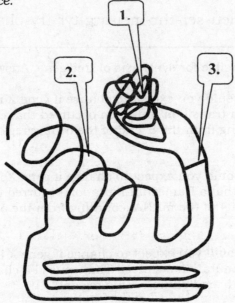

1.

2.

3.

4. What type of amino acids tend to be located on the outside (water side) of the molecule?

Concepts: overlapping genes, differential hnRNA splicing

Chs. 13, 15 Ques.34 Some viruses, as well as eukaryotes, have evolved different mechanisms for obtaining more than one kind of protein from a single transcription unit (a transcription unit simply being a stretch of DNA that is transcribed into a single primary RNA transcript). Describe two different mechanisms.

Sample Test Questions

> **Concepts: genetic regulation, positive vs. negative control**

Ch. 15 Ques.35 Depending on the regulatory system, in prokaryotes when the regulatory protein **is** or **isn't** bound to the DNA, the operon may be **on** or **off**. Fill in the chart below and give a brief explanation of your reasoning.

Relationship of Regulator Protein to DNA	Operator	
	Positive control	Negative control
is bound		
isn't bound		

> **Concepts: experimental strategies, action of nucleases, DNase restriction endonucleases**

Ch. 17 Ques.36 DNase is often used to map the locations where DNA-binding proteins (histones, RNA polymerases, transcription factors, *etc.*) interact with DNA. Restriction endonucleases are used to cut DNA for identification and cloning. Why are these two different enzyme classes used in these different ways?

> **Concepts: experimental strategies cDNA probes Southern blots electrophoresis restriction endonuclease analysis hybridization**

Ch. 17, 18 Ques.37 Assume that you have a cDNA clone for the gene causing retinoblastoma and that you prepare Southern blots probing DNA in cells from normal individuals and from children with retinoblastoma. Genomic DNA is prepared using the restriction endonuclease *Hind*III (the *Rb* gene contains four *Hind*III fragments as indicated below), and the following hybridization appears:

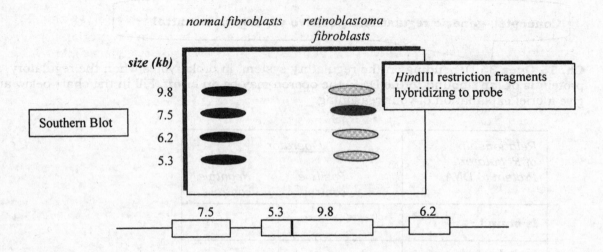

What does each band represent?

What conclusions can be drawn from these data?

Concepts: **experimental strategies, electrophoresis, restriction digestion, fragment analysis**

Ch. 17, 18, 19 Ques.38 The *thioredoxin* gene in bacteria aids in the necessary reduction of proteins. It encodes a protein of 108 amino acids and is contained in a 0.9 kb (*Pst*I/*Bam*HI) fragment. The gene for kanamycin resistance is contained in a 1.4 kb (*Bam*HI/*Pst*I) fragment. The restriction map (one orientation) of these two genes (flanked by *Bam*HI sites) in a plasmid vector is presented below.

(A)

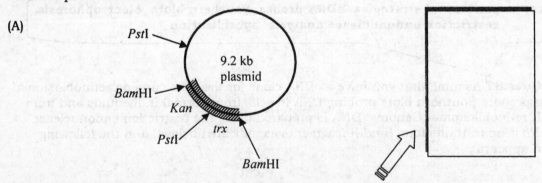

(a) Assume that the plasmid is restricted with the enzyme *Bam*HI. What would be the electrophoretic pattern of the cleaved fragments?

(b) Assume that the orientation given above is only a guess and that the *Bam* HI fragment containing the *trx* and *Kan* genes could possibly exist in the opposite orientation (B). What experiment would you perform to determine whether the orientation is as in (A) or (B)?

(B)

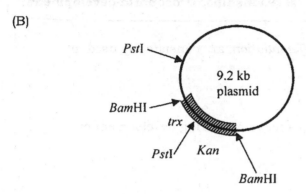

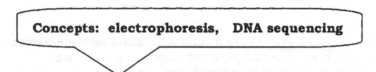

Concepts: electrophoresis, DNA sequencing

Chs. 17, 18, 19 Ques.39 The Maxam and Gilbert DNA sequencing procedure involves chemical reactions (methylation) and cleavages (piperidine) that produce ^{32}P-labeled DNA fragments. The chemical reagents can give rise to G, G+A, C, and C+T cleavages. These fragments are then separated on electrophoretic gels, and the sequence is read directly from the gel. A sample gel is given below. From this gel, provide the sequence of the DNA fragment.

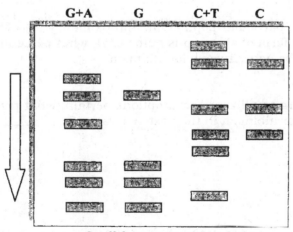

Small fragments at this end of gel

Concepts: determination, differentiation,, relationships, *Drosophila* development

Ch. 20 Ques.40 Two terms, *determination* and *differentiation*, are consistently used in discussions of development.

   (a) Provide a brief definition of each term.

   (b) Which, determination or differentiation, comes first during development of *Drosophila*, for example?

Concepts: variable gene activity hypothesis, genomic equivalence evidence for differential transcription

Ch. 20 Ques.41 Development may be defined as the attainment of a differentiated state. Given that all cells of a eukaryote probably contain the same complete set of genes, how do we currently explain development in terms of gene activity? What evidence supports your explanation?

Concepts: Hardy-Weinberg applications to gene maintenance of gene frequencies over time

Ch. 22 Ques.42 Assume that in a particular population, approximately 9% of the individuals show albinism. Knowing that this form of albinism is autosomal, what percentage of the individuals would be expected to be heterozygous for albinism?

Assuming that the Hardy-Weinberg equilibrium assumptions pertain, what percentage of individuals will be heterozygous for albinism in the next generation?

Concepts: factors which change gene frequencies, influence of inbreeding on gene frequencies

Chs. 22, 23 Ques.43 List and briefly describe factors that change gene frequencies in populations. Is inbreeding a factor in changing gene frequencies? Explain.

Concept: relationship between speciation and Hardy-Weinberg assumptions

Ch. 23 Ques.44 A *species* is often defined as a population of interbreeding, or potentially interbreeding, organisms reproductively isolated from other such populations. Given such an isolated population, will speciation (formation of a new species) occur if the Hardy-Weinberg assumptions are met?

Concepts: natural selection, speciation

Ch. 23 Ques.45 Assume there exists a group of organisms that is temporally or spacially isolated from other such groups. This group has evolved genetic differences from neighboring groups. Describe the process of speciation in terms of this genetically distinct group of organisms.

Concepts: conservation genetics, hybrid vigor, genetic diversity

Ch. 23, 24 Ques.46 Why is genetic diversity important for the long-term survival of a species? What are the factors that reduce genetic diversity? What is meant by the term *genetic erosion*?

Concepts: conservation genetics, hybridization, population dynamics

Ch. 24 Ques.47 What are the causes and consequences of *outbreeding depression* as related to conservation biology?

Sample Test Answers

The following answers should be examined AFTER you have attempted to completely resolve (on paper) the problem on your own. You will learn more by struggling with a solution over a period of time than by immediately searching out the correct solution in the answer book.

Ch. 1 Answer 1 lack of understanding of the genetic basis of variation and inheritance

Ch. 2 Answer 2 Gregor Mendel

Ch. 1 Answer 3 Genetics is a subdiscipline of biology concerned with the study of heredity and variation at the molecular, cellular, developmental, organismal, and populational levels.

Ch. 1 Answer 4 DNA, or deoxyribonucleic acid, is the hereditary material in eukaryotes and prokaryotes. Either DNA or RNA (ribonucleic acid) serves in viruses.

Ch. 1 Answer 5 homologous

Ch. 1 Answer 6 In mitosis, chromosome number remains constant, while in meiosis, chromosome number is reduced by half in the final products. In meiosis, there is pairing of homologous chromosomes.

Ch. 1 Answer 7 nitrogenous bases, phosphate, deoxyribose sugar

Chs. 2, 3 Answer 8 This question is intended to determine your understanding of mitosis, chromosome morphology, symbolism, the positioning of genes on chromosomes, and the changes in DNA content through the cell cycles. **(a)** Since the diploid chromosome number is six, there will be three bivalents, one involving metacentrics, and two involving acrocentrics in a primary oocyte. We can draw the chromosomes of the primary oocyte as follows:

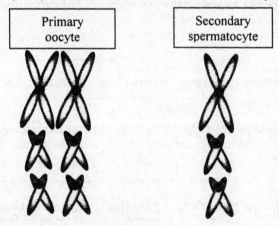

Since secondary spermatocytes arise after meiosis I, there should be only dyads, one metacentric and two acrocentric, and they should be aligned end-to-end as indicated in the above drawing .

(b) Given that there are about 20 picograms of DNA in a G1 nucleus, we would expect there to be 40pg in a G2 nucleus (after S phase) and 40pg to the point where homologous chromosomes separate in meiosis I. Secondary spermatocytes and secondary oocytes (as well as first polar bodies) should therefore, each have 20pg of DNA. After meiosis II the resulting nuclei should have 10pg each. If you understand events at interphase and in meiosis, this question is easy to answer. Carefully examine the figure below to understand events during interphase, as far as DNA content is concerned. Then examine the figures in Chapter 2 in this book to see how chromosomes behave in meiosis. From this information you should see the answers as follows:

Primary spermatocyte	= 40 pg
First polar body	= 20 pg
Secondary oocyte	= 20 pg
Ootid (in G1)	= 10 pg

It might be helpful to view changes in DNA content in graphic form:

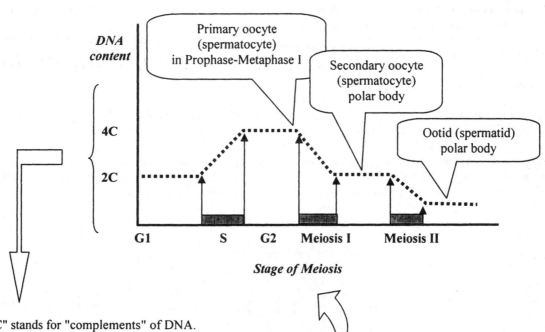

Stage of Meiosis

The "C" stands for "complements" of DNA.

Sketch chromosomes in the various stages listed above:

(c) If the mosquito is heterozygous for the recessive gene *wavy bristles* (*wb*) then it would have the genotype *Wb/wb*. Because there are four letters here representing the two genes, the slash between the symbols helps us to understand that there are only two genes being discussed.

We are asked to draw an acrocentric, mitotic metaphase chromosome complement in this heterozygous insect. We are expected to place the gene symbols on the chromosomes. Recall that there is no synapsis of homologous chromosomes in mitotic cells, therefore, the homologous chromosomes should not be placed side-by-side. Since sister chromatids are *identical* and homologous chromosomes are *similar*, we should draw the figure as follows:

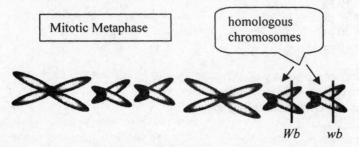

> **Common errors for Question 8:** incorrect number of chromosomes, incorrect chromosome morphology, metacentric, acrocentric, poor relationship of DNA content to cells, inappropriate symbols, inappropriate placement of genes

Chs. 2, 3 Answer 9 (a,b) Recall that a metacentric chromosome has "arms" of approximately equal length, while submetacentric and acrocentric chromosomes have arms of unequal length.

Metaphase I (primary oocyte): Homologous chromosomes are replicated and synapsed. There will be two X chromosomes present because oocytes occur in females. On the metacentric chromosomes (#1), place, such that sister chromatids are identical, the *Dd*. Place the + - alternatives on the X chromosomes.

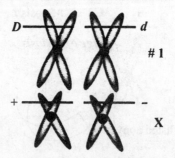

First polar body: The first polar body is a product of meiosis I, after homologous chromosomes have migrated to opposite poles. At this stage, dyads are present. Because females produce polar bodies, there should be an X chromosome present. Because the female is heterozygous, there are several possible answers. Note that there is only one representative of each allele for each gene pair.

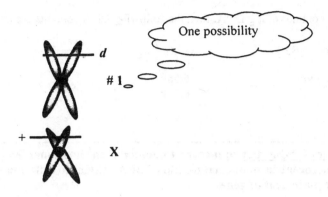

Secondary spermatocyte: A secondary spermatocyte will have the same chromosome configuration as a first polar body. Both are products of meiosis I and dyads should be present. Because spermatocytes occur in males, there will either be an X chromosome or a Y chromosome present. There are, therefore, two possible answers. Regarding the genetic constitution of these cells, as stated in the problem, we are to assume that the male is Rh⁻ and + for the *G6PD* locus. Since this locus is on the X chromosome, only one genotype (regarding the X chromosome) can be presented.

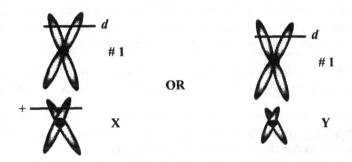

Secondary oocyte: Being a product of meiosis I, dyads will be present. Because oocytes occur in females, there should be an X (not a Y) chromosome present. The genetic labeling pattern for the secondary oocyte will be the same as for the first polar body.

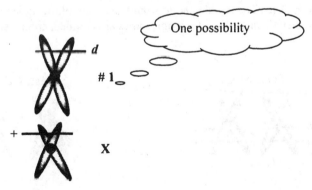

(c) If a G1 nucleus contains 6.5pg DNA, then the following DNA contents are expected:

Metaphase I (primary oocyte):	13pg
First polar body:	6.5pg
Secondary spermatocyte:	6.5pg
Secondary oocyte:	6.5pg

> **Common errors for Question 9:** incorrect number of chromosomes, incorrect chromosome morphology, metacentric, acrocentric, poor relationship of DNA content to cells, inappropriate symbols, inappropriate placement of genes

Ch. 2 Answer 10 (a) Since the cell contains only two chromosomes (2*n*=2) and there are two chromosomes pictured, it cannot represent a cell in the second phase (II) of meiosis. The chromosomes are telocentric, which means that the centromere is at the end of the chromosome. When pulled at anaphase, two sideways "Vs" or "< >" would be expected and the cell would be at the anaphase stage of meiosis I. The only other possibility to produce the "< >" figure would be a metaphase chromosome at anaphase of mitosis or anaphase II of meiosis. However, these possibilities are negated because the chromosomes are stated as being telocentric.

(b) In order to get the correct answer for the second part, one must consider that, because of the S-phase, at anaphase I the DNA complement is twice that of a G1 cell. Therefore, the correct answer is 16pg DNA.

> **Common errors for Question 10:** confusion on: significance of *telocentric*, significance of chromosome number, many students consider the chromosomes to be metacentric

Chs. 2, 3, 4 Answer 11 (a) The female parent would have the following labeled chromosomal symbolism (Remember that at meiotic metaphase I, chromosomes are doubled, condensed, and synapsed.):

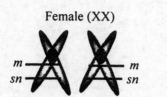

Female (XX)

m
sn

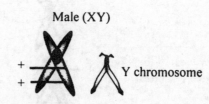

Male (XY)

+
+

Y chromosome

(b) In general, mitotic metaphase chromosomes are not synapsed, although in *Drosophila* mitotic chromosomes do pair. To avoid confusion and to be consistent with what is expected in other organisms, the mitotic chromosomes will not be drawn in the paired state.

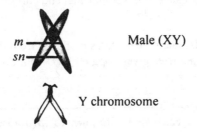

Male (XY)

Y chromosome

(c) All of the female offspring from the above cross should be heterozygous and phenotypically wild type. The one exceptional female could have resulted from maternal nondisjunction at meiosis I or II, thus producing an egg cell with two X chromosomes, each containing the *sn* and *m* genes. When fertilized by a sperm cell carrying the Y chromosome (along with the normal haploid set of autosomes) an $X^{sn\ m}X^{sn\ m}Y$ female is produced.

(d)

Female (XX)

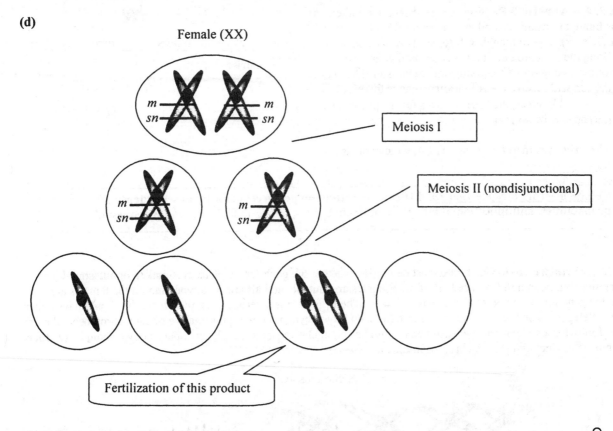

Meiosis I

Meiosis II (nondisjunctional)

Fertilization of this product

Common errors for Question 11: incorrect chromosome morphology, X and Y chromosomes, inappropriate symbols, inappropriate placement of genes, problems with meiotic nondisjunction

Ch. 2 Answer 12 (a) Since the chromosome numbers are given in *pairs*, recall that during meiosis each gamete contains one chromosome of each pair. If the red fox has 17 pairs of chromosomes, then each gamete will contain 17 chromosomes. For the Arctic fox, each gamete should contain 26 chromosomes. A zygote is produced from the union of the parental gametes; therefore, it should contain 43 chromosomes (17 + 26). It turns out that some such hybrids are viable, but are usually sterile because of developmental and chromosomal alignment and segregational problems at meiosis.

(b) If G1 nuclei contain 12pg and 8pg DNA, then the gametes produced from these organisms will contain 6 and 4pg DNA, respectively. Combining these gametes gives 10pg for a G1 cell. For a G2 cell there should be 20pg DNA.

> **Common errors for Question 12:** confusion with pairs of chromosomes, gametic chromosome number, confusion with uneven number of chromosomes, confusion with *somatic* cells

Chs. 3, 4, 5 Answer 13 Because the maternal grandfather was color-blind, the woman's mother is a carrier for this X-linked gene ($X^{Rg}X^{rg}$). The woman therefore has a 1/2 chance of inheriting the X^{rg} chromosome from her mother and a 1/2 chance of passing this X^{rg} chromosome to her son. The chance that the son will receive the X^{rg} chromosome is therefore 1/4 (1/2 X 1/2). However, the question asks for the probability that the son will be normal.

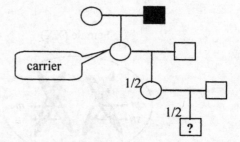

The answer is, therefore, 1 minus 1/4, which equals 3/4.

> **Common errors for Question 13:** difficulty in setting up pedigree, inability to see independent probabilities, multiplication of independent probabilities, seeing that the *normal* is requested

Chs. 3, 4, 5 Answer 14 (a) First, one must determine whether the gene for *tan body* is X-linked or autosomal (not on the sex chromosome). Because half of the F_2 males are mutant and half are wild type, and all the females are wild, the gene for *tan body* is behaving as X-linked. The F_1 female is heterozygous; therefore, she should have either of the alleles (t, t^+) on the one X chromosome (a secondary oocyte has one representative of each chromosomal pair) in the following arrangement. Because *Drosophila* has eight chromosomes, each secondary oocyte should have four chromosomes (including the X chromosome).

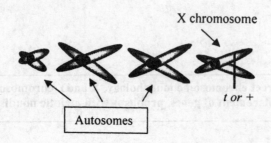

(b) A primary spermatocyte has the chromosomes in a doubled, condensed, and synapsed state. A tan-bodied male should have an X (containing a *t* gene) and a Y chromosome, as well as a diploid complement of autosomes.

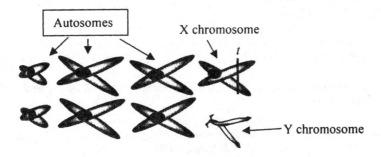

Common errors for Question 14: difficulty in recognizing X-linked inheritance, problems with placing genes on chromosomes, problems with visualizing genome

Ch. 3 Answer 15 First, assign gene symbols: *G* = gray, *gg* = white.

(a) Since there is an approximate 1:1 ratio in the progeny, the parental genotypes are *Gg* X *gg*.

(b) A 3:1 ratio is apparent, therefore the parental genotypes are *Gg* X *Gg*.

(c) Because there are no gray phenotypes and *gray* is the dominant allele, the parental genotypes must be *gg* X *gg*.

(d) Since there are no white types and the sample is sufficiently large, it is very likely that the parental genotypes are *GG* X *gg*.

Common errors for Question 15: students usually have only minor problems with this type of question, some careless, random mistakes

Chs 3, 4, 5 Answer 16 Set up the crosses with an appropriate symbol set such as the following:

h = hemophilia H = normal allele $I^A I^B$ = AB blood group $I^o I^o$ = O blood group.

Group A

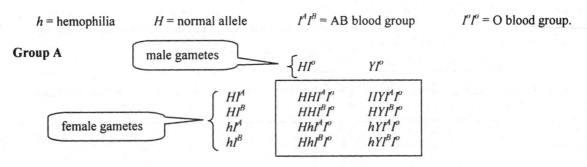

Collecting phenotypes gives:

1/4 female, normal, A blood (200)
1/4 female, normal, B blood (200)
1/8 male, normal, A blood (100)
1/8 male, normal, B blood (100)
1/8 male, hemophilia, A blood (100)
1/8 male, hemophilia, B blood (100)

Group B. In this example the forked-line method will be used. Consider what will be happening for the *hemophilia* locus independently from the blood group locus.

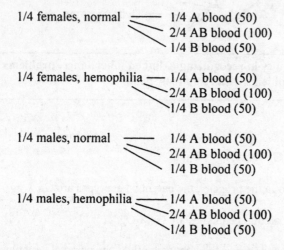

1/4 females, normal —— 1/4 A blood (50)
                        2/4 AB blood (100)
                        1/4 B blood (50)

1/4 females, hemophilia —— 1/4 A blood (50)
                           2/4 AB blood (100)
                           1/4 B blood (50)

1/4 males, normal —— 1/4 A blood (50)
                     2/4 AB blood (100)
                     1/4 B blood (50)

1/4 males, hemophilia —— 1/4 A blood (50)
                         2/4 AB blood (100)
                         1/4 B blood (50)

> **Common errors for Question 16**: difficulty with any dihybrid situation, X-linked with autosomal inheritance, incomplete dominance, calculating frequencies, observed numbers

Ch. 3 Answer 17 (a) An appropriate null hypothesis for this example would be that the observed (measured) values do not differ significantly from the predicted ratio of 1:1:1:1. One might also say that any deviation between the observed and predicted values is due to chance and chance alone.

(b) Because there are four classes being compared, there will be three degrees of freedom.

(c) Given that the Chi-square value of 20.00 is considerably greater than 7.82 (for three degrees of freedom) the null hypothesis should be rejected and the conclusion should be that the observed values differ significantly from the predicted values based on a 1:1:1:1 ratio.

> **Common errors for Question 17**: inability to see a 1:1:1:1 ratio, development of the expected ratios, interpreting probability values from table

Chs. 2, 5 Answer 18 In order for this type of fly to occur, the zygote must start out as a heterozygote in which both mutant genes are on one homologue and wild type alleles are on the other. In addition, one of the wild type chromosomes must get "lost" at the first mitotic division, thus making the female half $X^+ X^{w\ sn}$ and the other half $X^{w\ sn}$ O. The diagram below explains this situation.

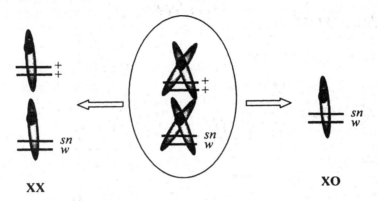

XX   **XO**

Because XX nuclei produce female tissue and XO nuclei produce male tissue, the phenotypes of the two sides are thus described. Developmentally, once the cleavage nuclei reach the peripheral areas of the egg to form a blastoderm, they become committed to their adult fate. Because there is little "wandering" of nuclei either during their migration to the egg periphery or after they reach the periphery, the male/female boundary is quite clean.

> **Common errors for Question 18:** difficulty in setting up the problem, dealing with mitotic nondisjunction, embryonic development of *Drosophila*

Chs. 2, 3, 21 Answer 19 At the *molecular level* one would consider that in discontinuous inheritance the gene products are acting fairly independently of each other, thereby providing a 9:3:3:1 ratio in a dihybrid cross, for example. Genotypic classes

$$A\_B\_,\ A\_bb,\ aaB\_,\ \text{and}\ aabb$$

can be clearly distinguished from each other because the gene products from the *A* locus produce distinct influences on the phenotypes as compared with those gene products from the *B* locus. Exceptions exist where epistasis and other forms of gene interaction occur. In discontinuous inheritance, one would consider each locus as providing a *qualitatively* different impact on the phenotype. For instance, even though the *brown* and *scarlet* loci interact in the production of eye pigments in *Drosophila*, each locus is providing qualitatively different input.

In continuous inheritance, we would consider each involved locus as having a quantitative input on the production of a single characteristic of the phenotype. In addition, although it may not always be the case, we would consider each gene product as being qualitatively similar. Under this model, the *quantity* of a particular set of gene products, influenced by a number of gene loci, determines the phenotypic characteristic.

Sample Test Answers

At the *transmission level* one sees "step-wise" distributions in discontinuous inheritance, but "smoother" or more bell-shaped distributions in continuous inheritance. For instance, in a dihybrid situation (*AaBb* X *AaBb*) where independent assortment holds, one would obtain a 9:3:3:1 ratio (assuming no epistasis, *etc.*) under a discontinuous mode, but a 1:4:6:4:1 ratio where genes (or gene products) are acting additively (continuous inheritance). Both patterns are formed from normal Mendelian principles of segregation, independent assortment, and random union of gametes. It is the manner in which the genes (or gene products) interact that distinguishes discontinuous from continuous inheritance.

> **Common errors for Question 19**: difficulty with "molecular level" of the question, confusion over differences and similarities relating discontinuous and continuous patterns

Chs. 2, 7 Answer 20 The basis of the solution is to recall that crossing over occurs at the "four-strand stage" (after the S-phase) and each chiasma involves only two of the four chromatids present in each tetrad. Therefore, for each chiasma only two of the four, or 1/2, of the chromatids are crossover chromatids.

Gene mapping basically is the process of dividing the number of crossover chromatids by the total number of chromatids. Since each chiasma involves only two of the four chromatids, the map distance must be half of the chiasma frequency. If there are 18 map units between two genes then the chiasma frequency would be 36%. If one examined 150 primary oocytes one would therefore expect to see 0.36 X 150, or 54, cells with a chiasma between the two loci.

> **Common errors for Question 20**: problem seeing relationships of chiasma and map units, problems "seeing" meiosis, visualization of crossing over

Ch. 4 Answer 21 The definition provided initially in the problem can be applied directly to the solution of this problem. The *genotype* of the mother determines the direction of coiling (phenotype) of the immediate offspring. In this case, one merely assigns the genotypes on the basis of normal Mendelian principles, then the phenotypes based on the genotype of the mother.

Notice that in Cross 2, the *Dd* has a sinistral phenotype. While this may confuse some students, remember that the phenotype is determined by the *maternal* genotype. When early developmental events are involved, often the maternal genotype will have a significant influence over those events because the mother makes the egg.

Cross #1:	*Offspring genotype(s):* Dd	*Offspring phenotype(s):* all sinistral
Cross #2:	*Offspring genotype(s):* Dd dd	*Offspring phenotype(s):* all dextral
Cross #3:	*Offspring genotype(s):* DD Dd dd	*Offspring phenotype(s):* all dextral

> **Common errors for Question 21**: When students are reminded of the nature of a maternal effect, that is, given a definition, there are very few errors. However, when they are asked to work the problem without the definition given, many have difficulty. Cross #2 causes most of the problems.

Ch. 7 Answer 22 The key to solving these types of "reverse mapping" problems is to keep in mind that a map unit is computed by the equation [# crossover types/total number (X 100)] and that if the map distance is given it is easy to determine the percentages of parental and crossover offspring. Remember that there are two classes of crossovers and two classes of parentals from each cross.

(a)   *AB/ab* = 40%, *ab/ab* = 40% (parentals)
             Ab/ab = 10%, *aB/ab* = 10% (crossovers)

(b)   *Pq/pq* = 25%, *pQ/pq* = 25% (parentals)
             PQ/pq = 25%, *pq/pq* = 25% (crossovers)

             Notice that this is independent assortment.

(c)   *DB/db* = 50%, *db/db* = 50% (all parentals)

(d)   *AB/ab* = 50%, *ab/ab* = 50% (all parentals)

The reason that there are all parentals and no crossovers in this cross is that there is no crossing over in male *Drosophila*. With no crossing over, the *AB/ab* chromosomes in the male are passed to gametes without crossovers.

> **Common errors for Question 22:** difficulty going from map units to offspring frequencies, failure to see that there are two parental and two crossover classes, careless mistakes

Ch. 8 Answer 23 (a) Disagree: The process being described refers to *transformation* not transduction. Transduction is *phage-mediated* recombination, whereas in transformation exogenous DNA is taken up as indicated in the statement.

(b) Agree: Viruses that can enter either the lytic or lysogenic cycle are called *temperate* viruses. During the process of lysogeny, the viral chromosome is integrated into the bacterial chromosome as stated.

(c) Disagree: This statement is fairly silly in that it states that phages are capable of producing bacteria. Regardless of the exposure to UV light, phages cannot produce bacteria. Ultraviolet light can cause induction of the lytic cycle, therefore phages, when lysogenic bacteria are exposed.

> **Common errors for Question 23:** carelessness in reading statements, confusion as to what terms mean: transduction, transformation, conjugation, lysogeny, temperate viruses

Chs. 9, 10, 11, 12, 13, 14 Answer 24 (a) DNA replicates in a semiconservative manner such that each daughter strand is "half-new" and 'half-old" in a particular pattern.

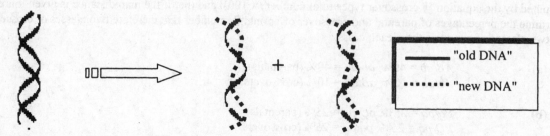

(b) The *Central Dogma of Biology* is based on the production (through transcription) of an RNA messenger from a DNA template and the subsequent "decoding" of that messenger by the process of translation.

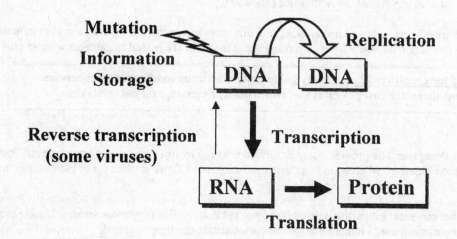

(c) The DNA template contains a sequence of nitrogenous bases that specifies a code from which amino acids are ordered in proteins. Through tautomeric shifts and a number of other natural factors (radiation, chemicals), changes can occur in that sequence of bases. Indeed, the mechanisms by which genes replicate themselves generate errors and leaves us with the conclusion that DNA is an inherently unstable molecule.

(d) Given the variety of organisms and the variation within organisms, there must be numerous, hundreds of millions, elementary factors that are inherited. DNA can provide for this variety by differences in the length and sequence of bases for each inherited functional unit. Given that there are four different types of bases, a sequence having merely ten bases would be capable of 4^{10} (over 1 million) different sequences.

> **Common errors for Question 24:** There are usually very few problems with this type of question, except that students often have difficulty clearly explaining that which they know in model form. Written descriptions tend to be more lists of examples rather than explanations of structures and/or processes.

Sample Test Answers

Chs. 9, 11 Answer 25 As discussed in the text, the rate of reassociation of melted DNA increases as the proportion of repetitive DNA increases. Such relationships are reflected in C_ot curves in which one plots the fraction of DNA reassociated against a logarithmic scale of C_ot values, which have the units (mole X sec/liter). Because denatured DNA strands that are repetitive have a higher likelihood of complementary interaction, the time of reassociation is less.

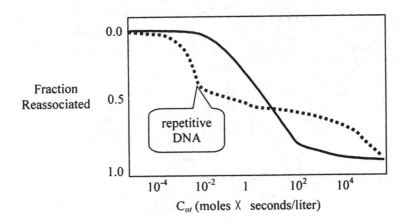

Common errors for Question 25: orientation (coordinates) of graph, significance of curve components, repetitive DNA fraction, unique fraction

Chs. 9, 10 Answer 26 (a) In this type of drawing, the various carbons of the sugar are readily apparent. It is the orientation and carbon numbering on the sugar that determines the 5'-3' orientation of the molecule. The bottom of the polymer has the 2' and 3' carbons projecting, while the top has the 5' carbon projecting. Therefore, the bottom, near the circle is the 3' end of the molecule.

(b) Notice that there is no vertical line protruding from the 2' carbon position in the drawing and that uracil (U) is present. The molecule must therefore be an RNA. **(c)** It is best to start this portion of the problem by roughly drawing the complementary strand, remembering that it will be antiparallel.

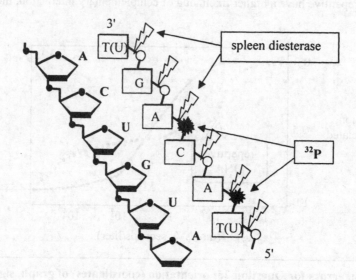

If it is a DNA complement, it will have thymine in place of uracil. There is no indication as to the complementary strand being RNA or DNA. Since all ATP's (or dATP's) have at their innermost phosphate a ^{32}P, make certain that they are properly labeled. Since spleen diesterase cleaves between the phosphate and the 5' carbon, the 5' neighbors (C, T or U) will be labeled with the ^{32}P.

(d) Since snake venom diesterase cleaves at the 3' position (between the phosphate and the 3' carbon), the originally labeled ATP (or dATP) will retain the label.

> **Common errors for Question 26:** 5' to 3' orientations, labeling of complementary strand, understanding enzyme cleavages

Ch. 10 Answer 27 Even though circular, in the context of this question, DNA from *E. coli* can be viewed in the following manner. Replication will occur semiconservatively and give the following sedimentation profile.

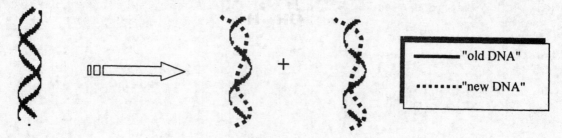

The heat treatment will cause the double-stranded structures to separate, giving the following strands and the profile as shown above.

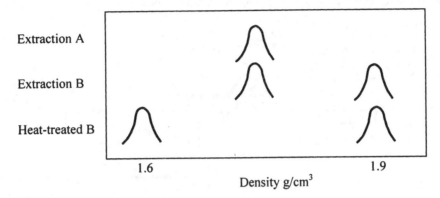

Ch. 10 Answer 28 (a) There will be two telocentric metaphase chromosomes in the drawing and each chromatid will be labeled.

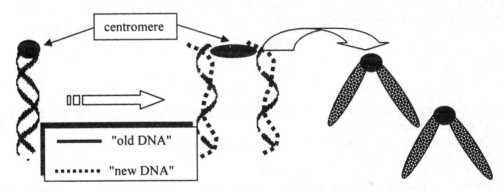

This autoradiographic pattern results because of semiconservative replication. Any cell that contains labeled chromosomes will have had its chromosomes pass through an S phase in the presence of label.

(b) Consider that the DNA was labeled with a dCTP having the innermost phosphate labeled. As this triphosphonucleoside is incorporated into the DNA, it will have the following relationship to its neighbors. *Snake venom diesterase* cleaves DNA at the 3' position meaning that it breaks the bond between the phosphate and the 3' carbon.

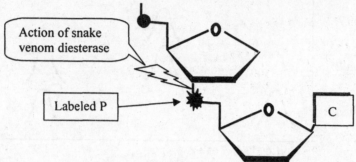

Therefore, the labeled phosphate remains attached to the 5' carbon of the cytosine nucleotide. The A+T/G+C ratio of 1.67 is of no consequence in answering this problem because all of the label remains attached to the cytosine.

Adenine_____   Guanine_____

Thymine_____   Cytosine <u>100%</u>

Common errors for Question 28: inappropriate labeling pattern, inability to draw telocentric chromosomes, understanding cleavage at 3' position, eliminating extraneous information

Ch. 10 Answer 29

1. This must be the *5' end* of the polymer because all synthesis of polymers is 5' to 3' and the head of the arrow is at the other end of the polymer.
2. The *leading strand* is that strand which is synthesized continuously.
3. A *DNA ligase* will join the nicks.
4. The *lagging strand* is the discontinuous strand.
5. The free end that is complementary to the 5' end at arrow #1 must be the 3' end. That being so, the complement to that 3' end would be 5'. Therefore the *5' end* is at arrow #5.
6. A *helicase* is involved in unwinding the DNA helix.
7. An *RNA primer* is synthesized to initiate DNA synthesis.
8. *DNA gyrase* functions to remove supercoils generated by unwinding the DNA helix.
9. *Single-stranded binding proteins* stabilize the template that is to be replicated.

Common errors for Question 29: determination of 5'- 3' polarity, naming of enzymes involved

Sample Test Answers

Chs. 12, 13 Answer 30 Overall, this is a drawing of simultaneous transcription and translation in which the RNA polymerase is moving from top to bottom, making an mRNA that is complementary to one of the two strands of DNA. Ribosomes have added to the nascent (newly forming) mRNA and what appear to be polypeptide chains are protruding from the ribosomes.

(1, 2) In answering this question remember that all synthesis of nucleic acids starts at the 5' end and finishes at the 3' end. Therefore, immediately label the end near point "B" with a 5'. The projecting strand is the nascent mRNA. Recall that all orientation of complementary strands is antiparallel and since the RNA polymerase is going from top-to-bottom (according to the arrow) the end of the DNA strand from which the mRNA is copied is the 3' end. Now, since the 3' end of the DNA template strand is identified, its DNA complementary end (at point "A") must be the 5' end.

(3) The codon-anticodon relationship is also antiparallel (based on hydrogen bonding) and since the 5' end of the mRNA is identified, letter "C" must be at the 5' end.

(4) While the diagram is *not to scale*, given the folded structure of the molecule and its position in the ribosome, consider the RNA nearest to letter "D" as tRNA.

(5) Remember that the 3' end of the tRNA holds the amino acid, therefore letter "D" is where the amino acid would be attached.

(6) The tRNA binds mainly to the large subunit of the ribosome, while the mRNA binds mainly to the small subunit of the ribosome. The question asks for the S value of the rRNA in that small subunit. Simultaneous transcription and translation occurs in prokaryotes only (not eukaryotes). The S value for the small subunit of a prokaryotic ribosome is 30S, but that value includes both rRNA and protein. The rRNA molecule, however, has an S value of 16, which is the correct answer.

(7) Since all of the ribosomes are moving along the same mRNA, the amino acid sequences are the same. Therefore, the amino acids nearest the letters "F" and "G" are the same.

> **Common errors for Question 30:** polarity of DNA and RNA strands, structure of ribosomes, overall understanding of translation

Chs. 12, 13, 14 Answer 31 One of the most frequent difficulties students have with this problem is remembering that the code is triplet and three bases in the mRNA code for each amino acid in a protein. The 5' end of the mRNA corresponds with the N-terminus of the amino acid chain.

(a) Transition mutations will cause amino acid substitutions. Counting over by "threes" from the N-terminus, the amino acid ile should be altered.

(b) Inserting a base between positions 3 and 4 will change the second amino acid; however, recall that acridine orange is a frameshift mutagen and insertion of a base will alter the reading frames for all "downstream" amino acids. Therefore, all amino acids in positions two (glu) through twelve will be influenced (excluding degeneracy).

(c) Nitrous acid causes base substitutions, therefore a mutation in the 11th base would influence the amino acid leu.

> **Common errors for Question 31:** counting amino acids as bases, not understanding what base changes do to amino acid sequences

Ch. 13 Answer 32 Notice that there are two mutant strains (cannot grow on minimal medium) and one wild type strain (t410). The best way to approach these types of problems, especially when the data are organized in the form given, is to realize that the substance (supplement) that "repairs," as indicated by a (+), a strain is after the metabolic block for that strain. In addition, and most importantly, the substance that "repairs" the highest number of strains either is the end product or is closest to the end product. Looking at the table, notice that supplement B "repairs" both the mutant strains. Therefore, it must be at the end of the pathway or at least after all the metabolic blocks (defined by each mutation). Supplement A "repairs" the next highest number of mutant strains (1), therefore, it must be second from the end. The pathway therefore would be as follows:

t409   *r3*

Precursor----⚡----> **A** --⚡-----> **B**

To determine the locations at which the strains block the pathway through mutation, apply a similar logic. A block that is "repaired" by all the supplements must be early in the pathway. A block that is "repaired" by only one supplement must be late in the pathway. A supplement that does not "repair" a strain is before that strain's metabolic block. Be certain not to introduce any "blocks" for the wild type strain.

> **Common errors for Question 32:** inability to construct a pathway, failure to see how additives "repair" mutant phenotypes, difficulty in assigning metabolic blocks in pathways

Ch. 13 Answer 33

1. hydrophobic cluster formed by interaction of hydrophobic amino acids

2. α helix formed from hydrogen bonds between components of the peptide linkage

3. covalent, disulfide bonds formed between cysteine residues

4. The polar amino acids will tend to orient to the outside of the protein where the charged R groups will interact with water.

> **Common errors for Question 33:** nature of hydrophobic clustering, understanding of α and β structures, polar side chains, and hydrophilic interactions

Chs. 13, 15 Answer 34 In some viruses, overlapping genes present a mechanism for providing two and sometimes more protein products from a single stretch of DNA. In eukaryotes, different sets of introns may be removed, thus providing for a variety of protein products from a single section of DNA. This process is often called *differential* or *alternative splicing.*

> **Common errors for Question 34:** Students often have difficulty in orienting *specific information* they have learned to a general question. If asked about overlapping genes, or differential hnRNA splicing, they would be able to develop an answer. Students sometimes confuse overlapping genes with the non-overlapping code.

Ch. 15 Answer 35 Any time a regulatory protein interacts with DNA and transcription is stimulated, it is called *positive* control. Any time a regulatory protein interacts with DNA and represses transcription, it is called *negative* control. In completing the chart, apply these simple rules.

Relationship of Regulator Protein to DNA	Operator	
	Positive control	*Negative control*
is bound	on	off
isn't bound	off	on

> **Common errors for Question 35:** confusion with positive and negative control, confusion with repressible and inducible systems

Ch. 17 Answer 36 DNase is a general term that includes a variety of exo- and endonucleases that cleave DNA from the ends or internally, respectively. Such cleavage is often irrespective of base sequence. If naked DNA is exposed to DNases, it is rapidly degraded to oligo- and mononucleotides. When protein is associated with DNA, it protects regions from degradation. Such protected regions can be analyzed as to base content. Restriction endonucleases cleave DNA at specific sequences often hundreds or thousands of base pairs apart. If one is interested in mapping protein binding sites, one would want to use an enzyme (a DNase) with frequent, yet relatively random cleavage characteristics, not restriction endonucleases.

> **Common errors for Question 36:** understanding overall strategy, differences between DNases, restriction endonucleases

Ch. 17, 18 Answer 37 Notice that the fragment sizes (in kb) on the left side of the figure match the *Hind*III restriction fragments that are hybridizing (cDNA probe + genomic fragment) to the radioactive probe. Each band, therefore, represents a region where the radioactive probe is "trapped" by complementary base pairing to single-stranded DNA fragments, which are bound to the filter. The smaller fragments migrate faster in the gel and, therefore, are in the bottom portion ,while the larger fragments are at the top, near the origin. Notice that the intensity of the bands from the normal individual is somewhat uniform, indicating that all the restriction fragments are found in equal amounts. However, the intensity of three of the bands from the patient with retinoblastoma are about half as dense as in the normal. One band (7.5 kb) has the same intensity as in the normal. Because humans are diploid organisms, with normally two copies of each gene, one may hypothesize that the individual with retinoblastoma has a heterozygous deletion of a portion of the retinoblastoma gene, which includes *Hind*III fragments (9.8, 6.2, and 5.3 kb). It is likely that the inheritance of such a deletion is instrumental in causing familial retinoblastoma.

> **Common errors for Question 37:** understanding of experimental design, cDNA probes, Southern blots electrophoresis, restriction endonuclease analysis, hybridization, recognition of deletion

Ch. 17, 18, 19 Answer 38 Below is a drawing of the expected product if either of the above plasmids (A) or (B) is restricted to completion with *Bam*HI. There should be a 2.3 kb fragment (1.4 + 0.9 kb) and the remainder (9.2 - 2.3 = 6.9). Notice that the 6.9 kb fragment migrates slower (higher in the gel) than the 2.3 kb fragment. Also notice that the intensity of the stain is less in the smaller band because there is less DNA to bind the stain.

(a)

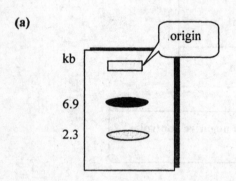

(b) To distinguish between the (A) and (B) orientations, one could make use of the change in position of the *Pst*I restriction site in the two orientations. First, estimate the number of kb in the two fragments resulting from *Pst*I restriction of orientation (A). Notice that in orientation (A) the *Pst*I fragments are approximately 2.4 (1.4 for the *Kan* gene + about 1.0) kb and 6.8 kb. In orientation (B) the sizes would be approximately 1.9 (0.9 for the *trx* gene + about 1.0) and 7.3 kb. With appropriate standards, these size differences could be distinguished on agarose gels.

> **Common errors for Question 38:** electrophoretic analysis, restriction enzyme analysis, experimental design

Chs. 17, 18, 19 Answer 39 It is a relatively simple procedure to determine the sequence of DNA from the gel given. Start at the bottom with the smallest fragments. As one reads up the gel, one is reading from the 5' to the 3' direction. In the first case, note that there is a band in both the G+A and G lanes. Read this as a "G" because if an "A" occurs, it would exist as a band *only* in the G+A lane. The sequence would be as follows: 5'-GTGGTCACGACT.

> **Common errors for Question 39:** reading the gel as the sequence, difficulty in dealing with G+A and C+T lanes, careless mistakes

Ch. 20 Answer 40 *Determination* is a significant, complex, yet poorly understood process whereby the specific pattern of genetic activity is initially established in a cell. This pattern will direct the developmental fate (differentiation) of that cell.

Differentiation is the process of cellular expression of the determined state. It is the complex series of genetic, morphological, and physiological changes that characterize the variety of adult cells.

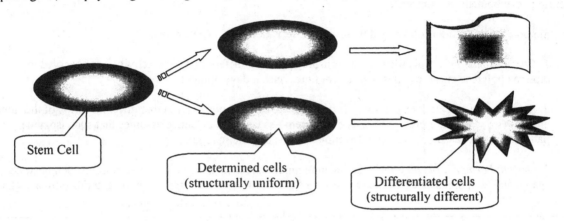

Stem Cell

Determined cells
(structurally uniform)

Differentiated cells
(structurally different)

(b) *Determination* occurs before *differentiation*. In *Drosophila*, determinative events are thought to occur about the time of blastoderm formation, when nuclei encounter the peripheral regions of the egg. *Differentiation* of most of the adult cells occurs during metamorphosis, some five to six days after embryogenesis (determination).

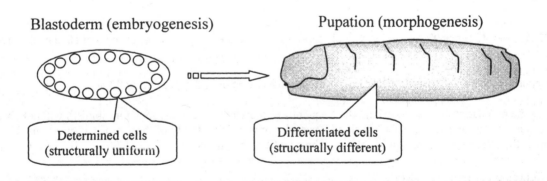

Blastoderm (embryogenesis)

Pupation (morphogenesis)

Determined cells
(structurally uniform)

Differentiated cells
(structurally different)

Common errors for Question 40: providing accurate definitions, failure to relate determination and differentiation to each other temporally

Ch. 20 Answer 41 The *variable gene activity hypothesis* of differentiation acknowledges the genomic equivalence of cells within an organism and assumes that of all the genes in a given cell type, only certain ones produce products, while the others are shut down and are not transcribed. Certain genes will be active in all cells, those *housekeeping* genes coding for vital cellular functions, while others will be differentially regulated in various cell types. Differential gene transcription occurs in both spatial (different cells of an organism) and temporal (different times during development) dimensions.

Support for this model is provided by several observations and experiments.

1. *Chromosome puffs*: Specific puff patterns, representing differential gene activity, are observed in dipteran polytene chromosomes at different times during development.

2. *Isozymes*: Differential gene activity is demonstrated by the observation that different forms of the same enzyme (isozymes) are present in cells of different tissues. This evidence assumes that such isozyme patterns are not caused by post-transcriptional forms of genetic regulation.

3. *Growth hormone*: *In situ* hybridization and immunochemical studies in mouse embryos demonstrate spatial and temporal aspects of the regulation of growth hormone transcripts in the anterior pituitary gland.

Common errors for Question 41: With a general question such as this, students sometimes have difficulty focusing on the area in their notes or in the text that relates to the question. Students may understand what is meant by the variable gene activity hypothesis, but not immediately see that it relates to the question. Students also have difficulty in relating a variety of experimental findings to a general theme.

Ch. 22 Answer 42 Since 9% of the individuals express the trait, the frequency (q) of the recessive gene would be 0.3.

The frequency of individuals that are heterozygous would be $2pq$ or $2(.3)(.7) = .42$ or 42%.

Because the population is in equilibrium, the frequency of individuals heterozygous for albinism will not change from generation to generation. Students should be aware of many deviations of these types of questions. The basic scheme is the Hardy-Weinberg equilibrium and the equations that apply.

Common errors for Question 42: application of the Hardy-Weinberg equations to an autosomal gene, failure to apply the Hardy-Weinberg equations in determining the frequency of heterozygous individuals, students often make the question harder than it is by forgetting that under equilibrium conditions, gene frequencies do not change

Ch. 22, 23 Answer 43 *Mutation*, while being an original source of genetic variability, is not usually considered to be a significant factor in changing gene frequencies.

Migration occurs when individuals move from one population to another. The influence of migration on changing gene frequencies is proportional to the differences in gene frequency between the donor and recipient populations. Organisms often migrate as a result of some stress. Those organisms suffering from the most stress are often those that leave. Therefore, they do not represent a random sample of the individuals in that home range.

Selection can be a significant force in changing gene frequencies. It results when some genotypic classes are less likely to produce offspring than others. Selection may be directional, stabilizing, or disruptive.

Genetic drift can be a significant force in changing gene frequencies in populations that are numerically small or have a small number of effective breeders. In such populations, random and relatively large fluctuations in gene frequency occur by "sampling error."

Inbreeding is not a significant factor in changing gene frequencies in populations, however, it will change zygotic or genotypic frequencies. The number of homozygotes will increase at the expense of the heterozygotes.

Common errors for Question 43: failure to provide a complete list, failure to briefly and adequately describe each term, failure to see that inbreeding does not, in itself, change gene frequencies

Ch. 23 Answer 44 Reproductive isolation can occur because of the introduction of geographic barriers or other dramatic changes in the environment that subdivide a population. Such factors facilitate speciation because gene flow is eliminated or at least restricted. With gene flow restricted, isolated populations can experience changes in gene frequencies when the Hardy-Weinberg assumptions are not met. Under Hardy-Weinberg equilibrium conditions where there is *random mating, no genetic drift, no selection, no mutation*, and *no migration*, gene frequencies will remain the same and speciation will not occur.

Common errors for Question 44: confusion as to what the question is asking, difficulty in relating information from one chapter to information contained in a different chapter

Ch. 23 Answer 45 Any circumstance or process that favors changes in gene frequencies has the potential of generating a new species.

Factors such as selection, migration, genetic drift, or even mutation, may be important in species formation. One would certainly include geographic and/or temporal isolation as major barriers to gene flow and thus, an important process in such formation.

Natural selection occurs when there is nonrandom elimination of individuals from a population. Since such selection is a strong force in changing gene frequencies, it should also be considered as a significant factor in species formation.

Common errors for Question 45: explanations of terms, general relationships among diverse phenomena

Ch. 23, 24 Answer 46 Genetic diversity provides for physiological and evolutionary plasticity in the sense that it allows populations a way of buffering habitat changes. Those species that have considerable genetic diversity are more able to respond as individuals through hybrid vigor and as populations by being able to shift gene frequencies (resulting from selection) to more adapted gene combinations. There are a number of factors that reduce genetic diversity including genetic drift, inbreeding, migration, founder effect and selection. Probably the most significant environmental factor driving loss of genetic diversity, by way of the factors mentioned above, is habitat loss. Genetic erosion is the loss of previously held genetic diversity.

Common errors for Question 46: generally students do well on such a question because most components are common sense, some difficulty with identifying factors associated loss of genetic diversity

Ch. 24 Answer 47 Outbreeding depression is caused by the introduction of less fit genes into a population or species. When breeding individuals are introduced into a host population, genes that are adapted to a different environment mingle with the existing, perhaps more adapted, genes. To a host population, outbreeding depression leads to an overall reduction in fitness and may threaten its survival. In many cases, because of the fragile state of some species, the negative outcome of outbreeding depression is overshadowed by the need to keep the species from extinction.

Common errors for Question 47: some students may struggle trying to identify exactly what is meant by outbreeding depression